Guide to the De-Identification of Personal Health Information

T0239823

OTHER INFORMATION SECURITY BOOKS FROM AUERBACH

Asset Protection through Security Awareness
Tyler Justin Speed
ISBN 978-1-4398-0982-2

The CISO Handbook: A Practical Guide to Securing Your Company
Michael Gentile, Ron Collette, and Thomas D. August
ISBN 978-0-8493-1952-5

CISO's Guide to Penetration Testing: A Framework to Plan, Manage, and Maximize Benefits
James S. Tiller
ISBN 978-1-4398-8027-2

The Complete Book of Data Anonymization: From Planning to Implementation
Balaji Raghunathan
ISBN 978-1-4398-7730-2

Cybersecurity: Public Sector Threats and Responses
Kim J. Andreasson, Editor
ISBN 9781-4398-4663-6

Cyber Security Essentials
James Graham, Editor
ISBN 978-1-4398-5123-4

Cybersecurity for Industrial Control Systems: SCADA, DCS, PLC, HMI, and SIS
Tyson Macaulay and Bryan L. Singer
ISBN 978-1-4398-0196-3

Cyberspace and Cybersecurity
George Kostopoulos Request
ISBN 978-1-4665-0133-1

Defense Against the Black Arts: How Hackers Do What They Do and How to Protect against It
Jesse Varsalone and Matthew McFadden
ISBN 978-1-4398-2119-0

The Definitive Guide to Complying with the HIPAA/HITECH Privacy and Security Rules
John J. Trinckes, Jr.
ISBN 978-1-4665-0767-8

Digital Forensics Explained
Greg Gogolin
ISBN 978-1-4398-7495-0

Digital Forensics for Handheld Devices
Eamon P. Doherty
ISBN 978-1-4398-9877-2

Electronically Stored Information: The Complete Guide to Management, Understanding, Acquisition, Storage, Search, and Retrieval
David R. Matthews
ISBN 978-1-4398-7726-5

FISMA Principles and Best Practices: Beyond Compliance
Patrick D. Howard
ISBN 978-1-4200-7829-9

Information Security Governance Simplified: From the Boardroom to the Keyboard
Todd Fitzgerald
ISBN 978-1-4398-1163-4

Information Technology Control and Audit, Fourth Edition
Sandra Senft, Frederick Gallegos, and Aleksandra Davis
ISBN 978-1-4398-9320-3

Managing the Insider Threat: No Dark Corners
Nick Catrantzos
ISBN 978-1-4398-7292-5

Network Attacks and Defenses: A Hands-on Approach
Zouheir Trabelsi, Kadhim Hayawi, Arwa Al Braiki, and Sujith Samuel Mathew
ISBN 978-1-4665-1794-3

PRAGMATIC Security Metrics: Applying Metametrics to Information Security
W. Krag Brotby and Gary Hinson
ISBN 978-1-4398-8152-1

The Security Risk Assessment Handbook: A Complete Guide for Performing Security Risk Assessments, Second Edition
Douglas Landoll
ISBN 978-1-4398-2148-0

The 7 Qualities of Highly Secure Software
Mano Paul
ISBN 978-1-4398-1446-8

Smart Grid Security: An End-to-End View of Security in the New Electrical Grid
Gilbert N. Sorebo and Michael C. Echols
ISBN 978-1-4398-5587-4

Windows Networking Tools: The Complete Guide to Management, Troubleshooting, and Security
Gilbert Held
ISBN 978-1-4665-1106-4

AUERBACH PUBLICATIONS
www.auerbach-publications.com
To Order Call: 1-800-272-7737 • Fax: 1-800-374-3401
E-mail: orders@crcpress.com

Guide to the De-Identification of Personal Health Information

Khaled El Emam

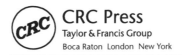

CRC Press
Taylor & Francis Group
Boca Raton London New York

CRC Press is an imprint of the
Taylor & Francis Group, an **informa** business

AN AUERBACH BOOK

CRC Press
Taylor & Francis Group
6000 Broken Sound Parkway NW, Suite 300
Boca Raton, FL 33487-2742

First issued in paperback 2020

© 2013 by Taylor & Francis Group, LLC
CRC Press is an imprint of Taylor & Francis Group, an Informa business

No claim to original U.S. Government works

ISBN-13: 978-1-4665-7906-4 (hbk)
ISBN-13: 978-0-367-65918-9 (pbk)

This book contains information obtained from authentic and highly regarded sources. Reasonable efforts have been made to publish reliable data and information, but the author and publisher cannot assume responsibility for the validity of all materials or the consequences of their use. The authors and publishers have attempted to trace the copyright holders of all material reproduced in this publication and apologize to copyright holders if permission to publish in this form has not been obtained. If any copyright material has not been acknowledged please write and let us know so we may rectify in any future reprint.

Except as permitted under U.S. Copyright Law, no part of this book may be reprinted, reproduced, transmitted, or utilized in any form by any electronic, mechanical, or other means, now known or hereafter invented, including photocopying, microfilming, and recording, or in any information storage or retrieval system, without written permission from the publishers.

For permission to photocopy or use material electronically from this work, please access www.copyright. com (http://www.copyright.com/) or contact the Copyright Clearance Center, Inc. (CCC), 222 Rosewood Drive, Danvers, MA 01923, 978-750-8400. CCC is a not-for-profit organization that provides licenses and registration for a variety of users. For organizations that have been granted a photocopy license by the CCC, a separate system of payment has been arranged.

Trademark Notice: Product or corporate names may be trademarks or registered trademarks, and are used only for identification and explanation without intent to infringe.

Library of Congress Cataloging-in-Publication Data

El Emam, Khaled.
    Guide to the de-identification of personal health information / author, Khaled El Emam.
        pages cm
        Includes bibliographical references and index.
        ISBN 978-1-4665-7906-4 (hardback)
        1. Medical records. 2. Information storage and retrieval systems--Medicine. 3. Confidential communications. I. Title.

R864.E43 2013
610.285--dc23   2013002174

Visit the Taylor & Francis Web site at
http://www.taylorandfrancis.com

and the CRC Press Web site at
http://www.crcpress.com

Contents

SECTION II UNDERSTANDING DISCLOSURE RISKS

Foreword

Personal health information comprises the most sensitive and intimate details of one's life, such as those relating to one's physical or mental health, and the health history of one's family. Intuitively, we understand the importance of protecting health information in order to ensure the confidentiality of such personal data and the privacy of the individual to whom it relates. Personal health information must also be accurate, complete, and accessible to health care practitioners in order to provide individuals with necessary health care. At a broader level, for secondary uses that go beyond the treatment of the individual, health-related data are needed for the benefit of society as a whole. These vitally important secondary uses include activities to improve the quality of care, health research, and the management of publicly funded health care systems.

As the information and privacy commissioner of Ontario, Canada, my role includes the oversight of health privacy legislation governing the collection, use, and disclosure of personal health information by organizations and individuals involved in the delivery of health care services. Ontario's Personal Health Information Protection Act (PHIPA) aims to respect an individual's right to privacy in relationship to his or her own personal health information while accommodating the legitimate need to access health information for well-defined purposes. PHIPA does this in part by establishing clear rules for the use and disclosure of personal health information for secondary purposes. The object of these rules is to maximize the benefits of both respecting personal privacy and making health information accessible for purposes that serve society as a whole.

My office has long championed a model that enables multiple goals. This process, which forms the basis of privacy by design, seeks to retire the traditional zero-sum paradigm, pitting individual privacy rights against broader societal interests, in favor of a doubly enabling positive-sum model in which both values are maximized. In the health sector, privacy by design addresses this issue by protecting the privacy of personal health information while at the same time making available quality health data for valuable secondary purposes. I am delighted to introduce this guide, which provides a practical, risk-based methodology for the de-identification of personal health information—an excellent example of the privacy by design approach in the health information context.

The de-identification of sensitive personal health information is one of our most valuable tools for protecting individual privacy. The routine de-identification or anonymization of personal health information can help health information custodians to comply with data minimization principles, incorporated in PHIPA, that require personal health information not to be collected, used, or disclosed if other information will serve the purpose, and that no more identified health information should be collected, used, or disclosed than is reasonably necessary to meet the purpose. Routine de-identification also helps to prevent privacy breaches in the case of loss, theft, or unauthorized access to personal health information.

At the same time, the de-identification of personal health information can enable the use of health data for important secondary purposes, such as health-related research. Done in a manner that significantly minimizes the risk of re-identification, while maintaining a level of data quality that is appropriate for the secondary purpose, the de-identification of personal health information embodies a privacy by design solution and rejects the traditional model's false dichotomy of privacy vs. data quality. By arguing persuasively for the use of de-identification as a privacy-enhancing tool, and setting out a practical methodology for the use of de-identification techniques and re-identification risk measurement tools, this book provides a valuable and much needed resource for all data custodians who use or disclose personal health information for secondary purposes. Doubly enabling, privacy-enhancing tools like these, that embrace privacy by design, will ensure the continued availability of personal health information for valuable secondary purposes that benefit us all.

Dr. Ann Cavoukian
Information and Privacy Commissioner of Ontario

Acknowledgments

Some of the materials in this book were based on peer-reviewed publications by myself and my colleagues. Where appropriate, I have referenced the originating publications. I also acknowledge and thank all of my coauthors on that earlier work.

This work was originally funded by the Office of the Privacy Commissioner of Canada under its contributions program. I thank the commissioner's office for this support, without which it would have been difficult to get this project started. Other sources of supportive funding for material included in this book are the Canadian Institutes of Health Research, the Natural Sciences and Engineering Research Council, the Canada Research Chairs Program, and the Public Health Agency of Canada through a number of contracts.

I thank the following diverse individuals who have contributed to our research and implementation of the concepts and methods in this book, for reviewing earlier drafts, and providing critical input throughout the last seven years that has shaped our approach to de-identification (in alphabetical order): Luk Arbuckle, Sadrul Chowdhury, Fida Dankar, Ben Eze, Anita Fineberg, Lisa Gaudette, Elizabeth Jonker, Gunes Koru, Sarah Lyons, Grant Middleton, Angelica Neisa, Michael Power, Hassan Quereshi, Sean Rose, Saeed Samet, Morvarid Sedhakar, and John Wunderlich.

Also, it is important to acknowledge our development teams at the Electronic Health Information Laboratory and Privacy Analytics, whose implementation of the metrics and concepts in this book have allowed us to apply them in many different health data releases over the last few years. These practical applications have informed much of our work. Finally, I thank Brian Dewar for his help in formatting and arranging the manuscript.

Glossary (Abbreviations and Acronyms)

AHRQ: Agency for Healthcare Research and Quality
AIDS: Acquired immune deficiency syndrome
CA: Confidentiality agreement
CFR: Code of Federal Regulations
CIHR: Canadian Institutes of Health Research
CR: Capture-recapture model
CTO: Chief technology officer
DC: Data custodian
DF: De-identified file
DHHS: Department of Health and Human Services
DNA: Deoxyribonucleic acid
DSA: Data sharing agreement
DSMB: Data Safety Management Board
EHR: Electronic health record: EMR: Electronic medical record
ePHI: Electronic personal health information
EU: European Union
FOIA: Freedom of Information Act
FOIPPA: Freedom of Information and Protection of Privacy Act
GAPP: Generally accepted privacy principles
GIC: Group Insurance Commission
GPS: Global positioning system
HAF: HIPAA authorization form
HCFA: Health Insurance Claim Form (The Centers for Medicare and Medicaid Services)
HIA: Health Information Act
HIPAA: Health Insurance Portability and Accountability Act
HITECH: Health Information Technology for Economic and Clinical Health Act
HIV: Human immunodeficiency virus
HPV: Human papillomavirus

HR: Human resources
ICD: International Statistical Classification of Diseases and Related Health Problems (codes)
IM: Information management
IP: Internet protocol (address)
IPC: Information and Privacy Commissioner
IRB: Institutional Review Board
ISO/IEC: International Organization for Standardization/International Electrotechnical Commission
ITRC: Identity Theft Resource Center
MCI: Mitigating controls assessment instrument
MITS: Management of information technology security
MRC: Medical Research Council (UK)
MRN: Medical record number
NCVHS: National Committee on Vital and Health Statistics
NDA: Non-disclosure agreement
NIH: National Institutes of Health
NIST: National Institutes of Standards and Technology
OCR: Optical character recognition
OECD: Organization for Economic Cooperation and Development
OLA: Optimal lattice anonymization
OSSPS: Operational Security Standard on Physical Security
PHI: Personal health information
PHIA: Personal Health Information Act
PHIPA: Personal Health Information Protection Act (Ontario)
PHIPA: Personal Health Information Protection and Access Act (New Brunswick)
PIA: Privacy impact assessment
PIPEDA: Personal Information Protection and Electronic Documents Act
PPHI: Protection of personal health information
PPIA: Protection of Personal Information Act
REB: Research Ethics Board
RFID: Radio frequency identification
SAS: Statistical Analysis Software
SEER: Surveillance epidemiology and end results
SID: State inpatient database
SNP: Single nucleotide polymorphism
SPSS: Statistical Package for the Social Sciences
SSHRC: Social Sciences and Humanities Research Council of Canada
SSL: Single sockets layer (protocol for encrypting information over the Internet)
SSN: Social security number
THIPA: The Health Information Protection Act

TRA: Threat and risk assessment
URL: Universal resource locator
USA PATRIOT Act: Uniting and Strengthening America by Providing Appropriate
    Tools Required to Intercept and Obstruct Terrorism Act
VA: Vulnerability assessment

Chapter 1

Introduction

There is great demand for data. This may be financial data, health data, Internet transaction or clickstream data, or it may be travel/movement data. Large volumes of data can now be analyzed quite efficiently to gain new insights on the phenomenon being modeled. Some have called ours the age of the algorithm and have heralded the rise of data science.

The purposes for demanding such data vary widely. For example, the data may be used to develop new services and products or improve the efficiency and effectiveness of existing ones, for research and public health purposes, or to inform or even change the behavior of the public. Access to data also promotes transparency and provides the citizenry with the means to ensure accountability in government and public agencies.

Our focus here is on health data. While many of the methods described and conclusions drawn over the next few chapters may be relevant and valid for other types of data, the context and all of the examples will be on health data only.

At a time when our health care system is under serious fiscal strain, and the population is aging with multiple chronic conditions, it is incumbent on us to use the vast quantities of health data that are being collected to find ways to address system inefficiencies and improve patient outcomes and patient safety. In fact, one can argue that not to do so would be irresponsible and counter to what the public expects and the public interest.

There is little question that providing greater access to data will have many benefits to society (for instance, see the general examples in [1]). Therefore, with this as our starting assumption, we will not discuss the benefits part of the equation here. Our focus will be on how to make health data more accessible in a responsible way by protecting the privacy of patients and remaining compliant with current legislation and regulations.

De-identification of personal data is an effective way to protect the privacy of patients when their data are used or disclosed, and is the topic of this book. There are other ways to responsibly share health information while protecting patient privacy, and we will also discuss some of these. However, we argue that there are compelling legal and practical reasons why de-identification should be considered as one of the main approaches to use. We then present a risk-based methodology for the de-identification of health information.

Currently there are no complete, documented, and repeatable methodologies for the de-identification of health data. While there is a community of practice in this area, the sharing of practical details within that community tends to be limited. The methodology described here is intended to fill that gap, and it is based on our experiences with the de-identification of health information since 2005.

Primary and Secondary Purposes

Identifiable health data can be used for primary purposes, such as providing patient care. This is distinct from secondary purposes. Secondary purposes are defined as "non-direct care use of personal health information (PHI) including but not limited to analysis, research, quality/safety measurement, public health, payment, provider certification or accreditation, and marketing and other business including strictly commercial activities" [2].

When data are used for secondary purposes, this sometimes means that the data already exist. The data have been collected for a primary purpose and are now in a database, such as an electronic medical record (EMR) or in an integrated data warehouse, and there is a desire to use or disclose it for a secondary purpose, say, a research project. Data can also be collected for secondary purposes, for example, when a survey is conducted for a public health initiative.

Many primary purposes require that the data be identifiable, and therefore de-identification is not a realistic option. For instance, when providing care to a patient, it is not possible to hide the identity of that patient during the encounter.

On the other hand, using and disclosing health data for secondary purposes will often *not* require that the patients be identifiable. For example, for many health services research studies the identity of patients is not necessary to perform the analysis, and it may not be necessary to have identifiable patient data for training medical students or for evaluating health plan performance.

But there will be situations where identity is also important. For example, a research study may need to contact patients who meet certain criteria to collect additional information. In such a case the identity of the patients would be needed to contact the patients. Alternatively, there may be a need to re-identify patients in a de-identified database. For example, a public health analysis may detect that certain patients have been exposed to a virus, say, those who traveled to a certain country, and would want to identify those individuals to contact them and perform follow-up interviews and tests, and for contact tracing. In such a case there needs to be a mechanism for re-identification under controlled conditions.

The Spectrum of Risk for Data Access

Data custodians can share health data with different degrees of access restrictions. At one extreme, they can make data available publicly with no access restrictions. For example, data can be made available by posting it on a website with no access controls. This option means that the data custodian imposes no constraints on who gets the data and what the data recipients do with those data. Data recipients may analyze the data by themselves or link them with other databases to create more detailed and richer data sets, which they may then also make publicly available. The custodian may not even know who has copies of the data at any point in time. Data recipients may be in the same country or halfway across the world, and they may be professional analysts or hobbyists and amateurs experimenting with the data.

An important caveat with the no-access-restrictions model is that the data custodian will not be able to manage the quality of the data analysis that is performed using the data. It will not be possible to ensure the verisimilitude of conclusions drawn by others from manipulations of the data—these conclusions may contest some of the custodian's own conclusions. These conclusions may put the data custodian in a negative light. While this is not a privacy issue, it often acts as a deterrent for the public disclosure of health information.

At the other extreme, the data custodian can disclose the health data under some restricted access regime. There are many ways in which this can be operationalized. The data recipient would have to sign a data sharing agreement and may have to go through regular audits to ensure that she has good security and privacy practices in place to handle the data. The audits may be conducted by the data custodian herself, or the data recipient may be required to conduct third-party audits and send the results of these audits to the data custodian on a regular basis.

Each of the above two approaches is suitable under different circumstances, and the option chosen will depend on factors such as the sensitivity of the data, as well as the data custodian's resources and their proclivity for risk. Clearly the former option allows much greater access to data and is the cheapest for the data custodian, as it does not require oversight of the data recipients. However, for data custodians that are risk averse and have resources to put into oversight, then the latter option may be more attractive.

Between these two ends of the spectrum there will be multiple possible options. The full spectrum of tradeoffs is illustrated conceptually in Figure 1.1. As shown, if we consider the data release as a transaction, the transaction risk does not have to be at one of the extremes. We will consider some examples to illustrate the spectrum.

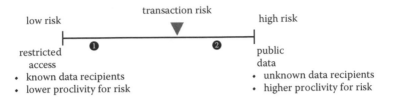

Figure 1.1   The tradeoffs for a data custodian in choosing the type of access to provide for data sets.

- A data custodian may be somewhat risk averse but does not have resources to provide significant oversight over data recipients. This means that she cannot really afford to conduct audits or enforce data sharing agreements. For instance, the data recipients may be researchers in other provinces/states/countries and the data custodian does not have the funds to conduct audits in other jurisdictions or halfway across the world. However, the data custodian may ask for third-party audits of the researchers' sites and practices, say, every three years. For such an organization transaction risk may be at point 1 in Figure 1.1.

- A data custodian may be running a public competition using her health data set. For example, this could be an analytics competition where the entrants have to build models using the data. However, the data custodian wants to create a deterrent against adversaries who may attempt to re-identify patients and contact them. Therefore all entrants must agree to terms of use for the data, and provide correct contact information. The data custodian is then prepared to legally pursue those who violate the terms rather than go and audit all data recipients (which would not be affordable because if the competition is successful, there could be thousands of entrants). In this case, the transaction risk would be around point 2 in Figure 1.1.

Once the transaction risk has been determined, even conceptually at this point, we need tools to manage that risk.

Managing Risk

De-identification methods provide a tool that allows data custodians to manage the transaction risk. This means that if a data custodian's transaction risk in Figure 1.1 is high, she can use de-identification methods to make it acceptable by reducing that risk. Even if the transaction risk is low, some de-identification would be needed because "low" does not mean "zero."

The amount of de-identification that is applied to a data set can be adjusted along a spectrum. As illustrated in Figure 1.2, the amount of de-identification can

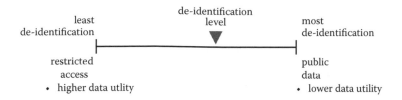

Figure 1.2   The use of de-identification to manage transaction risks.

be varied to manage the transaction risk. The rationale is easy to illustrate. One would not treat a public data release, on the web, the same way as the release to a trusted business or research partner. From a risk management perspective that would make no sense.

Consider Figure 1.3, which shows some of the tradeoffs. Following a balanced risk management approach, when the transaction risk is high, then more de-identification should be applied to the data to protect it, and when the transaction risk is low, then less de-identification is needed to protect the data.

A data custodian that always applied a lot of de-identification irrespective of the transaction risk would sometimes be conservative (quadrant 2) and sometimes have a risk-balanced outcome (quadrant 4). When he is conservative, it means that he unnecessarily incurs a high-cost burden to de-identify the data, and he will also unnecessarily use or disclose data that has a lower quality. The data custodian may also incur additional costs to ensure that the transaction risk is low, for example, by requiring a data sharing agreement with the data recipient. In quadrant 2 the data recipient has most likely invested in ensuring that its data management practices are strong, and so it will also incur some costs. Despite both the data recipient and the data custodian incurring a higher-cost burden, the data quality that is

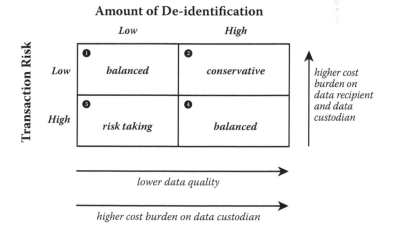

Figure 1.3   Tradeoffs from managing risk.

released is lower than it needs to be. This acts as a strong disincentive for the data recipient to invest in ensuring that the transaction risk is low.

Another common scenario is the data custodian who does not wish to incur any cost burden, and this puts him in quadrant 3. In that quadrant the data custodian is releasing high-quality data with a low amount of de-identification applied. There is also little cost incurred by the data recipient because he does not have to invest in improving their practices. However, the transaction risk is very high and it is not being managed. Operating in quadrant 3 can have significant negative legal, financial, and regulatory consequences on the data custodian. Let us consider some examples where a data release was in quadrant 3:

- With the intention of providing a real data set to be used by researchers working in the area of Internet search, AOL posted search queries from its clients on the web. *New York Times* reporters were able to re-identify one individual from these queries [3–5]. The bad publicity from this resulted in the CTO of the company resigning and the researcher who posted the data to lose his job.
- A Canadian national broadcaster aired a report on the death of a 26-year-old female taking a particular drug [6]. She was re-identified by the adverse drug reaction database released by Health Canada after matching with public obituary information. Subsequently, Health Canada restricted access to certain fields in the adverse drug event database that it releases, and litigation between the two organizations continued until 2008 in federal court.
- A re-identification attack on a movie ratings data set for a competition organized by Netflix [7] resulted in Netflix canceling a second competition and settling a class action lawsuit [8–10]. This had financial and reputational impacts on the organization.

A risk management approach would place the data custodian in quadrant 1 or 4. This concept of adjusting the level of de-identification to manage transaction risk will be explored in great detail and operationalized in the rest of the book.

There are two important implications from this risk-based approach to de-identification:

- The level of de-identification has an impact on data utility. The more de-identification that is applied, the lower the data utility. Here, reduced data utility means that the data have less information in them. Therefore, when the transaction risks are high, the data recipient will get lower utility level, and vice versa. Low data utility does not mean that analytics cannot be performed in the data. To the contrary, if de-identification is done properly, then the data are still useful for sophisticated data analysis. It is only when the de-identification is not optimized or not done adequately that data utility can be diminished significantly.

■ The level of de-identification is not fixed for all data sets and for all data recipients. The same data set may be de-identified to a different extent depending on the transaction risk. For example, if the transaction risk is low, the amount of de-identification performed on the data may be quite small. This is because there are other factors that are in place to manage the overall risk, like data sharing agreements, audits to ensure that the data recipient can manage health information, and the most sensitive fields not being released to the data recipient. Therefore the totality of de-identification and other activities ensure that the risk is acceptable and that the data release is being done responsibly.

A risk-based approach to de-identification is not entirely new. Many organizations that have been disclosing and sharing data have been doing risk assessments for more than two decades. They may not have articulated the risk assessment precisely or formally, and the whole process may have been experiential. However, they did consider some of the same factors that we will be covering here. Our contribution is in formalizing this process, providing well-defined metrics and ways to interpret them, and by applying it specifically to health care data sets.

What Is De-Identification?

De-identification is, in general, intended to protect against inappropriate disclosure of personal information. In the disclosure control literature, there are two kinds of disclosure that are of concern: identity disclosure and attribute disclosure [11, 12]. The first type of disclosure is when an adversary can assign an identity to a record in a data set. For example, if the adversary would be able to determine that record number 10 belongs to patient Joe Bloggs, then this is identity disclosure. The second type of disclosure is when an adversary learns a sensitive attribute about a patient in the database with a sufficiently high probability without knowing which specific record belongs to that patient [11, 13]. For example, assume that in a specific data set all males born in 1967 had a creatine kinease lab test (a test often given to individuals showing symptoms of a heart attack), as illustrated in Table 1.1. Let's assume that an adversary knows that Joe Bloggs has a record in Table 1.1. This adversary does not need to know which record belongs to Joe Bloggs to know that he had that test if Joe was born in 1967. This is an example of attribute disclosure.

We only focus on identity disclosure and protections against that. There are three very pragmatic reasons why we do so: (1) Existing legislation and regulations only require protection against identity disclosure when a data set is de-identified, (2) there are no publicly known re-identification attacks that involve attribute disclosure, and (3) protections against attribute disclosure would destroy data utility for most analytical purposes. We examine each of these in turn.

All the analysis leading up to the U.S. Department of Health and Human Services (DHHS) issuing the (HIPAA) Privacy Rule de-identification standards

Table 1.1 Example of a Data Set with Lab Test Results

Sex	Year of Birth	Lab Test
Male	1959	Albumin, serum
Male	1967	Creatine kinase
Female	1955	Alkaline phosphatase
Male	1959	Bilirubin
Female	1942	BUN/creatinine ratio
Female	1975	Calcium, serum
Female	1966	Free thyroxine index
Female	1987	Globulin, total
Male	1959	B-type natriuretic peptide
Male	1967	Creatine kinase
Male	1968	Alanine aminotransferase
Female	1955	Cancer antigen 125
Male	1967	Creatine kinase
Male	1967	Creatine kinase
Female	1966	Creatinine
Female	1955	Triglycerides
Male	1967	Creatine kinase
Female	1956	Monocytes
Female	1956	HDL cholesterol
Male	1978	Neutrophils
Female	1966	Prothrombin time
Male	1967	Creatine kinase

has focused on protections against identity disclosure [14, 15]. HIPAA does not address identifiability risks from attribute disclosure. The case is similar for the different federal and provincial privacy and health privacy laws in Canada and the EU. Some of these definitions will be examined later on.

Known re-identification attacks of personal information that have actually occurred are all identity disclosures [19], for example:

1. Reporters figured out which queries belonged to a specific individual from a database of web search queries publicly posted by AOL [3–5].
2. Students re-identified individuals in the Chicago homicide database by linking it with the social security death index [16].
3. At least one individual was believed to be re-identified by linking his or her movie ratings in a publicly disclosed Netflix file to another public movie ratings database [7].
4. The insurance claims records of the governor of Massachusetts were re-identified by linking a claims database sold by the state employees' insurer with the voter registration list [17].
5. An expert witness re-identified most of the records in a neuroblastoma registry [18, 19].
6. A national broadcaster matched the adverse drug event database with public obituaries to re-identify a 26-year-old girl who died while taking a drug and filmed a documentary on the drug afterwards [6].
7. An individual in a prescriptions record database was re-identified by a neighbor [20].
8. The DHHS in the United States linked a large medical database with a commercial database and re-identified a handful of individuals [21].

In all of these cases the privacy breach was to assign individual identities to records that were ostensibly de-identified.

Finally, we illustrate the impact of attribute disclosure on the ability to perform analysis using an example. Consider Table 1.2, which is a data set showing whether daughters of parents with a particular religious affiliation are being vaccinated against HPV. HPV is a virus that is known to cause cervical cancer, and existing vaccines have been shown to provide effective protection. However, the data suggest that parents affiliated with religion A are not likely to vaccinate their daughters because they do not believe they will engage in sexual activity that would cause an infection, or put another way, if they vaccinate them, then they are admitting that they will engage in sexual activity (which is something they believe is not or should not be true). The relationship is statistically significant (chi-square test, $p < 0.05$).

However, the data set in Table 1.2 also has a big risk of attribute disclosure. We now know that individuals affiliated with religion A are not likely to vaccinate their daughters: The no vaccination rate is 89%. This may be stigmatizing information in

Table 1.2   Relationship between HPV Vaccination and Affiliation with Religion A

	HPV Vaccinated	Not HPV Vaccinated
Religion A	5	40
Religion B	40	5

Table 1.3 Relationship between HPV Vaccination and Affiliation with Religion A after Suppressing Some Records in the Data Set

	HPV Vaccinated	Not HPV Vaccinated
Religion A	5	6
Religion B	6	5

that it exposes those girls to a higher rate of infection and transmission of the virus. It is not necessary to know that Joe Bloggs is even in the data set to be able to draw this conclusion, let alone knowing which record belongs to Joe.

In Table 1.3 we have suppressed some records and removed them from the data set. Now it is not possible to draw a conclusion that there is a relationship between these two variables (the chi-square test is not statistically significant). This also eliminates the risk from attribute disclosure. But because attribute disclosure often represents the key relationships that we want to detect in a data set, the reduction in attribute disclosure also directly removes those relationships from the data. Eliminating interesting relationships in the data set would not be a desirable outcome of a de-identification exercise.

In the above example we are also able to make inferences about individuals who are not in the data, and if the relationship is robust, these inferences will likely be accurate. This is the basis of statistics and data analysis. If we eliminate the ability to draw inferences about the population at large, then we have crippled data analytics.

Therefore, as defined in this book, when a data set is de-identified, then the probability of assigning a correct identity to one or more records in the data is very small.

Attribute disclosure can still be considered a privacy breach under certain conditions. Based on our experiences, regulators do consider attribute disclosure issues when deciding whether a data set should be released or not. However, de-identification methods are not the appropriate tools to manage such risks. Other governance and regulatory mechanisms would need to be put in place. For example, in a research context ethics boards make decisions on whether a particular research question about a specific population is stigmatizing, and whether or how such research needs to be conducted and communicated. Outside the research world there are no such well-defined governance mechanisms, and this is a gap that would need to be addressed moving forward. However, it is not a gap that we are addressing here.

Learning Something New

The discussion of attribute disclosure brings us to a consideration of "learning something new" about the individuals in the data or the population at large. Figure 1.4 illustrates the possible scenarios that we consider. The columns indicate whether we

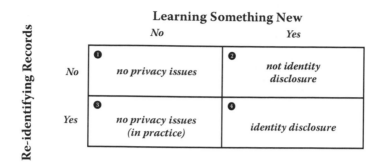

Figure 1.4 Situations where identity disclosure is relevant.

learn something new from the data, and the rows whether we can re-identify individuals in the data. For the latter, we do not make a distinction between whether new information learned is sensitive or not, or how sensitive it is. In quadrant 1 we do not learn anything new or re-identify individuals, so there would be no privacy concerns there, at least from the perspectives we are taking.

In quadrant 2 we learn something new about the individuals, but cannot re-identify their records. This is the classical attribute disclosure problem that we discussed above. While it is a potential privacy breach, it is not an identity disclosure issue.

The third quadrant is an interesting one. Here an individual is re-identified, but we do not learn something new about that individual. For example, consider a data set with two records about people who have had botulism, which is quite rare. Let's say that the data set has the age and gender of the individual, as well as the region of the country that they live in. Because it is rare and has a bad prognosis, these cases of botulism were also reported in the local media. An adversary then knows from the media that Joe Bloggs, who is male and 50, has botulism, and one of the records in the data set is for a 50-year-old male. In this case all of the information that exists in the data set is known by the adversary, and therefore the adversary learns nothing new. Strictly speaking, this is an identity disclosure problem because the adversary now knows that record number 2 in the data set is Joe Bloggs's, but the adversary does not learn anything new beyond what she used to re-identify the record. In practice, regulators have considered this not to be a disclosure of personal information. This is a pragmatic decision and makes a lot of common sense.

Finally, quadrant 4 is identity disclosure, and is the scenario that we focus on for the rest of this work.

The Status Quo

Today there are two distinct camps in the privacy community. One camp argues that current privacy protections through de-identification are inadequate and must therefore be abandoned en masse. This extreme view is counterbalanced by another extreme view arguing that the status quo is perfectly fine and nothing needs to change. Both camps have a strong vested interest in their positions. The former have developed new privacy protection models and methods, and would like them adopted quickly; they are pushing out the old to bring in the new. The latter have been practicing current de-identification methods for some time and would not want their work undermined by new approaches that claim to be superior.

We have taken a third view, which falls in the middle of these two camps. Our argument is that some aspects of current de-identification practices need to be updated, but the basic premise of existing standards is still sound and should not be abandoned. This viewpoint is driven both by the existing evidence and by pragmatism.

We will start off by examining the status quo in terms of de-identification practices. This will help you understand why improvements to the status quo are needed, and why we cannot just continue as we were.

Current approaches that are used for the de-identification of health data are exemplified by the two standards in the HIPAA Privacy Rule: (1) the Safe Harbor standard and (2) the statistical method (also known as the expert determination method).

The Safe Harbor standard (henceforth "Safe Harbor") is a precise method for the de-identification of health information. It stipulates the removal or generalization of 18 variables from a data set (see Sidebar 1.1). The certainty and simplicity of Safe Harbor makes it quite attractive for health information custodians when disclosing data without patient consent [22], and it is used quite often in practice. The statistical method requires an expert to certify that "the risk is very small that the information could be used, alone or in combination with other reasonably available information, by an anticipated recipient to identify an individual who is a subject of the information" (see Sidebar 1.2).

Sidebar 1.1: The 18 HIPAA Safe Harbor Elements

The following identifiers of the individual, or of relatives, employers, or household members of the individual, are removed:

1. Names
2. All geographic subdivisions smaller than a state, including street address, city, county, precinct, ZIP code, and their equivalent geocodes, except for the initial three digits of a ZIP code if, according to the current publicly available data from the Bureau of the Census:

    a. The geographic unit formed by combining all ZIP codes with the same three initial digits contains more than 20,000 people.

    b. The initial three digits of a ZIP code for all such geographic units containing 20,000 or fewer people is changed to 000.

3. All elements of dates (except year) for dates directly related to an individual, including birth date, admission date, discharge date, and date of death; and all ages over 89 and all elements of dates (including year) indicative of such age, except that such ages and elements may be aggregated into a single category of age 90 or older

4. Telephone numbers

5. Fax numbers

6. Electronic mail addresses

7. Social security numbers

8. Medical record numbers

9. Health plan beneficiary numbers

10. Account numbers

11. Certificate/license numbers

12. Vehicle identifiers and serial numbers, including license plate numbers

13. Device identifiers and serial numbers

14. Web universal resource locators (URLs)

15. Internet protocol (IP) address numbers

16. Biometric identifiers, including finger and voice prints

17. Full face photographic images and any comparable images

18. Any other unique identifying number, characteristic, or code

The catchall 18th element is "any other unique identifying number, characteristic, or code." Examples of interpretations of element 18 are clinical trial record numbers, unique keys that are derived from a date of birth or that are a hash value of a name and date of birth without a salt, and unique identifiers assigned to patients in electronic medical records.

Safe Harbor is relevant beyond the United States. For example, health research organizations in Canada choose to use the Safe Harbor criteria to de-identify data sets [23], Canadian sites conducting research funded by U.S. agencies need to comply with HIPAA [24], and international guidelines for the public disclosure of clinical trials data have relied on Safe Harbor definitions [25]. Therefore the validity and strength of Safe Harbor is of importance to a broad international community.

Sidebar 1.2: The Statistical Method in the HIPAA Privacy Rule

A covered entity may determine that health information is not individually identifiable health information if a person with appropriate knowledge of and experience with generally accepted statistical and scientific principles and methods for rendering information not individually identifiable:

- Applying such principles and methods, determines that the risk is *very small* that the information could be used, alone or in combination with other reasonably available information, by an anticipated recipient to identify an individual who is a subject of the information
- Documents the methods and results of the analysis that justify such determination

---

The statistical method definition of what is considered de-identified data is consistent with definitions in other jurisdictions. For example, the Article 29 Data Protection Working Party in the EU notes that the term *identifiable* should account for "all means likely reasonably to be used either by the controller or by any other person to identify the said person" [26], and Ontario's Personal Health Information Protection Act states that identifying information means "information that identifies an individual or for which it is reasonably foreseeable in the circumstances that it could be utilized, either alone or with other information, to identify an individual."

As we illustrate below, Safe Harbor does not provide adequate protection in that it is possible to re-identify records from data sets that meet the Safe Harbor standard. The statistical method is a much better starting point for a de-identification methodology.

Safe Harbor-Compliant Data Can Have a High Risk of Re-Identification

Out of the 18 elements, only elements 2 and 3 would be included in data sets that are disclosed. The remaining elements would have to be either removed or replaced with pseudonyms. Any other information that is not specified in Sidebar 1.1 can also be included in a data set, and the data set would be deemed compliant with the standard, for example, patient's profession, diagnosis codes, drugs dispensed, and laboratory tests ordered.

Below we describe common scenarios that can result in Safe Harbor-compliant data sets with a high risk of re-identification. To simplify these scenarios we assume that the data set is being disclosed publicly on the web. In such a case we assume that there is an adversary who will attempt a re-identification attack on the data.

The Adversary Knows Who Is in the Data

The Safe Harbor text does not explicitly state how re-identification risk is measured and what acceptable re-identification risk or the risk threshold is. However, the consultations and justifications provided by DHHS regarding Safe Harbor indicate that population uniqueness is the measure of re-identification risk that was being used in the analysis leading up to issuing the standard [14, 15]. Population uniqueness is defined as the proportion (or percentage) of individuals in the whole population who have unique values on the variables that can be used for re-identification.

There have been attempts at empirically measuring the actual re-identification risk of Safe Harbor data sets. One often cited analysis concluded that 0.04% of the U.S. population is unique in their gender, age in years, and first three digits of their ZIP code [27, 28]. Under an assumption that individuals in a data set are sampled with equal probabilities from the U.S. population, then a data set that meets the Safe Harbor requirements is expected to have a similar uniqueness value [29].

An important assumption being made here is that the adversary does not know who is in the data set. For example, if a particular data set is a random sample from the U.S. population, then it is reasonable to assume that an adversary would not know who is in that particular data set.

However, if the adversary does know who is in the data set, then the proportion of individuals that are unique can be much higher. Consider the small data set in Table 1.4 that is Safe Harbor compliant (it only includes age in years and the three digits of the ZIP code). All of the records in that data set are unique (i.e., 100% uniqueness) on age and ZIP3, which is quite different from the 0.04% value noted

Table 1.4 Example Data That Are Safe Harbor Compliant Where All Records Are Unique on Age and ZIP3

Gender	Age	ZIP3	Clinical Information (e.g., diagnosis)
M	55	112	Heart attack
F	53	114	Osteoporosis
M	24	134	Head injury

above. If the adversary knows that Tom is in this data set and knows Tom's age and the first three digits of his ZIP code, then Tom can be re-identified with certainty. In fact, the records of all three individuals, assuming that they are known to be in the data set, would be identifiable with certainty.

An adversary can know that an individual is in the data set under a number of different circumstances, for example:

1. Individuals may self-reveal that they are in the data set by mentioning that they are part of, say, a clinical trial to their colleagues or on their online social network.
2. It may be generally known whose records are in the data set, as in the case of an interview survey conducted in a company in which the participants missed half a day of work to participate. In such a case it is known within the company, and to an internal adversary, who is in the data set.
3. The data set may represent everyone in a particular group; for example, consider a registry on individuals with a rare and visible congenital anomaly in a particular state. If someone has that anomaly, then he would be in the registry with a high certainty, or if there is only one family doctor in a village, then all residents will be in a data set from that doctor's electronic medical record.

The Data Set Is Not a Random Sample from the U.S. Population

If a particular data set is a sample but it is not a random sample from the U.S. population, the percent of unique individuals can be quite high even for a data set that is Safe Harbor compliant. We will illustrate this with reference to the hospital discharge database for the state of New York for 2007. After cleaning, this database consists of approximately 1.5 million individuals who have been hospitalized. We took repeated 50% random samples from that data set. Any such sample drawn meets two criteria: (1) Hospitalized individuals in New York are not a random sample from the U.S. population, and (2) an adversary who knows that a patient has been hospitalized would not know if they are in the selected sample or not.

Our analysis shows that the expected percentage of unique individuals on gender, age in years, and the three-digit ZIP code was 0.71%, which is more than 17 times higher than the assumed Safe Harbor risk. If we restrict the cohort further to males over 65, then 0.91% are unique on these three variables, and males over 65 who were hospitalized for more than 14 days had a uniqueness of 4%, and those hospitalized more than 30 days had a uniqueness of 11.14%.

This example illustrates that if a particular cohort is not randomly selected from the U.S. population, the actual uniqueness can be dramatically higher than assumed, and it can be quite high in absolute terms as well. It would be fair to say that most health data sets are not random samples from the U.S. population, but rather they represent specific cohorts that can be quite different from the general population in their age and gender distribution.

Other Fields Can Be Used for Re-Identification

It is common for health data sets to have other kinds of fields that can be used for re-identification beyond the set included in Safe Harbor. Here we consider some examples of data elements that would pass the Safe Harbor standard but would still produce a data set with a high probability of re-identification.

First, Safe Harbor does not explicitly consider genetic data as part of the 18 fields to remove or generalize. There is evidence that a sequence of 30 to 80 independent single nucleotide polymorphisms (SNPs) could uniquely identify a single person [30]. There is also a risk of re-identification from pooled data, where it is possible to determine whether an individual is in a pool of several thousand SNPs using summary statistics on the proportion of individuals in the case or control group and the corresponding SNP value [31, 32].

Second, Safe Harbor does not consider longitudinal data. Longitudinal data contain information about multiple visits or episodes of care. For example, let us consider the state inpatient database for New York for the year 2007 again, which contains information on just over 2 million visits. Some patients had multiple visits and their ZIP code changed from one visit to the next. If we consider that the age and gender are fixed, and allow the three-digit ZIP code to change across visits (and the adversary knows those ZIP codes), then 1.8% of the patients are unique. If we assume that the adversary also knows the length of stay for each of the visits, then 20.75% of the patients are unique. Note that length of stay is not covered by Safe Harbor, and therefore can be included in the data set. Longitudinal information like the patient's three-digit ZIP code and length of stay may be known by neighbors, co-workers, relatives, and ex-spouses, and the public for famous people. As can be seen, there is a significant increase in uniqueness when the three-digit ZIP code is treated longitudinally, and a dramatic increase when other visit information is added to the data set.

Third, Safe Harbor does not deal with transactional data. For example, it has been shown that a series of International Statistical Classification of Diseases and Related Health Problems (ICD) diagnosis codes for patients makes a large percentage of individuals uniquely identifiable [33]. An adversary who is employed by the health care provider would have the diagnosis codes and patient identity, which can be used to re-identify records in a Safe Harbor-compliant data set.

Finally, other pieces of information that can re-identify individuals in free-form text and notes are not accounted for. The following actual example illustrates how the author used this information to re-identify a patient. In a series of medical records that had been de-identified using the Safe Harbor standard, there was one record about a patient with a specific (visible) injury. The notes mentioned the profession of the patient's father and hinted at the location of his work. This particular profession lists its members publicly. It was therefore possible to identify all individuals within that profession in that region. Searches through social networking sites allowed the identification of a matching patient (having the same surname) who posted the details of the specific injury during that specific period matching exactly the medical record. The key pieces of information that made re-identification possible were the father's profession and region of work. Profession is not part of the Safe Harbor list, and the region was broad enough to meet the ZIP code restrictions.

By specifying a precise and limited set of fields to consider, the Safe Harbor standard provides a simple "cookie cutter" approach to de-identification. However, it also ignores the many other fields that can be used to re-identify individuals, reducing its effectiveness at providing meaningful universal protections for different kinds of data sets.

Moving Forward beyond Safe Harbor

We have argued that the application of Safe Harbor cannot provide meaningful guarantees about the probability of re-identification except in the following very narrow circumstances: (1) The adversary does not know who is in the data, (2) the data are a simple random sample from the U.S. population, and (3) all variables in the data that can potentially be used for re-identification are covered by the 18 elements. It would be prudent for data custodians to evaluate carefully whether their data disclosures are consistent with these narrow criteria before using the Safe Harbor standard. But these are very narrow criteria indeed, and would only be met in few circumstances. The Safe Harbor standard cannot be seen as a broad and generally applicable standard because of its narrow scope of application. Even if the criteria are met, there is evidence that Safe Harbor results in data sets that have diminished utility for some important purposes, such as research and comparative effectiveness evaluation [34, 35].

We encounter data custodians who insist on using the Safe Harbor standard because it provides certainty, even if it does not provide meaningful protection. For example, the Safe Harbor standard is being used for longitudinal data and for free-form text where an adversary would know who is in the data set. This is the danger with a prescriptive regulation that has unlimited scope—it encourages and embeds poor practices.

The second standard in HIPAA, the statistical method, provides a better basis for a general risk-based de-identification methodology. However, as formulated, it leaves considerable room for interpretation: The specification of the scale and value for "very small," or multiple context-dependent values. This means that different experts may provide different, and possibly inconsistent, answers. It has been argued that the statistical standard is not used often in practice because it is perceived as not precise and too complex [36]. Furthermore, there have been concerns about the liability of the statisticians should the data be re-identified at a later point [37]. Precise guidance on both of these items would go a long way to ensuring that the application of the statistical standard is more protective of privacy under different scenarios and is repeatable when followed by different organizations. Public methodologies that are peer reviewed and open to scrutiny by the community can go a long way to ensure that the de-identification results are defensible.

In this book we provide a precise methodology for instantiating the statistical method.

Why We Wrote This Book

There are a number of reasons why we believed writing this book was important. These are enumerated as follows:

- There was a clear need to provide a more prescriptive process for the implementation of the "statistical method" in HIPAA. Given our critique of Safe Harbor, it was important to ensure that de-identification practices would meet certain quality standards through clear guidance to the community.
- There are examples of poor de-identification practices. Some we have already mentioned, such as AOL and Netflix in their public release of data [38]. While we do not claim that had they had this book, they would have done a better job, they at least would not have had an excuse for using poor de-identification practices.
- The Center for Democracy and Technology has promoted the idea of de-identification centers of excellence to serve as hubs of expertise and technology development to promote good practices in this area [39]. The material included here is intended to provide some practical information for such organizations.
- Many health information custodians are genuinely confused about what would be considered good practices for de-identification that are specific for health data. They would like to implement policies that will withstand scrutiny. The book can serve as the basis for developing and deploying risk-based de-identification policies.
- A group of experts convened by the Canadian Institute for Health Information and Canada Health Infoway developed a process guidance for de-identification that has been reviewed and found acceptable by large provincial data custodians and ministries [40]. This document, which is a *de facto* de-identification standard in Canada, covers basic concepts and metrics, but does not provide a detailed actionable process. Our book can serve as an implementation guide for that process standard.
- The disclosure control literature has good overviews of techniques that one can use [12, 41]. However, they do not provide a detailed methodology to follow in order to select and parameterize the techniques, many of the techniques they describe would not necessarily be adequate for health data, and many of them have not been applied on health data. For de-identification methods to be applied in practice, a coherent and repeatable methodology was needed that is known to work in practice in the health context.

Our concern was with the use and disclosure of individual-level health data. We discuss in detail the principles and methods that can be applied to ensure that the probability of assigning a correct identity to records in a data set is very small. We will also provide methods for determining what "very small" should be and what would be appropriate levels of access restrictions on these data.

Our approach is pragmatic and is based on our experiences with the use and disclosure of personal health information in Canada and the United States since 2005. We only present methods that work in practice and that we have found to be acceptable by the data analysis community. The objective is to give data custodians the tools to make decisions about the best way to use and disclose these data, but also ensure that the privacy of individuals is protected in a defensible way and that the resultant data can meet the analytic purpose of the use of disclosure.

We did not intend to write a literature review of the discipline of de-identification or disclosure control. There are already good reviews of statistical and computational disclosure control methods available [42, 43], and we did not wish to go over the same type of material. Rather, it is a selective assembly of practical information that can guide analysts in their efforts to create data sets with a known re-identification risk, and allow them to justifiably claim that the privacy concerns have been reasonably addressed. In practice, the issues that are not adequately addressed in the literature cause difficulties, such as how to measure re-identification risk in a defensible way and what is acceptable re-identification risk. These issues are covered here because they have to be in a real-world setting.

There were three audiences in mind when we wrote this book: (1) privacy professionals (for example, privacy officers, privacy lawyers, and those tasked with addressing privacy issues on research ethics boards), (2) policy makers and regulators, and (3) disclosure control professionals interested in risk measurement and management. To meet the needs of such a diverse group, the five sections of the book cover a broad set of legal, policy, and technical topics as follows:

Section I: The case for de-identifying personal health information. The first part of the book provides a detailed case for why de-identification is necessary and when it is advised to apply it when using and disclosing personal health information. This is essentially the business case for applying de-identification methods.

Section II: Understanding disclosure risks. In this part we situate and contextualize our risk-based methodology, and give a general overview of its steps. This part of the book gives important background.

Section III: Measuring re-identification risk. The measurement chapters explain in some detail how to measure re-identification risk. There are multiple dimensions to risk, and what is measured will depend on the assumptions made about re-identification attacks. Measurement is a critical foundation to our methodology.

Section IV: Practical methods for de-identification. The fourth part of the book explains how to go about applying transformations to data to reduce the risk of re-identification. We only focus on transformations that we know have worked on health information, rather than covering all possible approaches that have been published or proposed.

Section V: End matter. The book concludes with proofs and appendices of supporting materials.

The material is organized such that it needs to be read in order. With the exception of Section V, which consists of reference material, the first four parts of the book build on each other. And within the parts, the chapters also build on each other.

References

1. Yakowitz J. Tragedy of the commons. *Harvard Journal of Law and Technology*, 2011; 25.
2. Safran C, Bloomrosen M, Hammond E, Labkoff S, Markel-Fox S, Tang P, Detmer D. Toward a national framework for the secondary use of health data: An American Medical Informatics Association white paper. *Journal of the American Medical Informatics Association*, 2007; 14:1–9.
3. Hansell S. AOL removes search data on group of web users. *New York Times*, 2006: August 8.
4. Barbaro M, Zeller Jr. T. A face is exposed for AOL searcher no. 4417749. *New York Times*, 2006: August 9.
5. Zeller Jr. T. AOL moves to increase privacy on search queries. *New York Times*, 2006: August 22.
6. Federal Court (Canada). *Mike Gordon vs. the Minister of Health: Affidavit of Bill Wilson*. 2006.
7. Narayanan A, Shmatikov V. Robust de-anonymization of large sparse datasets. *Proceedings of the 2008 IEEE Symposium on Security and Privacy*. IEEE Computer Society, Los Namitos, CA, 2008.
8. Hunt N. Netflix prize update. 2010. http://blog.netflix.com/2010/03/this-is-neil-hunt-chief-product-officer.html. Archived at http://www.webcitation.org/6AM9lQYLI.
9. Singel R. Netflix spilled your Brokeback Mountain secret, lawsuit claims. *Wired*, 2009. http://www.wired.com/threatlevel/2009/12/netflix-privacy-lawsuit/. Archived at http://www.webcitation.org/6AM9qQqfR (accessed December 17).
10. *Doe v. Netflix*. United States District Court for the Northern District of California San Jose Division. 2009. http://www.wired.com/images_blogs/threatlevel/2009/12/doe-v-netflix.pdf. Archived at http://www.webcitation.org/6AM9xursz.
11. Skinner C. On identification dislcosure and prediction disclosure for microdata. *Statistics Neerlandica*, 1992; 46(1):21–32.
12. Subcommittee on Disclosure Limitation Methodology—Federal Committee on Statistical Methodology. *Report on statistical disclosure control*. Statistical Policy Working Paper 22. Statistical Policy Office, Office of Information and Regulatory Affairs, Office of Management and Budget, 1994.

13. Machanavajjhala A, Gehrke J, Kifer D. l-Diversity: Privacy beyond k-Anonymity. *Transactions on Knowledge Discovery from Data*, 2007; 1(1):1–47.
14. Department of Health and Human Services. Standards for privacy of individually identifiable health information. *Federal Register*, 2000. http://aspe.hhs.gov/admnsimp/final/PvcFR06.txt. Archived at http://www.webcitation.org/5tqU5GyQX.
15. Department of Health and Human Services. Standards for privacy of individually identifiable health information. *Federal Register*, 2000. http://aspe.hhs.gov/admnsimp/final/PvcFR05.txt. Archived at http://www.webcitation.org/5tqULb7hT.
16. Ochoa S, Rasmussen J, Robson C, Salib M. *Reidentification of individuals in Chicago's homicide database: A technical and legal study*. 2001. http://groups.csail.mit.edu/mac/classes/6.805/student-papers/spring01-papers/reidentification.doc. Archived at http://www.webcitation.org/5x9yE1e7L.
17. Sweeney L. k-Anonymity: A model for protecting privacy. *International Journal on Uncertainty, Fuzziness and Knowledge-Based Systems*, 2002; 10(5):557–570.
18. Appellate Court of Illinois—Fifth District. *The Southern Illinoisan v. Department of Public Health*. 2004. http://law.justia.com/cases/illinois/court-of-appeals-fifth-appellate-district/2004/5020836.html.
19. The Supreme Court of the State of Illinois. *Southern Illinoisan vs. the Illinois Department of Public Health*. 2006. http://www.state.il.us/court/opinions/supremecourt/2006/february/opinions/html/98712.htm (accessed February 1, 2011).
20. El Emam K, Kosseim P. Privacy interests in prescription records. Part 2. Patient privacy. *IEEE Security and Privacy*, 2009; 7(2):75–78. DOI: 10.1109/MSP.2009.47.
21. Lafky D. The Safe Harbor method of de-identification: An empirical test. Fourth National HIPAA Summit West, X2010. http://www.ehcca.com/presentations/HIPAAWest4/lafky_2.pdf. Archived at http://www.webcitation.org/5xA2HIOmj.
22. Mcgraw D. Building public trust in uses of Health Insurance Portability and Accountability Act de-identified data. *Journal of the American Medical Informatics Association*, 2012. DOI: 10.1136/amiajnl-2012-000936.
23. El Emam K. *Data anonymization practices in clinical research: A descriptive study*. Ottawa: Health Canada, Access to Information and Privacy Division, 2006.
24. UBC Clinical Research Ethics Board, Providence Health Care Research Ethics Board. *Interim guidance to clinical researchers regarding compliance with the US Health Insurance Portability and Accountability Act (HIPAA)*. University of British Columbia, 2003.
25. Hryanszkiewicz I, Norton M, Vickers A, Altman D. Preparing raw clinical data for publications: Guidance for journal editors, authors, and peer reviewers. *British Medical Journal*, 2010; 340:c181.
26. Article 29 Data Protection Working Party. Opinion 4/2007 on the concept of personal data: Adopted on 20th June. 2007. http://ec.europa.eu/justice_home/fsj/privacy/docs/wpdocs/2007/wp136_en.pdf. Archived at http://www.webcitation.org/5Q2YBu0CR.
27. National Committee on Vital and Health Statistics. *Report to the Secretary of the US Department of Health and Human Services on enhanced protections for uses of health data: A stewardship framework for "secondary uses" of electronically collected and transmitted health data*. 2007.
28. Sweeney L. Data sharing under HIPAA: 12 years later. Workshop on the HIPAA Privacy Rule's de-identification standard. 2010. http://www.hhshipaaprivacy.com/.
29. Skinner G, Elliot M. A measure of disclosure risk for microdata. *Journal of the Royal Statistical Society (Series B)*, 2002; 64(Part 4):855–867.

30. Lin Z, Owen A, Altman R. Genomic research and human subject privacy. *Science*, 2004; 305:183.
31. Homer N, Szelinger S, Redman M, Duggan D, Tembe W, Muehling J, Pearson J, Stephan D, Nelson S, Craig D. Resolving individuals contributing trace amounts of DNA to highly complex mixtures using high-density SNP genotyping microarrays. *PLOS Genetics*, 2008; 4(8):e1000167.
32. Jacobs K, Yeager M, Wacholder S, Craig D, Kraft P, Hunter D, Paschal J, Manolio T, Tucker M, Hoover R, Thomas G, Chanock S, Chatterjee N. A new statistic and its power to infer membership in a genome-wide association study using genotype frequencies. *Nature Genetics*, 2009; 41:1253–1257.
33. Loukides G, Denny J, Malin B. The disclosure of diagnosis codes can breach research participants' privacy. *Journal of the American Medical Informatics Association*, 2010; 17:322–327.
34. Clause S, Triller D, Bornhorst C, Hamilton R, Cosler L. Conforming to HIPAA regulations and compilation of research data. *American Journal of Health-System Pharmacy*, 2004; 61(10):1025–1031.
35. Peddicord D, Waldo A, Boutin M, Grande T, Luis Gutierrez J. A proposal to protect privacy of health information while accelerating comparative effectiveness research. *Health Affairs*, 2010; 29(11):2082–2090.
36. Beach J. *Health care databases under HIPAA: Statistical approaches to de-identification of protected health information.* DIMACS Working Group on Privacy/Confidentiality of Health Data, 2003.
37. American Public Health Association. *Statisticians and de-identifying protected health information for HIPAA.* 2005. http://www.apha.org/membergroups/newsletters/sectionnewsletters/statis/fall05/2121.htm.
38. El Emam K, Jonker E, Arbuckle L, Malin B. A systematic review of re-identification attacks on health data. *PLoS ONE*, 2011; 6(12).
39. Center for Democracy and Technology. *Encouraging the use of, and rethinking protections for de-identified (and "anonymized") health data.* 2009. https://www.cdt.org/files/pdfs/20090625_deidentify.pdf.
40. Health System Use Technical Advisory Committee—Data De-Identification Working Group. *"Best practice" guidelines for managing the disclosure of de-identified health information.* 2011. http://www.ehealthinformation.ca/documents/Data%20De-identification%20Best%20Practice%20Guidelines.pdf. Archived at http://www.webcitation.org/5x9w6635d.
41. Duncan G, Elliot M, Salazar-Gonzalez J-J. *Statistical confidentiality: Principles and practice.* New York: Springer, 2011.
42. Chen B-C, Kifer D, LeFevre K, Machanavajjhala A. Privacy preserving data publishing. *Foundations and Trends in Databases*, 2009; 2(1–2):1–167.
43. Fung BCM, Wang K, Chen R, Yu PS. Privacy-preserving data publishing: A survey of recent developments. *ACM Computing Surveys*, 2010; 42(4). DOI: 10.1145/1749603.1749605.

THE CASE FOR DE-IDENTIFYING PERSONAL HEALTH INFORMATION

Chapter 2

Permitted Disclosures, Consent, and De-Identification of PHI

In the following chapters we explain in great detail when and why it is important to create de-identified health data sets. There are legal, financial, and practical reasons for doing so. We start by providing some definitions and background information on health data flows.

Common Data Flows

The data flows that are relevant for this book are illustrated in Figure 2.1. The terms we use are often Ontario-specific, but there are almost always equivalents in other jurisdictions.

Personal heath information (PHI) is information about identifiable individuals. They may be, for example, patients, residents in a home, employees, students, or healthy clients. PHI may be collected from individuals directly or indirectly through reporters. An example of direct collection is when a patient completes a medical history form at a clinic. An example of indirect collection is in the case of an adverse drug reaction whereby a hospital or a physician may report the adverse reaction rather than the patient herself.

This PHI is collected by a custodian. A common example of a custodian would be a hospital. The custodian may have collected the information for a primary

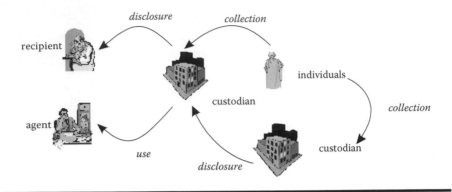

Figure 2.1 Basic data flow during a disclosure or use of PHI.

purpose, such as providing care to a patient. The custodian may have also collected the information explicitly for a secondary purpose, such as constructing a database of patients with diabetes for subsequent research.*

A custodian may disclose PHI to another custodian. For example, a hospital may disclose PHI to a public health agency. In such a case, the information is not coming directly from an individual, but indirectly through one (or possibly more) custodian.

An agent of the custodian may *use* the information for a secondary purpose. An agent is broadly defined as a person who acts on behalf of the custodian in respect of the personal information for the purposes of the custodian. For example, a data analyst employed by a hospital to produce reports on resource utilization would be an agent. Also, a subcontractor to the hospital performing work for the hospital would be considered an agent of the hospital. There is generally no legislative requirement to de-identify information that an agent uses and no requirement to obtain additional consent from the individuals/patients for such uses.

The custodian may also receive a request to *disclose* the information to a recipient for some secondary purpose. The recipient can be an individual (e.g., a researcher) or an organization (e.g., a pharmaceutical company). The recipient can also be internal or external to the custodian. For example, a researcher may be based within a hospital or can be an external researcher at a university or a government department requesting the information from the hospital.

Some PHI disclosures are mandatory and some are discretionary to the custodian. An example of a mandatory disclosure is reporting communicable diseases or reporting gunshot wounds in some jurisdictions. In these situations the disclosure of PHI is required.

---

* There are some exceptions. In Ontario "prescribed entities" hold information for secondary purposes, and strictly speaking, they are not considered health information custodians. In this book we will use the general term *data custodian* or just *custodian* to refer to health information custodians or prescribed entities for ease of presentation.

Otherwise, there are different types of recipients and purposes where disclosures of PHI are discretionary. However, the conditions for discretionary disclosure do vary. There are a set of permitted disclosures in Canadian privacy legislation where PHI may be disclosed without consent. Table 2.1 presents some examples of such permitted disclosures.

Other discretionary disclosures that are not explicitly permitted in legislation require that either consent be obtained from the individuals/patients or the information is de-identified. For example, in some jurisdictions the disclosure of PHI to a pharmaceutical company for marketing purposes requires that consent be obtained or that the information is deemed to be de-identified.

The Need for De-Identification

When de-identified, the data are no longer PHI. There is no legislative requirement to obtain consent for the use of de-identified information because it can no longer be connected to any particular individual or individuals. In order words, this information is no longer deemed to be personal once de-identified.

Therefore, to summarize, there are four scenarios to consider:

1. It is mandatory to disclose PHI to a recipient, and no consent is required.
2. PHI is used by an agent without consent.
3. It is permitted by legislation to disclose PHI to a recipient without consent under the discretion of the custodian.
4. The custodian *must* de-identify the PHI *or* obtain consent before disclosing the data to the recipient.

Disclosures under scenario 1 are outside our scope since they do not require any de-identification. Under those conditions patient identity is important in order to achieve the intended purpose. For example, for mandatory reporting of communicable diseases, public health may contact the affected individuals to investigate the outbreak or do contact tracing. In such circumstances knowing the identity of the individual is critical.

The case for de-identification of the information under each of the remaining three scenarios will vary. We address scenarios 2, 3, and 4 in the following chapters.

Table 2.1 Examples of Permitted Discretionary Disclosures of Personal Health Information in Canadian Jurisdictions

Purpose of Disclosure/Recipient	Mandatory (M)/ Discretionary (D)	Restrictions on Recipient	Legislation
For health or other programs: Eligibility to receive health care Audits or accreditation of the custodian QA activities Prescribed registries Medical officer of health under the Health Protection and Promotion Act (Ontario) for the purposes of that act Public health authority in Canada or another jurisdiction for a purpose substantially similar to that in the Health Protection and Promotion Act (Ontario)	D[a]	Restrictions or requirements in the regulations	PHIPA, ss.39(1)(2); Nfld. PHIA, s.39(1)(a); HIA, s.35(1)(f); Nfld. PHIA, s.39(4)(b); HIA, s.35(1)(g); Sask. THIPA, s.27(4)(g); O. Reg. 39/04 s.13 (registries); Nfld. PHIA s.39(4)(d); Nfld. PHIA, s.39(4)(e); Nfld. PHIA, s.39(4)(f); NB PHIPA, s.37(6)(b), (e), (f), (d) (registries)
Related to risks/care and custody: Eliminating or reducing significant risk of serious bodily harm to a person or group Penal/psychiatric institutions to assist in decision making regarding care and/or placements	D		PHIPA, s.40; HIA, s.35(1)(e); HIA, s.35(1)(m); Manitoba PHIA, s.22(2)(b); HIPA, s.27(4)(a); Nfld. PHIA, s.40(1); Nfld. PHIA, s.40(2); NB PHIPA, s.39(1); NS PHIA, s.38(1)(d)

Table 2.1 (continued)   Examples of Permitted Discretionary Disclosures of Personal Health Information in Canadian Jurisdictions

Purpose of Disclosure/Recipient	Mandatory (M)/ Discretionary (D)	Restrictions on Recipient	Legislation
Compliance with subpoena, warrant, court order	D		PHIPA, s.41(1)(d)(i); HIA, s.35(1)(i); NS PHIA s.38(1)(q) Manitoba PHIA s.22(2)(l); HIPA, s.27(2)(i); Nfld. PHIA, s.41(1)(b)
Disclosure for proceedings	D	Requirements or restrictions in the regulations (none currently prescribed in PHIPA)	PHIPA s.41(1); HIA, s.35(1(h); Manitoba PHIA, s.22(2)(k); THIPA, s.27(2)(i); Nfld. PHIA, s.41(2)(a); NB PHIPA, s.40(1),(2)
Disclosure to (potential) successor of custodian	D	Potential successor must enter into an agreement with the custodian re confidentiality and security of the PHI (PHIPA and NB PHIPA)	PHIPA, ss.42(1)(2); HIA, s.35(1)(q); Manitoba PHIA, s.27(4)(c); Nfld. PHIA, s.39(1)(i),(j); NB PHIPA, s.38(1)(i)(j)
Disclosures related to other acts	D		PHIPA, s.43; HIA, s.35(1)(p); Manitoba PHIA, s.22(2)(o); THIPA, s.27(2)(l); Nfld. PHIA, s.43

continued

Table 2.1 (continued)   Examples of Permitted Discretionary Disclosures of Personal Health Information in Canadian Jurisdictions

Purpose of Disclosure/Recipient	Mandatory (M)/ Discretionary (D)	Restrictions on Recipient	Legislation
Disclosures for research	D	Researcher must provide custodian with a research plan (as prescribed), obtain REB approval (as prescribed), and enter into a research agreement (PHIPA; HIA). Researcher is permitted to disclose information as prescribed (PHIPA).	PHIPA, s.44; O. Reg. 39/04, s.15 (REB requirements); s.16 (research plan requirements); s.17 (disclosure by researchers) HIA, ss.48–54 (note that the researcher may submit a proposal to an REB; it is not mandatory) Manitoba PHIA, s.24 (project must be approved by a health information privacy committee) (Reg. 245/97, s.8.1 and 8.2) or REB; agreement required (Reg. 245/97, s.8.3) PHIPA, s.29 (research ethics committee approval is required; research agreement is required)

Table 2.1 (continued)   Examples of Permitted Discretionary Disclosures of Personal Health Information in Canadian Jurisdictions

Purpose of Disclosure/Recipient	Mandatory (M)/ Discretionary (D)	Restrictions on Recipient	Legislation
Disclosures for research (continued)			Nfld. PHIA, s.44 (REB approval required under the Health Research Ethics Authority Act)
			Sask. THIPA, s.29; NS PHIA, s.56; NB PHIPA, s.43
Disclosure for planning and management of the health system: To prescribed entities for analysis or compilation of statistical information	D	Prescribed entity must have practices and procedures in place to protect privacy and maintain confidentiality; reviewed by the commissioner in Ontario	PHIPA, s.45; O. Reg. 39/04, s.18 (prescribed entities); Nfld. PHIA, s.39(1)(h)
For monitoring health care payments: To the minister on his/ her request To verify or monitor claims for payment for care funded in whole or in part by the ministry or LHIN	D		PHIPA, s.46; Nfld. PHIA, s.39(1)(b)

continued

Table 2.1 (continued) Examples of Permitted Discretionary Disclosures of Personal Health Information in Canadian Jurisdictions

Purpose of Disclosure/Recipient	Mandatory (M)/ Discretionary (D)	Restrictions on Recipient	Legislation
For analysis of the health system: At the minister's request (to a health data institute in PHIPA only) Management, evaluation, monitoring, allocation of resources, or planning	D	Minister must submit proposal to the commissioner for review and comment (PHIPA); subject to prescribed restrictions (none enacted for PHIPA)	PHIPA ss.47, 48; HIA s.46

[a] Note that all of the disclosures under Newfoundland and Labrador's Personal Health Information Act. PHIA ss.39, 41, and 43 are mandatory, as are those under s.37 of New Brunswick Personal Health Information Protection Act (PHIPA).

Chapter 3

Permitted Uses and Disclosures of Health Information

Uses of Health Information by an Agent

While agents are permitted to access PHI, it is often not necessary for them to have the data in identifiable form for them to perform their functions. When this is the case, it would be best to de-identify that information as a risk mitigation exercise. We consider three attack scenarios by an agent: (1) an insider inadvertently or maliciously causing a data breach, (2) an insider determining the identity of individuals, and (3) risks of breaches at subcontractors. Under these three scenarios, if the data used by the agent were de-identified, then the risks and impact on the data custodian would be significantly reduced.

Privacy and security breaches by insiders are relatively common [1–5]. In a recent survey a quarter of health care IT professionals identified a data breach by an internal person within the past year [6]. Internal breaches come from people who have (or recently had) legitimate access to the data, but whose behavior jeopardizes the organization's security and privacy. One survey found that 27% of breaches were due to insiders [7]. In a 2007 Computer Security Institute survey, 59% of the respondents claimed that they witnessed abuse of the network resources by an insider [8], and the 2009 survey shows that a significant percentage of monetary losses from breaches were due to malicious and nonmalicious insiders [9]. These could involve employees who have access to critical data and engage in unauthorized explorations; they could be individuals who join an organization with the intent to commit some kind of fraud, or some naïve employees who lose their laptop after they put sensitive information on it. There are also increasing cases of ex-employees taking or keeping personal information about clients/patients and other employees after they leave their employer (because they were laid off, resigned, or were fired) [10]. Recent analyses of breach data indicate that 20% are internal breaches [11]; 34% of security and IT leadership in organizations worldwide estimated that the likely source of security incidents in the last year was an employee, and 16% responded that it was an ex-employee [12], and in the United States and Canada, approximately 24% of data breaches in medical establishments (including hospitals and health insurance claims processors) are due to insiders, and 32% of breaches involving medical records are due to insiders (between January 2007 and June 2009) [13]. Overall, investigators reported a rapid increase in offenses committed by insiders [14].

Furthermore, insider breaches can be ongoing for a long time without the custodians being aware of them [15]. There is evidence that the detection of the vast majority of data breaches is passive—they are detected by third parties who then inform the custodian [11, 16, 17]. One recent survey found that 41% of breaches are reported by the patients themselves [18]. Therefore a custodian may not be aware that breaches involving his data have occurred at the time, and there may be some time lag before he becomes aware. This gives insiders a significant opportunity to leak information.

The type of attacks from the inside can have a huge impact on the organization. It was reported that an outside attack costs the organization on average $56,000, while an insider breach costs on average $2.7 million [14].

Subcontractors are also agents, and they may get personal health information from the custodian without consent. Consider a hospital network that has developed a system to provide its patients with Internet access to their electronic health records. The hospital has subcontracted the work to perform quality control for this software to a testing company across town. The testing company needs realistic patient data to test the software, for example, to make sure that the software can handle large volumes of patient records, that it displays the correct information to each patient, and so on. The testing company would be considered an agent of the hospital, and therefore it can obtain identifiable patient records without consent for the purpose of software testing. Giving the testing company PHI potentially exposes the hospital to additional risk if there is an inadvertent disclosure of this data (e.g., a breach at the testing company's site). It is always preferable from a risk management perspective to minimize the number of people who have access to PHI, and making that information available to the whole test team should be avoided if possible. According to the DHHS in the United States, one quarter of reported breaches affecting more than 500 records were at a business associate as of mid-July 2011.

If data sets used by custodians or their subcontractors are not de-identified properly, insiders have a unique ability to re-identify the records in these data sets. The main reason is that they would have access to more background knowledge than other adversaries. For example, in the United States, genotype and phenotype data collected from health care provider institutions for genome-wide association studies are being made more broadly available [19]. A recent study has demonstrated how an insider from one of the source institutions can re-identify patients in the DNA database with certainty [20].

In one recent example, hospital pharmacy records were being disclosed to a commercial data broker [21]. This data set included information about when the patient was admitted, his or her gender, age, residential geographic information, and admission and discharge dates. Such detailed information would not be considered de-identified even though patient names were removed. A neighbor who was working at the hospital was able to re-identify a record using prior knowledge about a patient, revealing the patient's diagnoses and prescriptions [21].

Disclosing Identifiable Data When Permitted

It should be noted that even in cases where reporting of PHI without consent by providers is *mandatory*, there is a considerable amount of underreporting due to privacy concerns (for example, for some communicable diseases) [22–34]. Therefore in cases where disclosure is discretionary, it would not be surprising to see that there is reluctance by providers to disclose personal information as well [34]. Drivers of that reluctance include (1) the impact of the disclosure on the patient-physician relationship, (2) the impact on public trust of the custodian, and (3) potential for litigation.

In such cases the custodian may consider de-identification anyway. This, of course, makes sense only if the purpose can be satisfied without having identifiable information. In practice, achieving many purposes does not require identifiable information. A good example of that is in the research context.

A research ethics board (REB) determines whether custodians can disclose PHI to researchers, and whether that information needs to be de-identified. REBs have total discretion to make that decision. In practice, most REBs will require that either consent from the patients be sought if the information needs to be identifiable or the disclosed information is adequately de-identified [35]. However, because of the discretionary nature of this type of disclosure, they may also allow identifiable information to be disclosed without consent under certain conditions.

For instance, consider the situation where a researcher is collecting clinical information from electronic health records (EHRs) and wants to link it with data in a provincial administrative database. The linking will not work if the EHR data are de-identified. In that case the REB may allow identifiable information to be disclosed for the purpose of linking without requiring the consent of the patients. The REB may then require the de-identification of the linked data.

References

1. Stolfo S, Bellovin S, Herkshop S, Keromytis A, Sinclair S, Smith S. *Insider attack and cyber security.* New York: Springer Verlag, 2008.
2. Kowalski E, Cappelli D, Moore A. *Insider threat study: Illicit cyber activity in the information technology and telecommunications sector.* Carnegie Mellon University and the United States Secret Service, 2008. http://www.cert.org/archive/pdf/insiderthreat_it2008.pdf. Archived at http://www.webcitation.org/5ir1TiKMS.
3. Randazzo M, Keeney M, Kowalski E, Cappelli D, Moore A. *Insider threat study: Illicit cyber activity in the banking and finance sector.* Carnegie Mellon University and the United States Secret Service, 2004. http://www.cert.org/archive/pdf/bankfin040820.pdf. Archived at http://www.webcitation.org/5ir1hY5Uk.
4. Keeney M, Kowalski E, Cappelli D, Moore A, Shimeall T, Rogers S. *Insider threat study: Computer system sabotage in critical infrastructure sectors.* Carnegie Mellon University and the United States Secret Service, 2005. http://www.cert.org/archive/pdf/insidercross051105.pdf. Archived at http://www.webcitation.org/5ir1rwVOF.
5. Kowalski E, Conway T, Keverline S, Williams M, Cappelli D, Willke B, Moore A. *Insider threat study: Illicit cyber activity in the government sector.* Carnegie Mellon University and the United States Secret Service, 2008. Available from http://www.cert.org/archive/pdf/insiderthreat_gov2008.pdf. Archived at http://www.webcitation.org/5ir25mBaS.
6. Kroll Fraud Solutions. *HIMSS analytics report: Security of patient data.* 2008. http://www.mmc.com/knowledgecenter/Kroll_HIMSS_Study_April2008.pdf. Archived at http://www.webcitation.org/5ipdyMtNJ.
7. *CSO Magazine.* 2006 e-crime watch survey. U.S. Secret Service, Carnegie Mellon University, and Microsoft Corporation, 2006.
8. Predd J, Hunker J, Bulford C. Insiders behaving badly. *IEEE Security and Privacy,* 2008; 6(4):66–70.
9. CSI. *14th Annual CSI computer crime and security survey.* 2009.
10. Ponemon Institute. *Data loss risks during downsizing.* 2009.
11. Verizon Business Risk Team. *2009 data breach investigations report.* 2009.
12. PriceWaterhouseCoopers. *Safeguarding the new currency of business: Findings from the 2008 global state of information security study.* 2008.
13. El Emam K, King M. *The data breach analyzer.* 2009. http://www.ehealthinformation.ca/dataloss.
14. Shaw E, Ruby K, Jerrold M. *The insider threat to information systems.* Department of Defense Security Institute, 1998.
15. Melodia M. Security breach notification: Breaches in the private sector: "Harm" in the litigation setting. Security Breach Notification Symposium, 2009.
16. Verizon Business Risk Team. *2008 data breach investigations report.* 2008.
17. Verizon Business Risk Team. *2010 data breach investigations report.* 2010.

18. Ponemon Institute. *Benchmark study of patient privacy and data security.* 2010.
19. National Institutes of Health. *Policy for sharing of data obtained in NIH supported or conducted genome-wide association studies (GWAS).* 2007. http://grants.nih.gov/grants/guide/notice-files/NOT-OD-07-088.html. Archived at http://www.webcitation.org/5iqujgEyy.
20. Loukides G, Denny J, Malin B. Do clinical profiles constitute privacy risks for research participants? Proceedings of the AMIA Symposium, 2009.
21. El Emam K, Dankar F, Vaillancourt R, Roffey T, Lysyk M. Evaluating patient re-identification risk from hospital prescription records. *Canadian Journal of Hospital Pharmacy*, 2009; 62(4):307–319.
22. Cleere R, Dougherty W, Fiumara N, Jenike C, Lentz J, Rose N. Physicians' attitudes toward venereal disease reporting. *JAMA*, 1967; 202(10):117–122.
23. Jones J, Meyer P, Garrison C, Kettinger L, Hermann P. Physician and infection control practitioner HIV/AIDS reporting characteristics. *American Journal of Public Health*, 1992; 82(6):889–891.
24. Konowitz P, Petrossian G, Rose D. The underreporting of disease and physicians' knowledge of reporting requirements. *Public Health Reports*, 1984; 99(1):31–35.
25. Gelman A, Vandow J, Sobel N. Current status of venereal disease in New York City: A survey of 6,649 physicians in solo practice. *American Journal of Public Health*, 1963; 53:1903–1918.
26. Marier R. The reporting of communicable diseases. *American Journal of Epidemiology*, 1977; 105(6):587–590.
27. Scatliff J. Survey of venereal disease treated by Manitoba physicians in 1972. *Canadian Medical Association Journal*, 1974; 110:179–182.
28. AbdelMalik P, Boulos M, Jones R. The perceived impact of location privacy: A web-based survey of public health perspectives and requirements in the UK and Canada. *BMC Public Health*, 2008; 8(156).
29. Drociuk D, Gibson J, Hodge J. Health information privacy and syndromic surveillance systems. *Morbidity and Mortality Weekly Report*, 2004; 53(Suppl.):221–225.
30. Rushworth R, Bell S, Rubin G, Hunter R, Ferson M. Improving surveillance of infectious disease in New South Wales. *Medical Journal of Australia*, 1991; 154:828–831.
31. Johnson R, Montano B, Wallace E. Using death certificates to estimate the completeness of AIDS case reporting in Ontario in 1985–87. *Canadian Medical Association Journal*, 1989; 141:537–540.
32. Rothenberg R, Bross D, Vernon T. Reporting of gonorrhea by private physicians: A behavioral study. *American Journal of Public Health*, 1980; 70(9):983–986.
33. Wojcik R, Hauenstein L, Sniegoski C, Holtry R. Obtaining the data. In *Disease surveillance: A public health informatics approach*, ed. J Lombardo and D Buckeridge. Hoboken, NJ. 2007.
34. El Emam K, Mercer J, Moreau K, Grava-Gubins I, Buckeridge D, Jonker E. Physician privacy concerns when disclosing patient data for public health purposes during a pandemic influenza outbreak. Under second review in *BMC Public Health*, 2010.
35. Willison D, Emerson C, Szala-Meneok K, Gibson E, Schwartz L, Weisbaum K. Access to medical records for research purposes: Varying perceptions across research ethics boards. *Journal of Medical Ethics*, 2008; 34:308–314.

Chapter 4

The Impact of Consent

In some cases the custodian does not have the option to disclose identifiable information without consent because there are no exceptions in the legislation. However, there will be situations where obtaining consent is not possible or practical. For example, in a health research context some of the reasons why obtaining patient consent may not be practicable include:

1. Making contact with a patient to obtain consent may reveal the individual's condition to others against his or her wishes. For example, sending a letter or leaving voice mails may alert spouses or co-inhabitants to a condition that they did not know the target individual had.
2. The size of the population represented in the data may be too large to obtain consent from everyone. This speaks to practical costs in meaningfully obtaining consent.
3. Many patients may have relocated or died, making it impossible or very difficult to obtain consent.
4. There may be a lack of existing or continuing relationship with the patients to go back and obtain consent. This makes it difficult to find an acceptable way to approach individuals to seek consent.
5. There may be a risk of inflicting psychological, social, or other harm by contacting individuals and/or their families in delicate circumstances, for example, if contacting a family brings back memories of the death of a child.
6. It may be difficult to contact individuals through advertisements and other public notices because the population is geographically distributed or no information was collected about their language.
7. Undue hardship may be caused by the additional financial, material, human, organizational, or other resources required to obtain consent.

In those instances the disclosure of personal information would not be permissible, and de-identification provides the only practical option for disclosure (assuming that the purpose can be achieved with the de-identified information).

However, even if obtaining consent was possible and practical, there have been strong concerns about the negative impact of consent requirements, for example, on the ability to conduct health research [1–18]. Consent may have a severe adverse consequence on the quality of the information. A primary reason is that individuals who consent tend to be different on many characteristics than those who do not consent (e.g., on age, gender, socioeconomic status, whether they live in rural or urban areas, religiosity, disease severity, and level of education) [19]. These differences can result in biased findings when the information is analyzed or used [20]. In such circumstances a strong case can be made for not seeking consent and de-identifying the information instead (again, assuming that the de-identified information will achieve the purpose of the disclosure).

In addition to the compelling evidence for the difference between consenters and non-consenters, seeking consent does result in a reduction of the number of individuals who agree to provide data or allow their data to be used. This reduction can be substantial, and has consequences on the cost and timeliness of an analysis.

Consider an example where a hospital is disclosing prescription data to a researcher. The hospital can make the case that it is not practical to obtain consent from the patients for this disclosure. The cost and delays of prospectively administering the additional consent forms for all admitted patients may be difficult to justify, and it would be quite time-consuming to do so retroactively for historical data. Therefore the hospital would have to de-identify the prescription data before disclosure.

In one study [19], which we summarize here, we performed two systematic reviews of the literature to identify the impact of consent on the process and outcomes of health research. We focused on health research because that is where the most detailed investigations of the impact of consent have been performed.

The first review focused on systematic reviews already conducted in the context of recruiting participants in clinical trials. Therefore it was effectively a review of systematic reviews. The reason we reviewed systematic reviews was because this question, in the context of clinical trials, had already been studied extensively and there were already a number of systematic reviews that were done. The second systematic review focused on original research investigating the impact of consent models on observational studies, including studies that use pre-existing databases.

Differences between Consenters and Non-Consenters in Clinical Trials

We wanted to identify and summarize studies examining differences between patients who consent to participate in clinical trials and those who do not. Because of the large number of articles that have investigated this issue, we limited our examination to meta-analyses and systematic reviews that have already been conducted.

Out of the 22 articles identified, two were promoted to the second systematic review due to their focus on observational health research, rather than clinical trials. Fifteen articles that provided information pertinent to patient characteristics were summarized. The other five articles were excluded from the summary, as they focused on physician factors and/or study design characteristics and their impact on consent and recruitment. A summary of the findings is provided in Table 4.1.

The evidence is therefore quite compelling that consenters in clinical trials are different on important demographic characteristics. Of course, one would not suggest waiving the consent requirement in interventional clinical trials. However, it is also important to be cognizant of this effect, which could work to bias results.

The Impact of Consent on Observational Studies

We also examined the impact of consent on observational studies. Some studies seek consent from the patient at the point of data collection in order to use the data for a specific purpose. For example, Hollander et al. collected primary source data by way of patient interviews in their emergency room-based survey on domestic abuse [36]. Consent was requested from patients prior to their participation in the interview.

Other studies seek consent at the point of data collection for the primary analysis and also for linkage to medical records or for subsequent specific or general disclosures of the original data for secondary purposes. For example, the study by Young et al. involved both primary data collection from patients and the use of data from existing databases, which are typically linked to the primary source data. In Young's study, patients were sent a survey questionnaire that included a request for consent to data linkage [37]. Survey answers were then linked to medical record data if consent was provided. Tu et al. provide an example of multiple consent requirements in their study of the Canadian Stroke Network Registry [38]. The researchers requested consent from eligible patients to be included in the registry, which would appear to be consent for primary data collection; however, the consent forms included a request for consent to both primary data collection and use of existing medical chart data, along with linkage to existing administrative databases, as well as the aggregation and release of data to external organizations [38]. Therefore the subjects in this study were asked for consent to primary data collection along with the secondary use of various existing databases, including medical records and administrative records, for linkage to the primary data, as well as to the subsequent disclosure of the information gathered in the registry itself.

Requesting consent at the point when data will be disclosed for secondary purposes is another approach. For example, in the study by Yawn et al. patients visiting an outpatient clinic were asked for consent to the use of their existing medical record data for research purposes [39].

Table 4.1   Summary of Patient Characteristics That Differ between Consenters and Non-Consenters in Clinical Trials

Bias Factors due to Consent	*Explanations*
Age [21–27]	Youth consent is hindered by parental consent requirements.
	The findings for adults are contradictory: In some studies older adults are found to be more likely to consent, and in other cases younger adults are found to be more likely to consent.
	One review looking exclusively at participation in the elderly (65+) found that the elderly are less likely to consent or be asked to participate in clinical trials [21].
Sex [22, 24–28]	Women of childbearing age are historically excluded from clinical trials.
	Males are generally found to be more likely to participate.
Socioeconomic background/status (SES) [22, 24, 26, 29]	Studies are contradictory, showing high consent levels for those of low SES in some studies [22], but low rates for those with low SES who are also a part of a minority group (i.e., ethnic minorities [26, 29] and women).
	In cancer trials, consent rates were found to be low for those with lower SES [24].
Ethnicity/race [23, 24, 26, 28–33]	Those from the ethnic majority are more likely to consent/participate than those of an ethnic minority.
	Ethnic minorities may be offered fewer opportunities to participate [26].
Location [24, 26]	Those in rural locations/communities were found to be less likely to participate as opposed to those in urban areas.
Education [22, 25]	A lower level of education was shown generally to increase consent vs. a higher level of education.
Language [26]	Those who speak the predominant language are more likely to consent or be asked to participate in trials vs. those who do not speak the language.

Table 4.1 (continued)   Summary of Patient Characteristics That Differ between Consenters and Non-Consenters in Clinical Trials

Bias Factors due to Consent	Explanations
Religiosity [26, 30]	One review found that religiosity decreased consent in some studies and increased consent in others [30].
	On the other hand, another review found no literature on religious barriers in trials, indicating that there has not been much research conducted in this area [26].
Health [21, 23, 24, 27, 29, 33–35]	Generally, the research shows that low/no co-morbidity increases the likelihood of participation.
	As the stages of one's disease progress (early–late), consent becomes less likely.
	One article presents contradictory evidence: that later stage disease/more co-morbidity increases participation [27] in prevention trials, and those with a healthy lifestyle are more likely to participate [27].
Social support [27, 34]	Inadequate social support indicates greater consent in some studies [27] but lower consent in others [34].

Whether consent is sought for a primary analysis, data linkage, possible future disclosure, or disclosure of pre-existing records, and whether it is sought at the time of collection or disclosure, will likely have an impact on our main outcomes. However, it was not possible to differentiate these effects from the articles. Therefore we report overall results.

Impact on Recruitment

Thirty-one articles reported lower recruitment rates as a result of consent requirements [36–67], and one reported no significant difference in recruitment due to consent requirements [68]. Three studies focusing on opt-in vs. opt-out methods have found that opt-out consent strategies generally produce significantly higher consent rates than opt-in strategies [44, 45, 63]. Junghans et al. found that 50% of opt-out patients participated, as opposed to 38% in the opt-in group [44]. Trevena et al. had similar findings with opt-in consent requirements producing a recruitment

Table 4.2 Recruitment Rate for Opt-In vs. Opt-Out Consent

Study	Sample	Consent Rate for Opt-In Method	Consent Rate for Opt-Out Method
Jacobsen et al. [63]	2,463	78%	97%
Junghans et al. [44]	510	38%	50%
Trevena et al. [45]	152	47%	67%

rate of 47% and opt-out producing a higher recruitment rate of 67% [45]. Lastly, Jacobsen et al. found that when results were analyzed in accordance with opt-in methods, the consent rate was 78%. However, when non-responders were considered to have provided opt-out consent, in accordance with the applicable Minnesota legislation—the law allows for passive consent (opt-out) in cases where patients have been notified about the study by mail on at least two occasions and told that their records may be released should the patient not object—the consent rate increased by 17.5% to 95.5% [63]. Results of these studies are outlined in Table 4.2.

Twenty-eight studies focusing on explicit consent (opt-in or opt-out) vs. implied consent found that studies with implied consent tended to have elevated recruitment rates. Three of these studies involved a direct comparison between the participation rates of groups requiring explicit informed consent and those using implied consent for observational health research. These researchers found that participation was higher in the implied condition when informed consent requirements were waived [41–43]. Ten studies presenting evidence of bias found that a request for explicit opt-in consent to record review, or linkage of study data to medical records, decreased participation in surveys and other observational studies [37, 39, 49, 51, 52, 54–56, 58, 61]. Two studies focusing on population-based cohorts both found that the requirement of explicit consent negatively affected the participation rates [50, 60]. Six studies examining participation in registries found that when explicit consent requirements were instated, the result was lower participation by patients [38, 48, 53, 57, 59, 62, 66, 67]. Even when opt-out consent methods were employed, the participation rate still decreased in one registry by 6.6% [62]. Three studies found that the requirement of obtaining explicit consent prior to contact from researchers worked to decrease participation rates [40, 47, 64]. Hollander et al. found that asking for explicit written informed consent led to lower recruitment rates (82%) as opposed to asking for a verbal "okay" (92%) [36]. Cheung et al. had similar findings in their mental health research. When patients were asked for consent, the participation rate decreased by 15.1% [65]. Finally, Beebe and colleagues looked at the impact of consent on survey response rate. They compared a group receiving a HIPAA authorization form (HAF) with a postal survey to that of a group receiving only the survey questionnaire and found that the group that was sent the HAF had a lower response rate (39.8%) than the group that was sent the survey alone (55%) [46]. The results from these studies are outlined in Table 4.3.

Table 4.3   Recruitment Rate for Explicit Consent Models vs. Implied Consent Models

Study	Sample	Response Rate	Consent Rate (% of sample)
Al-Shahi et al. [50]	187	59%	59%
Armstrong et al. [42]	1,221 (pre), 967 (post)	96% in pre-HIPAA period, 35% in post-HIPAA	34% provided written consent in post-HIPAA period
Angus et al. [40]	10,000	20%	25%[a]
Beebe et al. [46]	6,939	55% no HAF,[b] 40% with HAF	40%
Brown et al. [58]	1,612	71.5%	71.5%
Bryant et al. [60]	22,652	100%	52%
Buckley et al. [61]	1,269	69%	45%
Chertow et al. [57]	1,243	100%	51.9%
Cheung et al. [65]	73	85%	85%
Dunn et al. [49]	42,812	65%	32% to follow-up, 42% to medical record review
Dziak et al. [64]	~3,000	82% (mean of all sites)	94% (mean of opt-out sites), 63% (opt-in site)
Ford [62]	820	61%[c]	93%
Harris et al. [54]	2,276	75%	69%
Hess et al. [66]	86	100%	55% for RRP, 49% for PSL[d]
Hollander et al. [36]	3,466	87%	92% verbal okay, 82% written informed consent
Huang et al. [51]	15,413	95% complete responses	84%
Korkeila et al. [55]	52,739	40%	37%

continued

Table 4.3 (continued)   Recruitment Rate for Explicit Consent Models vs. Implied Consent Models

Study	Sample	Response Rate	Consent Rate (% of sample)
Krousel-Wood et al. [43]	177	21.5% prewaiver, 57% postwaiver	21.5%
Nelson et al. [41]	4,647	58% at sites with no consent, 39% with oral consent, 27% with written consent	39% (oral consent), 27% (written consent)
Peat et al. [56]	8,984	68%	25% to follow-up; 27% to medical record linkage
Schwartz et al. [53], Phipps et al. [48]	2,164	84%	58%
Tu et al. [38]	7,108	54% (phase I/II)	Phase I: 39%, phase II: 51%
Vates et al. [67]	14,330	35%	28%
Ward et al. [47]	2,804	37%	16%
Woolf et al. [52]	1,229	83%	60.5%
Yawn et al. [39]	15,997	94%	91%
Yawn et al. [59]	391	98%	98%
Young et al. [37]	39,883	52%	49%

Note: Response rate is the percentage of sample that responded either prior to or following consent. Consent rate pertains only to the percentage of the sample that provided explicit consent.

[a] The response rate is lower than the consent rate because of the requirement to obtain consent prior to participants being sent the survey questionnaire.

[b] HAF stands for HIPAA authorization form.

[c] This was an opt-out study, which is why the response rate is lower than the consent rate. Fifty-four percent of those contacted responded with written consent, though it was not required, and 6.6% responded in order to opt out.

[d] RRP stands for research registry project, and PSL stands for prospective subjects list.

Impact on Bias

Twenty-seven studies found a considerable difference in sociodemographic and/or health features between non-consenters and consenters, as well as between opt-in participants and opt-out participants, thereby indicating the presence of selection bias [37–40, 42–46, 48–55, 60–63, 65, 66, 69–73]. The variables most often cited were age, sex, race/ethnicity, marital status, education level, socioeconomic status, physical and mental functioning, lifestyle factors, health/disease factors like diagnosis or disease stage/severity, and mortality rate. Table 4.4 outlines in which areas each study showed evidence of bias. Two studies in our review found no difference in demographic variables between consenters and non-consenters in observational health research [36, 56].

Fifteen studies examined the age differences of consenters and non-consenters. Of these, ten studies [37, 39, 40, 42, 43, 52, 63, 71–73] showed that younger patients were more likely to refuse consent or not respond. Conversely, five studies found that older patients were more likely not to consent [38, 48, 49, 51, 53, 70].

Sex was another factor that tended to differ between consenters and non-consenters. Of the studies that looked at the sex differences [39, 43, 48, 52, 53, 61, 69, 71], seven found that women were more likely to refuse consent than men. Conversely, four studies found that women were more likely to give consent than men [40, 49, 60, 73]. Three of the ten studies found that the consent trends among the sexes tended to reverse in the elderly [40, 49, 71]. Interestingly, the study of survey response rate conducted by Beebe et al. provided contradictory results, showing no bias in the consenters group. They found that males were significantly over-represented in the group of respondents that received their survey questionnaire only (in comparison with population values), while no significant overrepresentation was found in the group in which active consent was sought by way of a HIPAA authorization form along with the questionnaire [46].

Of the four articles examining race as a factor in consent, all found that African Americans were less likely than Caucasians to participate in observational health research [42, 43, 52, 72].

Marital status was looked at in five studies. Four of these studies found that unmarried people were less likely to consent to participate and/or more likely to discontinue participation [37, 42, 51, 72]. Young et al. found that marital status was also tied to age, with younger consenters being less likely to be married and older consenters being more likely to be married [37]. The fifth study, by Hess et al., found that consenters to a research registry project were less likely to be divorced or widowed than non-consenters [66].

Differences in level of education were found in five studies. Four studies in our review found that those with lower education levels were less likely to provide active consent [37, 45, 48, 53, 72]. The study by Trevena and colleagues compared opt-in and opt-out consent methods and found that opt-out conditions included more

Table 4.4 Reported Evidence of Sociodemographic Differences between Consenters and Non-Consenters, or Opt-In vs. Opt-Out Participants

Study	Age	Sex	Race	Marital Status	Education Level	SES	Health	Lifestyle Factors	Functioning
Al-Shahi et al. [50]							X		
Armstrong et al. [42]	X		X	X			X		
Angus et al. [40]	X	X				X			
Beebe et al. [46]							X	X	
Bolcic-Jankovic et al. [71]	X	X							
Bryant et al. [60]		X							
Buckley et al. [61]		X					X	X	
Cheung et al. [65]							X		
DiMattio [72]	X		X	X	X	X	X		
Dunn et al. [49]	X	X					X		
Ford [62]							X		
Harris et al. [54]						X	X		

	1	2	3	4	5	6	7	8
Hess et al. [66]			X			X		
Huang et al. [51]	X		X	X		X		X
Jacobsen et al. [63]			X	X		X		X
Jaskiw et al. [70]			X			X		X
Jousilahti et al. [73]		X	X			X		X
Junghans et al. [44]	X	X	X			X		X
Korkeila et al. [55]		X	X			X		X
Krousel-Wood et al. [43]							X	X
Schwartz et al. [53], Phipps et al. [48]			X		X		X	X
Stang et al. [69]			X			X	X	X
Trevena et al. [45]		X	X		X			X
Tu et al. [38]	X		X			X		X
Woolf et al. [52]	X		X			X		X
Yawn et al. [39]			X			X		X
Young et al. [37]			X	X	X	X		X

participants with lower levels of education vs. opt-in conditions [45]. Alternately, one study showed that those with higher education levels were less likely to consent [51].

In terms of socioeconomic status, five studies found a difference between consenters and non-consenters, reporting the status of consenters to be higher than that of non-consenters [37, 40, 51, 54, 72]. One study found that in an elderly population, those who were employed or retired were more likely to consent to participate, whereas those participants who discontinued their involvement in the studies were more likely to have a low income [72].

Health factors also appeared to influence consent, as consent patterns varied within studies depending on the patients' health status and/or diagnosis. Twenty-two studies found evidence of bias related to health factors, as well as mortality [37–39, 42, 44–46, 48–50, 52–55, 61–63, 65, 66, 69, 70, 72, 73]. One article looking at consenters in a case-control study found that healthy patients who were approached to become control subjects were less likely to participate (68% participation rate) than case patients with the disease under study (80%) [69]. Another survey-based study found that general health was significantly better in survey respondents who were sent a consent form, as opposed to survey respondents who were sent the questionnaire alone [46]. Conversely, Harris et al. found that consenters generally reported poorer physical and mental health [54]. The severity of the disease was found to be a factor in two studies that found consent was greater in patients who had more severe illness/higher stage disease [52, 62]. Conversely, the study by Cheung et al. found that consenters were less severely ill but had a longer duration of illness than non-consenters [65]. In a medical records study by Young et al. it was found that older consenters reported lower use of GP services than did non-consenters [37]. However, in a review of nursing studies focusing on an elderly population, it was found that those with a higher number of hospitalizations were more likely to participate in observational research [72]. In terms of mortality, five studies found a higher mortality rate in non-consenters vs. consenters [37, 38, 42, 50, 73].

Lifestyle and risk factors were found to differ between consenters and non-consenters and opt-in vs. opt-out participants in six studies. Two studies found that consenters and opt-in participants were more likely to display risk factors, such as smoking, family history of disease, etc. [45, 55]. Four studies found the opposite trend, with consenters displaying fewer risk factors [44, 46, 61, 73]. Also, in terms of physical and mental functioning, three studies found that consent tended to be lower in those with lower mental and/or physical functioning [38, 44, 51]. Woolf et al., in their secondary use study, found the opposite trend, with higher participation in patients who had poorer physical function [52].

Impact on Cost

In our review, six studies found that costs increased with an increase in requirements for consent [38, 41, 42, 47, 48, 53]. In particular, staffing costs were found to increase due to the demands that obtaining consent can put on research staff [42, 48, 53, 67].

Impact on Time

Three studies found a negative impact of consent requirements on the time needed to conduct a study [38, 48, 53, 64]. Tu et al. found that the workload for nurse recruiters was especially heavy due to the requirements of gaining consent from each patient [38]. Schwartz and colleagues found that many personnel hours were required in order to obtain consent from potential patients, while the consent rate in turn was only 58% [53]. Lastly, it was found by Dziak et al. that the time required for their study increased due to variation in institutional review board (IRB) review requirements, as well as consequent consent requirements at the study sites [64].

References

1. Ness R. Influence of the HIPAA Privacy Rule on health research. *Journal of the American Medical Association*, 2007; 298(18):2164–2170.
2. Institute of Medicine. *Health research and the privacy of health information—The HIPAA Privacy Rule.* 2008. http://www.iom.edu/CMS/3740/43729.aspx.
3. Institute of Medicine. *Effect of the HIPAA Privacy Rule on health research: Proceedings of a workshop presented to the National Cancer Policy Forum.* 2006.
4. Association of Academic Health Centers. *HIPAA creating barriers to research and discovery.* 2008.
5. Wilson J. Health Insurance Portability and Accountability Act Privacy Rule causes ongoing concerns among clinicians and researchers. *Annals of Internal Medicine*, 2006; 145(4):313–316.
6. Walker D. *Impact of the HIPAA Privacy Rule on health services research.* Abt Associates Inc. for the Agency for Healthcare Research and Quality, 2005.
7. Hanna K. The Privacy Rule and research: Protecting privacy at what cost? *Research Practitioner*, 2007; 8(1):4–11.
8. Association of American Medical Colleges. Testimony on behalf of the Association of American Medical Colleges before the National Committee on Vital and Health Statistics Subcommittee on Privacy. 2003.
9. Friedman D. HIPAA and research: How have the first two years gone? *American Journal of Opthalmology*, 2006; 141(3):543–546.
10. Nosowsky R, Giordano T. The Health Insurance Portability and Accountability Act of 1996 (HIPAA) Privacy Rule: Implications for clinical research. *American Medical Review*, 2006; 57:575–590.
11. Hiatt R. HIPAA: The end of epidemiology, or a new social contract? *Epidemiology*, 2003; 14(6):637–639.
12. Erlen J. HIPAA—Implications for research. *Orthopaedic Nursing*, 2005; 24(2):139–142.
13. Kulynych J, Korn D. The effect of the new federal medical Privacy Rule on research. *New England Journal of Medicine*, 2002; 346(3):201–204.

14. O'Herrin J, Fost N, Kudsk K. Health Insurance Portability and Accountability Act (HIPAA) regulations: Effect on medical record research. *Annals of Surgery*, 2004; 239(6):772–778.

15. National Cancer Institute, National Cancer Advisory Board. *The HIPAA Privacy Rule: Feedback from NCI cancer centers, cooperative groups and specialized programs of research excellence (SPOREs)*. 2003.

16. Shalowitz D. Informed consent for research and authorization under the Health Insurance Portability and Accountability Act Privacy Rule: An integrated approach. *Annals of Internal Medicine*, 2006; 144(9):685–688.

17. Academy of Medical Sciences. *Personal data for public good: Using health information in medical research*. 2006.

18. Steinberg M, Rubin E. *The HIPAA Privacy Rule: Lacks patient benefit, impedes patient growth*. Association of Academic Health Centers, 2009.

19. El Emam K, Dankar F, Issa R, Jonker E, Amyot D, Cogo E, Corriveau J-P, Walker M, Chowdhury S, Vaillancourt R, Roffey T, Bottomley J. A globally optimal k-anonymity method for the de-identification of health data. *Journal of the American Medical Informatics Association*, 2009; 16:670–682.

20. Harris MA, Levy AR, Teschke KE. Personal privacy and public health: Potential impacts of privacy legislation on health research in Canada. *Canadian Journal of Public Health*, 2008; 2008:293–296.

21. Townsley CA, Selby R, Siu LL. Systematic review of barriers to the recruitment of older patients with cancer onto clinical trials. *Journal of Clinical Oncology*, 2005; 23(13):3112–3124.

22. Ellis PM. Attitudes towards and participation in randomised clinical trials in oncology: A review of the literature. *Annals of Oncology*, 2000; 11(8):939–945.

23. Rendell JM Merritt RK, Geddes J. Incentives and disincentives to participation by clinicians in randomised controlled trials [review]. *Cochrane Database of Systematic Reviews*, 2007(2).

24. Ford JG, Howerton MW, Bolen S, Gary TL, Lai GY, Tilburt J, Gibbons MC, Baffi C, Wilson RF, Feuerstein CJ, Tanpitukpongse P, Powe NR, Bass EB. *Knowledge and access to information on recruitment of underrepresented populations to cancer clinical trials*. Evidence Report 122. AHRQ Evidence Based Practice Program, 2007.

25. Donovan JL, Brindle L, Mills N. Capturing users' experiences of participating in cancer trials. *European Journal of Cancer Care*, 2002; 11(3):210–214.

26. Hussain-Gambles M, Leese B, Atkin K, Brown J, Mason S, Tovey P. Involving South Asian patients in clinical trials. *Health Technology Assessment*, 2004; 8(42):iii–109.

27. Britton A, McKee M, Black N, McPherson K, Sanderson C, Bain C. Threats to applicability of randomised trials: Exclusions and selective participation. *Journal of Health Services and Research Policy*, 1999; 4(2):112–121.

28. McDaid C, Hodges Z, Fayter D, Stirk L, Eastwood A. Increasing participation of cancer patients in randomised controlled trials: A systematic review. *Trials*, 2006; 7:16.

29. Cox K, McGarry J. Why patients don't take part in cancer clinical trials: An overview of the literature. *European Journal of Cancer Care*, 2003; 12(2):114–122.

30. Yancey AK, Ortega AN, Kumanyika SK. Effective recruitment and retention of minority research participants. *Annual Review of Public Health*, 2006; 27:1–28.

31. Lai GY, Gary TL, Tilburt J, Bolen S, Baffi C, Wilson RF, Howerton MW, Gibbons MC, Tanpitukpongse TP, Powe NR, Bass EB, Ford JG. Effectiveness of strategies to recruit underrepresented populations into cancer clinical trials. *Clinical Trials*, 2006; 3(2):133–141.

32. UyBico SJ, Pavel S, Gross CP. Recruiting vulnerable populations into research: A systematic review of recruitment interventions. *Journal of General Internal Medicine*, 2007; 22(6):852–863.

33. Hughes C, Peterson SK, Ramirez A, Gallion KJ, McDonald PG, Skinner CS, Bowen D. Minority recruitment in hereditary breast cancer research. *Cancer Epidemiology, Biomarkers and Prevention*, 2004; 13(7):1146–1155.

34. Mills EJ, Seely D, Rachlis B, Griffith L, Wu P, Wilson K, Ellis P, Wright JR. Barriers to participation in clinical trials of cancer: A meta-analysis and systematic review of patient-reported factors. *Lancet Oncology*, 2006; 7(2):141–148.

35. Howerton MW, Gibbons MC, Baffi CR, Gary TL, Lai GY, Bolen S, Tilburt J, Tanpitukpongse TP, Wilson RF, Powe NR, Bass EB, Ford JG. Provider roles in the recruitment of underrepresented populations to cancer clinical trials. *Cancer*, 2007; 109(3):465–476.

36. Hollander JE, Schears RM, Shofer FS, Baren JM, Moretti LM, Datner EM. The effect of written informed consent on detection of violence in the home. *Academic Emergency Medicine*, 2001; 8(10):974–979.

37. Young AF, Dobson AJ, Byles JE. Health services research using linked records: Who consents and what is the gain? [see comment]. *Australian and New Zealand Journal of Public Health*, 2001; 25(5):417–420.

38. Tu J, Willison D, Silver F, Fang J, Richards J, Laipacis A, Kapral M. Impracticability of informed consent in the registry of the Canadian Stroke Network. *New England Journal of Medicine*, 2004; 350(14):1414–1421.

39. Yawn BP, Yawn RA, Geier GR, Xia Z, Jacobsen SJ. The impact of requiring patient authorization for use of data in medical records research. *Journal of Family Practice*, 1998; 47(5):361–365.

40. Angus VC, Entwistle VA, Emslie MJ, Walker KA, Andrew JE. The requirement for prior consent to participate on survey response rates: A population-based survey in Grampian. *BMC Health Services Research*, 2003; 3(1):21.

41. Nelson K, Rosa E, Brown J, Manglone C, Louis T, Keeler E. Do patient consent procedures affect participation rates in health services research? *Medical Care*, 2002; 40(4):283–288.

42. Armstrong D, Kline-Rogers E, Jani S, Goldman E, Fang J, Mukherjee D, Nallamothu B, Eagle K. Potential impact of the HIPAA Privacy Rule on data collection in a registry of patients with acute coronary syndrome. *Archives of Internal Medicine*, 2005; 165:1125–1129.

43. Krousel-Wood M, Muntner P, Jannu A, Hyre A, Breault J. Does waiver of written informed consent from the institutional review board affect response rate in a low-risk research study? *Journal of Investigative Medicine*, 2006; 54(4):174–179.

44. Junghans C, Feder G, Hemingway H, Timmis A, Jones M. Recruiting patients to medical research: Double blind randomised trial of "opt-in" versus "opt-out" strategies. *British Medical Journal*, 2005; 331(940).

45. Trevena L, Irwig L, Barratt AEM. Impact of privacy legislation on the number and characteristics of people who are recruited for research: A randomised controlled trial. *Journal of Medical Ethics*, 2006; 32(8):473–477.
46. Beebe T, Talley N, Camilleri M, Jenkins S, Anderson K, Locke R. The HIPAA authorization form and effects on survey response rates, nonresponse bias, and data quality: A randomized community study. *Medical Care*, 2007; 45(10):959–965.
47. Ward H, Cousens S, Smith-Bathgate B, Leitch M, Everington D, Will R, Smith P. Obstacles to conducting epidemiological research in the UK general population. *British Medical Journal*, 2004; 329:277–279.
48. Phipps E, Harris D, Brown N, Harralson T, Brecher A, Polansky M, Whyte J. Investigation of ethnic differences in willingness to enroll in a rehabilitation research registry: A study of the Northeast Cognitive Rehabilitation Research Network. *American Journal of Physical Medicine and Rehabilitation*, 2004; 83(12):875–883.
49. Dunn KM, Jordan K, Lacey RJ, Shapley M, Jinks C. Patterns of consent in epidemiologic research: Evidence from over 25,000 responders. *American Journal of Epidemiology*, 2004; 159(11):1087–1094.
50. Al-Shahi R, Vousden C, Warlow C. Bias from requiring explicit consent from all participants in observational research: Prospective, population based study. *British Medical Journal*, 2005; 331:942.
51. Huang N, Shih SF, Chang HY, Chou YJ. Record linkage research and informed consent: Who consents? *BMC Health Services Research*, 2007; 7:18.
52. Woolf S, Rothemich S, Johnson RE, Marsland D. Selection bias from requiring patients to give consent to examine data for health services research. *Archives of Family Medicine*, 2000; 9:1111–1118.
53. Schwartz MF, Brecher AR, Whyte J, Klein MG. A patient registry for cognitive rehabilitation research: A strategy for balancing patients' privacy rights with researchers' need for access. *Archives of Physical Medicine and Rehabilitation*, 2005; 86(9):1807–1814.
54. Harris T, Cook DG, Victor C, Beighton C, DeWilde S, Carey IE. Linking questionnaires to primary care records: Factors affecting consent in older people. *Journal of Epidemiology and Community Health*, 2005; 59(4):336–338.
55. Korkeila K, Suominen S, Ahvenainen J, Ojanlatva A, Rautava P, Helenius H, Koskenvuo M. Non-response and related factors in a nation-wide health survey. *European Journal of Epidemiology*, 2001; 17(11):991–999.
56. Peat G, Thomas E, Handy J, Wood L, Dziedzic K, Myers H, Wilkie R, Duncan R, Hay E, Hill J, Lacey R, Croft P. The Knee Clinical Assessment Study—CAS(K). A prospective study of knee pain and knee osteoarthritis in the general population: Baseline recruitment and retention at 18 months. *BMC Musculoskeletal Disorders*, 2006; 7:30.
57. Chertow G, Pascual M, Soroko S, Savage B, Himmelfarb J, Ikizler T, Paganini E, Mehta R, PICARD. Reasons for non-enrollment in a cohort study of ARF: The Program to Improve Care in Acute Renal Disease (PICARD) experience and implications for a clinical trials network. *American Journal of Kidney Disease*, 2003; 42(3):507–512.
58. Brown J, Jacobs DJ, Barosso G, Potter J, Hannan P, Kopher R, Rourke M, Hartman T, Hase K. Recruitment, retention and characteristics of women in a prospective study of preconceptional risks to reproductive outcomes: Experience of the Diana Project. *Paediatric and Perinatal Epidemiology*, 1997; 11(3):345–358.
59. Yawn B, Gazzuola L, Wollan P, Kim W. Development and maintenance of a community-based hepatitis C registry. *American Journal of Managed Care*, 2002; 8(3):253–261.

60. Bryant H, Robson P, Ullman R, Friedenreich C, Dawe U. Population-based cohort development in Alberta, Canada: A feasibility study. *Chronic Diseases in Canada*, 2006; 27(2):51–59.
61. Buckley B, Murphy A, Byrne M, Glynn L. Selection bias resulting from the requirement for prior consent in observational research: A community cohort of people with ischaemic heart disease. *Heart*, 2007; 93(9):1116–1120.
62. Ford H. The effect of consent guidelines on a multiple sclerosis register. *Multiple Sclerosis*, 2006; 12(1):104–107.
63. Jacobsen S, Xia Z, Campion M, Darby C, Plevak M, Seltman K, Melton L. Potential effect of authorization bias on medical records research. *Mayo Clinic Proceedings*, 1999; 74(4):330–338.
64. Dziak K, Anderson R, Sevick MA, Weisman CS, Levine DW, Scholle SH. Variations among institutional review board reviews in a multisite health services research study. *Health Services Research*, 2005; 40(1):279–290.
65. Cheung P, Schweitzer I, Yastrubetskaya O, Crowley K, Tuckwell V. Studies of aggressive behaviour in schizophrenia: Is there a response bias? *Medicine Science and the Law*, 1997; 37(4):345–348.
66. Hess R, Matthews K, McNeil M, Chang CH, Kapoor W, Bryce C. Health services research in the privacy age. *Journal of General Internal Medicine*, 2005; 20(11): 1045–1049.
67. Vates JR, Hetrick JL, Lavin KL, Sharma GK, Wagner RL, Johnson JT. Protecting medical record information: Start your research registries today. *Laryngoscope*, 2005; 115(3):441–444.
68. Shah S, Harris TJ, Rink E, DeWilde S, Victor CR, Cook DG. Do income questions and seeking consent to link medical records reduce survey response rates? A randomised controlled trial among older people. *British Journal of General Practice*, 2001; 51(464):223–225.
69. Stang A, Ahrens W, Jockel KH. Control response proportions in population-based case-control studies in Germany. *Epidemiology*, 1999; 10(2):181–183.
70. Jaskiw GE, Blumer TE, Gutierrez-Esteinou R, Meltzer HY, Steele V, Strauss ME. Comparison of inpatients with major mental illness who do and do not consent to low-risk research. *Psychiatry Research*, 2003; 119(1–2):183–188.
71. Bolcic-Jankovic D, Clarridge BR, Fowler Jr. FJ, Weissman JS. Do characteristics of HIPAA consent forms affect the response rate? *Medical Care*, 2007; 45(1):100–103.
72. DiMattio MJ. Recruitment and retention of community-dwelling, aging women in nursing studies. *Nursing Research*, 2001; 50(6):369–373.
73. Jousilahti P, Salomaa V, Kuulasmaa K, Niemela M, Vartiainen E. Total and cause specific mortality among participants and non-participants of population based health surveys: A comprehensive follow up of 54 372 Finnish men and women. *Journal of Epidemiology and Community Health*, 2005; 59:310–315.

Chapter 5

Data Breach Notifications

Many jurisdictions have breach notification laws that require notifications to be sent to the individuals affected, regulators, attorneys general, and/or the media when a data breach occurs. Table 5.1 is a summary of the types of personal information that require notification in the state laws in the United States. As can be seen, only five states and one terriroty actually require breach notification if health information is involved (Arkansas,* California,† Missouri,‡ New Hampshire,§ Texas,¶ and Puerto Rico**). This does not totally absolve health information custodians from the notification requirement, as many medical records also contain other types of information, such as financial information, which is covered by other state laws. More recently the Health Information Technology for Economic and Clinical Health (HITECH) Act†† added national breach notification requirements for health information, making it necessary for the DHHS to report the number of notified breaches to Congress on an annual basis.

Benefits and Costs of Breach Notification

Some of the benefits of breach notification laws include a small reduction in the incidence of identity theft [1], the public feels more comfortable with the collection

---

* See Arkansas Civil Code §4-110-101 *et seq.*
† See California Civil Code, Sections 1798.80–1798.84.
‡ See Missouri Revised Statutes, c. 407, Merchandising Practices, Section 407.1500.
§ See New Hampshire Statutes, Title XXX, Chapter 332-I.
¶ See Texas Business and Commercial Code, Section 521, *et seq.*
** See Laws of Puerto Rico, Title 10, Section 4051, *et seq.*
†† The HITECH Act consists of Division A, Title XIII and Division B, Title IV of ARRA.

Table 5.1   Definitions of Personal Information in State Breach Notification Laws[a]

State	Personal Information Definition
Alaska	First name/first initial and last name plus one of the following: Social security number, driver's license number, or financial account number/credit card number/debit card number with security code/access code/password.
Arizona	First name/first initial and last name plus one of the following: Social security number, driver's license number, nonoperating ID license number, or financial account number/credit card number/debit card number with security code/access code/password.
Arkansas	First name/first initial and last name plus one of the following: Social security number, driver's license number/ Arkansas ID card number, financial account number/credit card number/debit card number with security code/access code/password, or any identifiable medical information.
California	First name/first initial and last name plus one of the following: Social security number, driver's license number/ California ID card number, financial account number/credit card number/debit card number with security code/access code/password, medical information (i.e., medical history), or health insurance information.
Colorado	First name/first initial and last name plus one of the following: Social security number, driver's license number/ID card number, or financial account number/ credit card number/debit card number with security code/access code/password.
Connecticut	First name/first initial and last name plus one of the following: Social security number, driver's license number/ Connecticut ID card number, or financial account number/ credit card number/debit card number with security code/access code/password.
Delaware	First name/first initial and last name plus one of the following: Social security number, driver's license number/ Delaware ID card number, or financial account number/ credit card number/debit card number with security code/access code/password.

Table 5.1 (continued)   Definitions of Personal Information in State Breach Notification Laws[a]

State	Personal Information Definition
District of Columbia	First name/first initial and last name plus one of the following: Social security number, driver's license number/ District of Columbia ID card number, or credit card number or debit card number.
Florida	First name/first initial and last name plus any one of the following: Social security number, driver's license number/ Florida ID card number, financial account number/credit card number/debit card number with security code/access code/password.
Georgia	First name/first initial and last name plus one of the following: Social security number, driver's license number/ Georgia ID card number, financial account number/credit card number/debit card number, or security code/access code/password. Any of these pieces of information should be considered personal information on its own if it could be used for the purpose of identity theft without needing the individual's name.
Hawaii	First name/first initial and last name plus one of the following: Social security number, driver's license number/ Hawaii ID card number, financial account number/credit card number/debit card number or security code/access code/password that would permit access to a financial account.
Idaho	First name/first initial and last name plus one of the following: Social security number, driver's license number/ID card number, or financial account number/ credit card number with security code/access code/password.
Illinois	First name/first initial and last name plus one of the following: Social security number, driver's license number/ Illinois ID card number, or financial account number/credit card number/debit card number with security code/access code/password.

continued

Table 5.1 (continued)   Definitions of Personal Information in State Breach Notification Laws[a]

State	Personal Information Definition
Indiana	First name/first initial and last name or social security number plus one of the following: Driver's license number/Indiana ID card number, credit card number, or financial account number/debit card number with security code/access code/password.
Iowa	First name/first initial and last name plus one of the following: Social security number, driver's license number/government-issued ID number, financial account number/credit card number/debit card number with security code/access code/password, electronic identifier/routing code with a security code/access code/password that would allow access to a financial account, or biometric data (i.e., fingerprints)/other unique physical or digital representation of biometric data.
Kansas	First name/first initial and last name plus one of the following: Social security number, driver's license number/Kansas ID card number, financial account number/credit card number/debit card number, and/or security code/access code/password.
Louisiana	First name/first initial and last name plus one of the following: Social security number, driver's license number, or financial account number/credit card number/debit card number with security code/access code/password.
Maine	First name/first initial and last name plus one of the following: Social security number, driver's license number/Maine ID card number, financial account number/credit card number/debit card number, and/or account passwords/PI numbers/other access codes. Any of these pieces of information should be considered PI on its own if it could be used for the purpose of identity theft without needing the individual's name.
Maryland	First name/first initial and last name plus one of the following: Social security number, driver's license number, financial account number/credit card number/debit card number with security code/access code/password, or taxpayer ID number.

Table 5.1 (continued)   Definitions of Personal Information in State Breach Notification Laws[a]

State	Personal Information Definition
Massachusetts	First name/first initial and last name plus one of the following: Social security number, driver's license number/ Massachusetts ID card number, or financial account number/credit card number/debit card number with security code/access code/password.
Michigan	First name/first initial and last name plus one of the following: Social security number, driver's license number/ Michigan ID card number, or demand deposit/financial account number/credit card number/debit card number with security code/access code/password.
Minnesota	First name/first initial and last name plus one of the following: Social security number, driver's license number/ Minnesota ID card number, or financial account number/ credit card number/debit card number and security code/access code/password.
Mississippi	First name/first initial and last name plus one of the following: Social security number, driver's license number/ Mississippi ID card number, or financial account number/ credit card number/debit card number with security code/access code/password.
Missouri	First name/first initial and last name plus one of the following: Social security number, driver's license number/ government-issued ID number, financial account number/ credit card number/debit card number with security code/access code/password, electronic identifier/routing code with a security code/access code/password that would allow access to a financial account, medical information (i.e., medical history), or health insurance information.
Montana	First name/first initial and last name plus one of the following: Social security number, driver's license number/ Montana or tribal ID card number, or financial account number/credit card number/debit card number with security code/access code/password.

continued

Table 5.1 (continued) Definitions of Personal Information in State Breach Notification Laws[a]

State	Personal Information Definition
Nebraska	First name/first initial and last name plus one of the following: Social security number, driver's license number/state ID card number, financial account number/credit card number/debit card number with security code/access code/password, electronic identifier/routing code with a security code/access code/password that would allow access to a financial account, or biometric data (i.e., fingerprints).
Nevada	First name/first initial and last name plus one of the following: Social security number, driver's license number/ID card number, financial account number/credit card number/debit card number and security code/access code/password.
New Hampshire	First name/first initial and last name plus one of the following: Social security number, driver's license number/government ID card number, or financial account number/credit card number/debit card number with security code/access code/password.
New Jersey	First name/first initial and last name plus one of the following: Social security number, driver's license number/state ID card number, or financial account number/credit card number/debit card number with security code/access code/password.
New York	First name/first initial and last name plus one of the following: Social security number, driver's license number/nondriver ID card number, or financial account number/credit card number/debit card number with security code/access code/password.
North Carolina	First name/first initial and last name plus one of the following: Social security number, driver's license number/state ID card number/passport number, financial account numbers, credit card numbers, debit card numbers, PIN, digital signature, numbers or information that can be used to access financial resources, biometric data, or fingerprints. Also, certain information would be considered PI (in conjunction with name) if it allowed access to financial resources: electronic ID numbers, email name/address, Internet account numbers/ID names, parent's legal surname prior to marriage, or passwords.

Table 5.1 (continued)   Definitions of Personal Information in State Breach Notification Laws[a]

State	Personal Information Definition
North Dakota	First name/first initial and last name plus one of the following: Social security number, driver's license number, nondriver ID card from department of transportation, financial account number/credit card number/debit card number with security code/access code/password, date of birth, mother's maiden name, employee number, or electronic signature.
Ohio	First name/first initial and last name plus one of the following: Social security number, driver's license number/ state ID card number, financial account number/credit card number/debit card number with security code/access code/password. This does not include publically available information, information printed in media reports, or information distributed by charitable/nonprofit organizations.
Oklahoma	First name/first initial and last name plus one of the following: Social security number, driver's license number/ state ID card number, or financial account number/credit card number/debit card number with security code/access code/password.
Oregon	First name/first initial and last name plus one of the following: Social security number, driver's license number/state ID card number, ID number issued by another country, passport number/U.S.-issued ID number, or financial account number/ credit card number/debit card number with security code/ access code/password.
Pennsylvania	First name/first initial and last name plus one of the following: Social security number, driver's license number/ state ID card number, or financial account number/credit card number/debit card number with security code/access code/password.
Rhode Island	First name/first initial and last name plus one of the following: Social security number, driver's license number/ state ID card number, or financial account number/credit card number/debit card number with security code/access code/password.

continued

Table 5.1 (continued) Definitions of Personal Information in State Breach Notification Laws[a]

State	Personal Information Definition
South Carolina	First name/first initial and last name plus one of the following: Social security number, driver's license number/state ID card number, financial account number/credit card number/debit card number with security code/access code/password, other numbers that would allow access to financial accounts, or unique government/regulatory-issued number.
Tennessee	First name/first initial and last name plus one of the following: Social security number, driver's license number/state ID card number, or financial account number/credit card number/debit card number with security code/access code/password.
Texas	First name/first initial and last name plus one of the following: Social security number, driver's license number/government-issued ID card number, financial account number/credit card number/debit card number with security code/access code/password, information related to the physical or mental health of the individual, provision of health care, or payment for health care provided.
Utah	First name/first initial and last name plus one of the following: Social security number, driver's license number/state ID card number, or financial account number/credit card number/debit card number with security code/access code/password.
Vermont	First name/first initial and last name plus one of the following: Social security number, driver's license number/nondriver ID card number, financial account numbers/credit card numbers/debit card numbers if they can be used without additional information or access codes, or account passwords, ID numbers, or access codes for financial accounts.
Virginia	First name/first initial and last name plus one of the following: Social security number, driver's license number/state ID card number, or financial account number/credit card number/debit card number with security code/access code/password.

Table 5.1 (continued) **Definitions of Personal Information in State Breach Notification Laws**[a]

State	Personal Information Definition
Washington	First name/first initial and last name plus one of the following: Social security number, driver's license number/ state ID card number, or financial account number/credit card number/debit card number with security code/access code/password.
West Virginia	First name/first initial and last name plus one of the following: Social security number, driver's license number/ state ID card number, or financial account number/credit card number/debit card number with security code/access code/password.
Wisconsin	First name/first initial and last name plus one of the following: Social security number, driver's license number/ state ID card number, financial account number/credit card number/debit card number, or security code/access code/password, DNA profile, or biometric data.
Wyoming	First name/first initial and last name plus one of the following: Social security number, driver's license number/ state ID card number, financial account number/credit card number/debit card number with security code/access code/password, tribal ID card, or government-issued ID card number.

Source: Gidari A, Reingold B, Lyon S, *Security Breach Notification: State Laws Chart. Update*, Perkins Coie LLP, 2010. With permission.

[a] The highlighted states cover medical information.

of personal information if breach notification laws are in place [2, 3], and timely notification gives individuals a chance to reduce the damage from the breach (e.g., possibly minimize financial losses) [4].

In general, it is not necessary to notify if the data are de-identified. This is because de-identified data will almost certainly not include the data elements in Table 5.1, and would ensure that the probability of inferring them is low. Organizations that de-identify their data would avoid the negative consequences of breach notification that are detailed below.

Breach notifications themselves can have negative impacts on the custodians and the individuals affected. It has been argued that medical data breaches may potentially be eroding the public's trust in health information custodians in general [5, 6], which means decreased loyalty and higher churn among the customer base. One survey found that 58% of respondents who had self-reported that they received

Table 5.2 Costs across Various Industries

Year	Avg. per Person	Organizational Avg.
2011	$194	$5,501,889
2010	$214	$7,241,899
2009	$204	$6,751,451
2008	$202	$6,655,758
2007	$197	$6,355,132
2006	$182	$4,789,637
2005	$138	$4,541,429

Source: Data from Ponemon Institute, *2009 Annual Study: Cost of a Data Breach*, Traverse City, MI: Ponemon Institute, 2010; Ponemon Institute, *2010 Annual Study: U.S. Cost of a Data Breach*, Traverse City, MI: Ponemon Institute, 2011; Ponemon Institute, *2011 Cost of a Data Breach Study: United States*, Traverse City, MI: Ponemon Institute, 2012.

a notification of a data breach involving their personal data said that the breach event diminished their trust and confidence in the organization [7]. Nineteen percent of the same respondents indicated that they have already discontinued or plan to discontinue their relationship with the organization because of the breach, and a further 40% said that they might discontinue their relationship [7].

Furthermore, there are direct costs associated with breach notification. A summary of these costs based on existing data is provided in Table 5.2.

Cost of Data Breach Notifications to Custodian

The costs to the data custodians of a breach notification can be substantial. Listed corporations, on average, suffer a loss in their share price after the announcement of a security breach [9–14]. In effect, markets punish organizations for the increased business, reputation, and liability risks when personal and confidential data are inappropriately disclosed. After a breach, there are also costs associated with investigations, the notification itself, litigation, redress, and compensation, as well as productivity losses due to dealing with the breach [14, 15, 23]. Recently, regulators and courts in the United States and the UK have started imposing fines on organizations after particularly egregious breaches, repeat offenses, or to set examples [16–22].

Below we present some data on the costs of breaches to custodians. Some of the results are of health data and some are not specific to health care. In the latter case

Table 5.3   Direct and Indirect Costs per Breach

Year	Direct Costs	Indirect Costs
2011	$59	$135
2010	$73	$141
2009	$60	$144
2008	$50	$152

Source: Data from Ponemon Institute, *2010 Annual Study: U.S. Cost of a Data Breach,* Traverse City, MI: Ponemon Institute, 2011; Ponemon Institute, *2011 Cost of a Data Breach Study: United States,* Traverse City, MI: Ponemon Institute, 2012.

the numbers are still illustrative because health information custodians do hold large amounts of financial information as well.

Various studies in the United States that attempted to compute these costs are summarized in Table 5.3. These estimates include the cost of breach detection and escalation, notification, *ex-post* response (e.g., credit monitoring offered to victims), and lost business. Among multiple industries, health care was on the higher end of the scale in terms of breach costs from 2008 to 2011 [15, 25–27, as shown in Table 5.4]. Privacy Rights Clearinghouse reported the breach of 39.5 million electronic health records in the United States between 2005 and 2008. In the two-year period between 2010 and 2011, a reported 18 million Americans had their electronic health information breached [28]. Although the cost of a breach across industries declined in 2011, the Ponemon Institute has reported an increase in the economic impact for their benchmark health care organizations; the average cost increasing from $2,060,174 per health care organization in 2010 [23] to $2,243,700 in 2011 [24].

Lost business continues to consume the largest portion of the cost of a breach across industries, at $3,007,015 (54.7%) in 2011 [27]. In 2010, the cost due to lost business was $4,536,380, or 39% of the average total organizational cost of a breach [26]. In 2008 and 2009, lost business made up 43% and 40% of the average total organizational cost of a breach. Broken down by industry, abnormal customer churn rates were highest in the health care (6%, 7%) and pharmaceutical (6%, 8%) industries in both 2009 and 2010 (respectively) [26]. In 2011, health care experienced the third highest churn rates (4.2%) behind the communications (5.2%) and financial (5.6%) industries [27].

Costs similar to those in the United States were found in the UK, as summarized in Table 5.5. The costs due to lost business made up an even higher percentage

Table 5.4 Costs by Selected Industries

Year	Industry	Avg. per Person
2011 [27]	Health care	$240
	Services	$185
	Financial	$247
2010 [26]	Health care	$301
	Services	$301
	Financial	$353
2009 [25]	Health care	$294
	Services	$256
	Financial	$249
2008 [15]	Health care	$282
	Services	$283
	Financial	$240

Source: Data from Ponemon Institute, *Fourth Annual U.S. Cost of Data Breach Study*, Traverse City, MI: Ponemon Institute, 2009; Ponemon Institute, *2009 Annual Study: Cost of a Data Breach*, Traverse City, MI: Ponemon Institute, 2010; Ponemon Institute, *2010 Annual Study: U.S. Cost of a Data Breach*, Traverse City, MI: Ponemon Institute, 2011; Ponemon Institute, *2011 Cost of a Data Breach Study: United States*, Traverse City, MI: Ponemon Institute, 2012.

of the overall costs of a breach in the UK. In 2010, lost business accounted for 42% of the breach costs, up from 2009 (41%) and down slightly from 2008 (45%) [29].

One international study, covering multiple industries, included "catastrophic breaches" only—the smallest breach reported on involved 2,520 records, and the largest involved 101,000 records [30]. These costs are summarized in Table 5.6. Another study has found that the total annual costs for identity fraud have increased since 2007, when it reached a five-year low of $45 billion. In 2008 it increased to $48 billion and in 2009 to $54 billion [31]. The annual cost of Medicare fraud was estimated in 2010 to be $60 billion per year [28].

Information from the Federal Trade Commission-sponsored surveys on identity theft in 2003 and 2004, as reported by the Progress and Freedom Foundation, indicates that the annual cost of identity theft was approximately $55 billion: $50 billion for business and $5 billion for consumers [14]. The average cost of one incident of identity theft was found to be $4,800 for business and $500 for the individual [14]. In the 2006 FTC survey, the average individual loss per incident was $371 [32].

Table 5.5   Costs Across Various Industries

Year	Avg. per Person	Organizational Avg.
2010	£71	£1,903,265
2009	£65	£1,681,561
2008	£60	£1,725,639

Source: Ponemon Institute, 2010 Annual Study: U.K. Cost of a Data Breach, Traverse City, MI: Ponemon Institute, 2011. With permission.

Table 5.6   Cost of a Breach in Five Countries across Various Industries

Year	Country	Avg. per Person	Organizational Avg.
2009	United States	$204	$6,751,451
	United Kingdom	$98	$2,565,702
	Germany DE	$177	$3,444,898
	France	$119	$2,532,122
	Australia	$114	$1,832,732

Source: Ponemon Institute, Five Countries: Cost of Data Breach, Traverse City, MI: Ponemon Institute, 2010. With permission.

Data Breach Trends

A summary of breaches that have been notified is provided in Sidebar 5.1. The trend of rising breaches shown in Sidebar 5.1 is consistent with other data. There is evidence of rising self-reports of breaches among health information custodians [23, 33–35], and of a lack of preparedness to manage breach risks [23, 33, 35].

These numbers are likely undercounts of actual breaches that are occurring. There is clear evidence that data custodians were not disclosing all of the breaches that they discover [36, 37]. A recent survey found that 38% of responding health care providers do not notify their patients when there is a breach [23]. Another survey reported that only 11% of organizations report security breaches, even though 29% experienced inappropriate disclosure of employee or customer data [38]. An analysis of 141 confirmed breaches found that two-thirds were not disclosed [39], and an analysis of incidents on breach notification lists found that a large percentage of data custodians do not report breaches to the states [40]. There are additional examples of failure to notify in a timely manner in nonhealth contexts [41–43]. Such a discrepancy has been one of the arguments used against the effectiveness of current breach notification laws in the United States [44].

Furthermore, custodians may not be aware of breaches that are occurring. Data breaches by insiders are relatively common and increasing [39, 45–48]. Insider breaches can be ongoing for a long time without the custodians being aware of them [59]. Furthermore, there is evidence that the detection of the vast majority of data breaches is passive—they are detected by third parties who then inform the custodian [39, 55, 60]. One recent survey found that 41% of breaches are reported by the patients themselves [23].

Sidebar 5.1: The Number of Notified Breaches in the United States

We have recently examined the trends in U.S. breach reporting in more detail. The methodology for estimating notified breaches for 2007–2009 is described in more detail in Chapter 22.

Our numbers indicate that there was an increase in disclosed large breaches between 2007 and 2008, which is consistent with claims made by some analysts that medical data breaches are on the rise [61–63]. However, there was a drop of 44% from 2008 to 2009. Small breaches dropped between 2007 and 2008 and remained at approximately the same level into 2009. A summary of the results is shown in the table below.

	2007 (est.)	2008 (est.)	2009 (est.)	2010
<500 records	147	112	110	>25,000
≥500 records	85	95	53	207

The 2007–2009 numbers include all breaches from health information custodians, and not only those of PHI. The 2010 numbers include only PHI breaches. Given that 2007–2009 had a broader coverage, one would expect the numbers to be higher than 2010. However, during most of 2007–2009 only state breach notification laws applied, many of which did not require the reporting of PHI breaches, whereas in 2010, the national breach notification law that covered PHI was in effect. This explains the dramatic rise in reported breaches in 2010, and suggests that the state laws were not effective in identifying PHI breaches.

Some states have a risk-based trigger that involves the custodian applying a test to determine whether a breach poses a significant risk of financial, reputational, or other harm to the individual [64, 65]. Custodians may avoid the potentially negative consequences of breach notification by convincing themselves that their particular situation is exempt or does not trigger notification. Some analysts have commented that data custodians are getting better acquainted with the requirements of breach notification laws, and therefore are less likely to announce minor incidents [66], suggesting that custodians are being more nuanced in their notification practices.

Given that in practice it is extremely difficult to demonstrate harm [67] and that class action lawsuits seeking damages have demonstrated that individual rights for compensation do not exist [59, 68], some custodians may feel reduced exposure if they do not notify after evaluating a risk-based trigger. Furthermore, it has been argued that risk-based triggers leave the notification decision in the hands of the custodian who is naturally biased toward a low risk decision [36, 69], and that they create an incentive to expend little effort doing the risk assessment lest a thorough assessment create an obligation to notify [65].

Custodians may also be reluctant to notify out of fear of the consequences, for instance, to avoid damaging their reputation as a consequence of the negative publicity [61]. For example, a 2006 survey by the Computer Security Institute and the FBI indicates that only 25% of organizations reported security breaches to law enforcement, and 15% reported them to legal counsel [70]. The main reason provided for not reporting was concern about negative publicity [70]. The 2008 version of that survey showed similar numbers, with the top reasons for not reporting including concerns about bad publicity and the perception that the incidents were "too small to bother reporting" [71].

There *are* penalties for a failure to comply with state breach notification laws, which vary from state to state. Many permit enforcement by state attorneys general. Some states, such as Arizona, Arkansas, Connecticut, and Florida, allow civil penalties. At the extreme end of penalties, some states (e.g., Arkansas and Connecticut) allow for the termination of the right to conduct business in the state. If there is a real risk of penalties for not reporting, then this may be a disincentive for custodians not to report even if a breach passes a trigger. Some have argued that without enforcement of penalties few organizations would disclose a breach because of the potential bad publicity [72].

State breach notification laws did not commit resources to increase the probability of apprehension and conviction for the failure to notify; therefore, for a custodian, the cost of compliance can be higher than the cost of sanctions, making the decision not to notify the lowest-cost decision [68]. There is also a mixed perception by health information custodians about the strength of enforcement of breach notification requirements [33], which may dilute the incentive to notify. While there have been penalties levied for the breaches themselves [73], we are aware of only one recent penalty for not reporting a breach [37], and this is under appeal [74]. There is one case in New York where a settlement was reached for slow notification, but the fine was only to recover costs, and the custodian did notify, albeit the delay was considered unacceptable [41]. In another recent case the Indiana attorney general is suing a health insurer for a delay in notifying consumers of a breach, although it is not known whether this will result in penalties or a settlement [75].

To explore further whether there have been unreported penalties, we identified states that had breach notification laws the longest and that have the highest penalties (suggesting that they take not notifying more seriously): Florida (law came into effect in 2005 and penalty of $500,000 for not notifying), Utah (law came into effect in 2007 and penalties of $2,500 per consumer, up to $100,000, for not notifying), Virginia (law came into effect in 2008 with penalty of $150,000 for not notifying), and Michigan (law came into effect in 2007 and maximum penalties of $750,000 for not notifying). For these states we sent a Freedom of Information Act (FOIA) request to the attorneys general to get information on any penalties or fines that they have levied for not notifying a breach pursuant to the state breach notification laws. At the time of writing Michigan, Utah, and Virginia had responded, indicating that there have been no penalties thus far.

Of course, increased enforcement of the breach notification requirement for health information by DHHS may change the incentives to notify over time.

The Value of Health Data

One question that is often raised is why an adversary would be interested in health information to start off with? Even if there is a breach of health data, what could the possible harm be to individuals from that breach? In fact, health data can be quite valuable to adversaries from a financial perspective. Below we review some examples.

Financial Information in the Health Records

Adversaries will try to get access to health data if the records have financial information in them (e.g., information used for billing purposes) or information that is useful for financial fraud, for example, date of birth, address, and mother's maiden name. In some cases in the United States the medical record may contain social security numbers (SSNs) (which are often used as a unique identifier). All of this information is useful for committing financial crimes. In general, one individual's identity information is not worth that much in the underground market. For a self-assessment that may surprise you, try this tool from Symantec.* Therefore records with such information are only useful in large quantities to make it worthwhile for

---

* See http://www.everyclickmatters.com/victim/assessment-tool.html.

adversaries. This means that adversaries would be interested in databases of records rather going after a single individual's records.

Financial Value of Health Records

It has been estimated that the percentage of fraud resulting from the exposure of health data, versus other kinds of data, has increased from 3% in 2008 to 7% in 2009 [76]. Furthermore, health information is exploitable for fraud four times longer than other types of information [76]. One reason is the limited life span of credit card information: Once the affected individual discovers errant transactions or the financial institution detects it, then the card is canceled. It takes longer to detect fraud using health information. Health care fraud consists of filing false patient claims to insurers or government agencies that provide services and collecting the payouts. Furthermore, health information that can help adversaries purchase prescription drugs and then resell them would be valuable (such as prescriptions and insurance information) [77]. Physician information can be used to write fake prescriptions.

As illustrated in Figures 5.1 and 5.2, there is a market for health information, with buyers seeking data and sellers looking for buyers. Of course, such data dumps are not as useful if they are de-identified.

Medical Identity Theft

In the case of medical records, even if they do not have information in them that is suitable for financial fraud, if your record has information about your health insurance, then it can be very valuable. It is easier for fraudsters, illegal immigrants, the

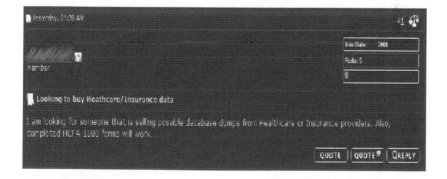

Figure 5.1   A screen shot from an underground market site whereby a user is asking for medical claims data. The text says, "I am looking for someone that is selling possible database dumps from Healthcare or Insurance providers. Also, completed HCFA 1500 forms will work." (From RSA, *Cybercrime and the Healthcare Industry*, 2010. With permission.)

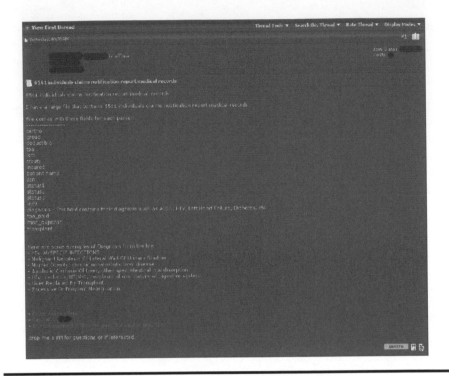

Figure 5.2 A post in an underground market site seeking buyers for medical records on more than 6,000 patients. The opening line says, "I have a large file that contains 6561 individuals claims notification report medical records" and proceeds to detail some of the fields, which include SSN and diagnosis. (From RSA, *Cybercrime and the Healthcare Industry*, 2010. With permission.)

uninsured, wanted criminals, and drug abusers to commit medical identity theft if they get access to individuals' identity and medical insurance information.

Medical identity theft entails someone getting health care in your name. This is most likely to happen because a person has no insurance because they cannot afford it or because they cannot get it (illegal immigrants, or individuals running from the law) [77–86]. Medical records have been used by terrorist organizations to target law enforcement personnel and intimidate witnesses [87, 88]. The inclusion of medical information with the identity information in such records can be further monetized by criminals through extortion of the data custodian by requesting large ransoms for the data [89, 90]. A good example of that happening in Canada occurred in Alberta, where a fraudster was creating new identities, including passports and health insurance cards, in the names of Canadian children who died a few decades prior. There are known cases of uninsured Americans, for example, buying these identities and coming to Canada to receive expensive medical care for free [91].

Monetizing Health Records through Extortion

Personal records are a good source of revenue if you are in the extortion business. One example is Express Scripts, a pharmacy benefits management company that was hacked by extortionists who threatened to publicize clients' personal information.[*] The company was using production data containing personal information for software testing, and there was a breach on the testing side of the business. Unfortunately, using production data for testing is common. The initial extortion attempt was based on the breach of 75 records. It turned out later that 700,000 individuals may have been affected by the breach.[†]

Another example is the recent extortion attempt in which an extortionist demanded $10 million after hacking into a database of prescription records at the Virginia Department of Health Professions.[‡] This database was intended to allow pharmacists and health care professionals to track prescription drug abuse, such as incidents of patients who go "doctor shopping" to find more than one doctor to prescribe narcotics. The ransom note is shown in Figure 5.3.

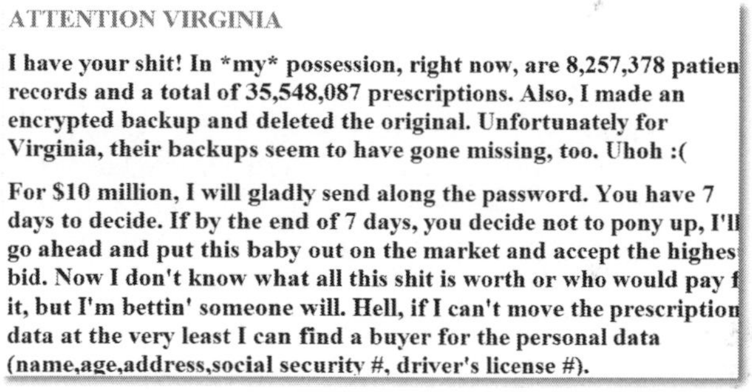

> ATTENTION VIRGINIA
>
> I have your shit! In *my* possession, right now, are 8,257,378 patien
> records and a total of 35,548,087 prescriptions. Also, I made an
> encrypted backup and deleted the original. Unfortunately for
> Virginia, their backups seem to have gone missing, too. Uhoh :(
>
> For $10 million, I will gladly send along the password. You have 7
> days to decide. If by the end of 7 days, you decide not to pony up, I'll
> go ahead and put this baby out on the market and accept the highes
> bid. Now I don't know what all this shit is worth or who would pay f
> it, but I'm bettin' someone will. Hell, if I can't move the prescription
> data at the very least I can find a buyer for the personal data
> (name,age,address,social security #, driver's license #).

Figure 5.3   A screen shot of the home page of the Virginia Prescription Monitoring Program with the ransom note.

---

[*] See the story at http://www.ehealthinformation.ca/blogs/extortion_plot_threatens.mht.
[†] See the story at http://www.computerworld.com/s/article/9138723/Express_Scripts_700_000_notified_after_extortion.
[‡] See the story at http://ehip.blogs.com/ehip/2009/05/hacker-threatens-to-expose-health-data-demands-10m.html.

References

1. Romanosky S, Telang R, Acquisti A. Do data breach disclosure laws reduce identity theft? Seventh Workshop on the Economics of Information Security, 2008.
2. EKOS Research Associates. *Health information and the Internet: Part of rethinking the information highway study.* 2005.
3. EKOS Research Associates. *Electronic health information and privacy survey: What Canadians think.* For Health Canada, Canada Health Infoway, and the Office of the Privacy Commissioner of Canada, 2007.
4. FTC. *2006 identity theft survey report.* 2007.
5. Robeznieks A. Privacy fear factor arises. *Modern Healthcare*, 2005; 35(46):6.
6. Becker C, Taylor M. Technical difficulties: Recent health IT security breaches are unlikely to improve the public's perception about the safety of personal data. *Modern Healthcare*, 2006; 38(8):6–7. PMID: 16515213.
7. Ponemon L. National survey on data security breach notification. 2005. http://www.ehealthinformation.ca:5051/documents/Security_Breach_Survey.pdf. Archived at http://www.webcitation.org/5uyiAJgNm (accessed May 1, 2010).
8. Gidari A, Reingold B, Lyon S. *Security breach notification: State laws chart. Update.* Perkins Coie LLP, 2010.
9. Acquisti A, Friedman A, Telang R. Is there a cost to privacy breaches? An event study. ICIS 2006 Proceedings, 2006.
10. Garg A, Curtis J, Halper H. Quantifying the financial impact of IT security breaches. *Information Management and Computer Security*, 2003; 11(2):74–83. DOI: 10.1108/09685220310468646.
11. Campbell K, Lawrence G, Loeb M, Zou L. The economic cost of publicly announced information security breaches. *Journal of Computer Security*, 2003; 11:431–448.
12. Cavusoglu H, Mishra B, Raghunathan S. The effect of Internet security breach announcements on market value of breached firms and Internet security developers. *International Journal of Electronic Commerce*, 2004; 9(1):69–104.
13. Andoh-Baidoo F, Amoako-Gyampah K, Osei-Bryson K-M. How Internet security breaches harm market value. *IEEE Security and Privacy*, 2010; 8(1):36–42. DOI: 10.1109/MSP.2010.37.
14. Lenard T, Rubin P. An economic analysis of notification requirements for data security breaches. 2005. http://www.pff.org/issues-pubs/pops/pop12.12datasecurity.pdf. Archived at http://www.webcitation.org/5uyj6flIy (accessed May 1, 2010).
15. Ponemon Institute, *Fourth annual U.S. cost of data breach study.* 2009. Ponemon Institute LLC: Traverse City, MI. http://www.ponemon.org/local/upload/fckjail/generalcontent/18/file/2008-2009%20US%20Cost%20of%20Data%20Breach%20Report%20Final.pdf. Archived at http://www.webcitation.org/5uyitZrR4 (accessed May 1, 2010).
16. Information Commissioner's Office. *Information commissioner's guidance about the issue of monetary penalties prepared and issued under Section 55C(1) of the Data Protection Act 1998.* 2010. http://www.ico.gov.uk/upload/documents/library/data_protection/detailed_specialist_guides/ico_guidance_monetary_penalties.pdf. Archived at http://www.webcitation.org/5uyjHJvFN (accessed May 1, 2010).
17. Ornstein C. Kaiser hospital fined $250,000 for privacy breach in octuplet case. *Los Angeles Times*, May 15, 2009.

18. FSA fines Nationwide over laptop theft. ComputerWeekly.com. 2007. http://www. computerweekly.com/Articles/2007/02/15/221780/fsa-fines-nationwide-over-laptop-theft.htm. Archived at http://www.ehealthinformation.ca/blogs/fsa_fines_nationwide. mht (accessed May 1, 2010).

19. The Associated Press. Seattle company agrees to pay $100,000 HIPAA fine. *Seattle Post-Intelligencer*, 2008. Archived at http://www.ehealthinformation.ca/blogs/seattle_company_agrees.mht (accessed May 1, 2010).

20. OCR shines a harsh light on data breaches. *Health Data Management*, 2010. http:// www.healthdatamanagement.com/issues/18_5/ocr-shines-a-harsh-light-on-data-breaches-40156-1.html (accessed May 2, 2010).

21. Vijayan J. Court gives preliminary OK to $4m consumer settlement in Heartland case. *Network World*, 2010. http://www.networkworld.com/news/2010/050710-court-gives-preliminary-ok-to.html (accessed July 7, 2010).

22. Mosquera M. *Civil rights office steps up health privacy enforcement.* 2010. http://www. govhealthit.com/newsitem.aspx?nid=73735 (accessed May 13, 2010).

23. Ponemon Institute. *Benchmark study of patient privacy and data security.* 2010.

24. Ponemon Institute, *Second Annual Benchmark Study on Patient Privacy & Data Security.* 2011, Ponemon Institute LLC: Traverse City, MI.

25. Ponemon Institute. *2009 annual study: Cost of a data breach.* Traverse City, MI: Ponemon Institute, 2010.

26. Ponemon Institute. *2010 annual study: U.S. cost of a data breach.* Traverse City, MI: Ponemon Institute, 2011.

27. Ponemon Institute, *2011 Cost of Data Breach Study: United States,* Ponemon Intitute LLC: Traverse City, MI, 2012.

28. American National Standards Institute, *The Financial Impact of Breached Protected Health Information.* American National Standards Institute: Washington, DC, 2012.

29. Ponemon Institute. *2010 annual study: U.K. cost of a data breach.* Traverse City, MI: Ponemon Institute, 2011.

30. Ponemon Institute. *Five countries: Cost of data breach.* Traverse City, MI: Ponemon Institute, 2010.

31. Javelin Strategy & Research. *2010 identity fraud survey report.* Pleasanton, CA: Javelin Strategy & Research, 2010.

32. Synovate. *2006 identity theft survey report.* McLean, VA: Federal Trade Commission, 2007.

33. HIMSS Analytics. *2009 HIMSS analytics report: Evaluating HITECH's impact on healthcare privacy and security.* HIMSS, 2009.

34. HIMSS Analytics. *2010 HIMSS analytics report: Security of patient data.* HIMSS, 2010.

35. Identity Force. *Spring 2010 national survey of hospital compliance executives.* 2010.

36. Schwartz M. ITRC: Why so many data breaches don't see the light of day. *Dark Reading*, 2010. http://www.darkreading.com/security/attacks/showArticle. jhtml?articleID=225702908. Archived at http://www.webcitation.org/5sdi4aNei.

37. Clark C. *Hospital fined $250,000 for not reporting data breach.* HealthLeaders Media, 2010. http://www.healthleadersmedia.com/page-1/TEC-256217/Hospital-Fined-250000-For-Not-Reporting-Data-Breach. Archived at http://www.webcitation. org/5sdW86ElH (accessed September 10, 2010).

38. Claburn T. Most security breaches go unreported. *InformationWeek*, 2008. http:// www.informationweek.com/news/security/attacks/showArticle.jhtml?articleID= 209901208. Archived at http://www.webcitation.org/5tkTiKRxt.

39. Verizon Business Risk Team. *2010 data breach investigations report*. 2010.
40. Staring into the abyss: How many breaches go unreported? 2010. http://www.databreaches.net/?p=14330. Archived at http://www.webcitation.org/5tkYXBuzg.
41. New York Attorney General. 540,000 New Yorkers and owner of personal data not properly notified that their personal information was at risk. 2007. http://www.ag.ny.gov/media_centre/2007/apr/apr26a_07/html. Archived at http://www.webcitation.org/5t2K9iiYy (accessed May 1, 2010).
42. Circuit Court for Davidson County, Tennessee. *Raymond T. Throckmorton III, Timothy T. Ishii, and Regina Newson v. Metropolitan Government of Nashville and Davidson County, the Wackenhut Corporation, and Specialized Security Consultants, Inc.* 2008.
43. Georgia USDC-NDo. *Keith Irwin v. RBS Worldplay, Inc.* 2009.
44. Cate F. *Information security breaches: Looking back and thinking ahead.* Centre for Information Policy Leadership, Hunton & Williams LLP, 2008.
45. Stolfo S, Bellovin S, Herkshop S, Keromytis A, Sinclair S, Smith S. *Insider attack and cyber security.* New York: Springer Verlag, 2008.
46. Kowalski E, Cappelli D, Moore A. *Insider threat study: Illicit cyber activity in the information technology and telecommunications sector.* Carnegie Mellon University and the U.S. Secret Service, 2008. http://www.cert.org/archive/pdf/insiderthreat_it2008.pdf. Archived at http://www.webcitation.org/5ir1TiKMS.
47. Randazzo M, Keeney M, Kowalski E, Cappelli D, Moore A. *Insider threat study: Illicit cyber activity in the banking and finance sector.* Carnegie Mellon University and the U.S. Secret Service, 2004. http://www.cert.org/archive/pdf/bankfin040820.pdf. Archived at http://www.webcitation.org/5ir1hY5Uk.
48. Keeney M, Kowalski E, Cappelli D, Moore A, Shimeall T, Rogers S. *Insider threat study: Computer system sabotage in critical infrastructure sectors.* Carnegie Mellon University and the U.S. Secret Service, 2005. http://www.cert.org/archive/pdf/insidercross051105.pdf. Archived at http://www.webcitation.org/5ir1rwVOF.
49. Kowalski E, Conway T, Keverline S, Williams M, Cappelli D, Willke B, Moore A. *Insider threat study: Illicit cyber activity in the government sector.* Carnegie Mellon University and the U.S. Secret Service, 2008. http://www.cert.org/archive/pdf/insiderthreat_gov2008.pdf. Archived at http://www.webcitation.org/5ir25mBaS.
50. Kroll Fraud Solutions. *HIMSS analytics report: Security of patient data.* 2008. http://www.mmc.com/knowledgecenter/Kroll_HIMSS_Study_April2008.pdf. Archived at http://www.webcitation.org/5ipdyMtNJ.
51. *CSO Magazine.* 2006 e-crime watch survey. U.S. Secret Service, Carnegie Mellon University, and Microsoft Corporation, 2006.
52. Predd J, Hunker J, Bulford C. Insiders behaving badly. *IEEE Security and Privacy,* 2008; 6(4):66–70.
53. CSI. *14th annual CSI computer crime and security survey.* 2009.
54. Ponemon Institute. *Data loss risks during downsizing.* 2009.
55. Verizon Business Risk Team. *2009 data breach investigations report.* 2009.
56. PriceWaterhouseCoopers. *Safeguarding the new currency of business: Findings from the 2008 global state of information security study.* 2008.
57. El Emam K, King M. *The data breach analyzer.* 2009. http://www.ehealthinformation.ca/dataloss.
58. Shaw E, Ruby K, Jerrold M. *The insider threat to information systems.* Department of Defense Security Institute, 1998.

59. Melodia M. Security breach notification: Breaches in the private sector: "Harm" in the litigation setting. Security Breach Notification Symposium, 2009.
60. Verizon Business Risk Team. *2008 data breach investigations report*. Verizon, 2008.
61. Pear R. Tighter medical privacy rules sought. *New York Times*, 2010. http://www.nytimes.com/2010/08/23/health/policy/23privacy.html?_r=3. Archived at http://www.webcitation.org/5sFCJ6vcM (accessed August 22, 2010).
62. Day G, Kizer K. *Stemming the rising tide of health privacy breaches*. Booz Allen Hamilton, 2009.
63. Worthen B. New epidemic fears: Hackers. *Wall Street Journal*, 2009.
64. Lessemann D. Once more unto the breach: An analysis of legal, technological, and policy issues involving data breach notification statutes. Howard University School of Law, 2009.
65. Burdon M, Reid J, Low R. Encryption safe harbours and data breach notification laws. *Computer Law and Security Review*, 2010; 26(5):520–534. DOI: 10.1016/j.clsr.2010.07.002.
66. Sullivan R. The changing nature of U.S. card payment fraud: Industry and public policy options. *Federal Reserve Bank of Kansas City Economic Review*, 2010; QII:101–133.
67. Romanosky S, Acquisti A. Privacy costs and personal data protection: Economic and legal perspectives of ex ante regulation, ex post liability and information disclosure. *Berkeley Technology Law Journal*, 2009; 24(3):1060–1100.
68. Winn J. Are better security breach notification laws possible ? *Berkley Technology Law Journal*, 2009; 24.
69. Geiger H. *HHS' new harm standard for breach notification*. Centre for Democracy and Technology, 2009. http://blog.cdt.org/2009/09/11/hhs%E2%80%99-new-harm-standard-for-breach-notification/. Archived at http://www.webcitation.org/5sdhrGevT.
70. Gordon L, Loeb M, Lucyshyn W, Richardson R. *CSI/FBI computer crime and security survey*. CSI/FBI, 2006.
71. Richardson R. *CSI computer crime and security survey*. CSI/FBI, 2008.
72. CSI/FBI. *CSI/FBI computer crime and security survey*. CSI/FBI, 2005.
73. Clark C. Six major patient record breaches draw $675,000 in penalties. HealthLeaders Media, 2010. http://www.healthleadersmedia.com/content/LED-252360/Six-Major-Patient-Record-Breaches-Draw-675000-In-Penalties. Archived at http://www.webcitation.org/5sdW0JX7D.
74. Vijayan J. Hospital appeals $250,000 fine for late breach disclosure. *CompterWorld*, 2010. http://www.computerworld.com/s/article/9184679/Hospital_appeals_250_000_fine_for_late_breach_disclosure. Archived at http://www.webcitation.org/5seoQsqPR.
75. Indiana AG sues WellPoint for breach. *Health Data Management*, 2010. http://www.healthdatamanagement.com/news/wellpoint-breach-lawsuit-indiana-attorney-general-41280-1.html. Archived at http://www.webcitation.org/5twF6iXo5.
76. RSA. *Cybercrime and the healthcare industry*. 2010.
77. Man accused of forging prescriptions for 15,000 painkiller pills. CBC, 2009. http://www.cbc.ca/canada/calgary/story/2009/02/19/cgy-pharmacy-oxycontin-fraud.html. Archived at http://www.webcitation.org/5uxHyiAp6 (accessed May 1, 2010).
78. Dixon P. *Medical identity theft: The information crime that can kill you*. World Privacy Forum, 2006.
79. Messmer E. Health care organizations see cyberattacks as growing threat. *Network World*, 2008. http://www.infoworld.com/print/32801. Archived at http://www.webcitation.org/5uxGim78f (accessed May 1, 2010).

80. Wereschagin M. Medical ID theft leads to lengthy recovery. *Pittsburgh Tribune-Review*, 2006. http://www.pittsburghlive.com/x/pittsburghtrib/news/cityregion/s_476326. html. Archived at http://www.webcitation.org/5uxGsaBlB (accessed May 1, 2010).
81. *United States of America v. Fernando Ferrer Jr. and Isis Machado*. 06-60261. U.S. District Court, Southern District of Florida, 2006.
82. Bogden D. Las Vegas pharmacist charged with health care fraud and unlawful distribution of controlled substances. U.S. Department of Justice, U.S. Attorney, District of Nevada, 2007. http://lasvegas.fbi.gov/dojpressrel/pressrel07/healthcarefraud022307. htm. Archived at http://www.webcitation.org/5uxH2MTsw (accessed May 1, 2010).
83. Diagnosis: Identity theft. *BusinessWeek*, 2007. http://www.businessweek.com/magazine/ content/07_02/b4016041.htm. Archived at http://www.webcitation.org/5uxH8VEHj (accessed May 1, 2010).
84. Booz Allen Hamilton. *Medical identity theft: Environmental scan*. 2008. http://www. hhs.gov/healthit/documents/IDTheftEnvScan.pdf. Archived at http://www.webcitation. org/5uxHJAOcC (accessed May 1, 2010).
85. Lafferty L. Medical identity theft: The future threat of health care fraud is now. *Journal of Health Care Compliance*, 2007; 9(1):11–20.
86. Bird J. The uninsured turn to fraud. *Charlotte Business Journal*, 2009. http://charlotte.biz-journals.com/charlotte/stories/2009/11/16/focus1.html?b=1258347600%5E2432371. Archived at http://www.webcitation.org/5lOoTAT1N (accessed May 1, 2010).
87. "Dissident operation" uncovered. BBC News, July 2, 2003. http://news.bbc.co. uk/1/low/northern_ireland/3038852.stm. Archived at http://www.webcitation.org/ 5Wd0DNdAZ (accessed May 1, 2010).
88. McGuigan C, Browne M. Hospital leak linked to witness in LVF case. *Belfast Telegraph*, August 2007. http://www.sundaylife.co.uk/news/article2896291.ece. Archived at http:// www.webcitation.org/5Wd0LZKEG (accessed May 1, 2010).
89. Kravets D. Extortion plot threatens to divulge millions of patients' prescriptions. Wired, 2008. http://www.wired.com/threatlevel/2008/11/extortion-plot/. Archived at http://www.webcitation.org/5hKiktSWV (accessed May 1, 2010).
90. Krebs B. Hackers break into Virginia health professions database, demand ransom. *Washington Post*, 2009. http://voices.washingtonpost.com/securityfix/2009/05/hack-ers_break_into_virginia_he.html. Archived at http://www.webcitation.org/5hKisjsS4 (accessed May 1, 2010).
91. Pendleton J. *The growing threat of medical identity theft in Canada*. Electronic Health Information and Privacy, 2008.

Chapter 6

Peeping and Snooping

In his 2009 article, Peter Swire describes a growing phenomenon in relation to electronic medical records—peeping. He outlines three types of peeping in his article: "the gaze, the gossip and the grab" [1]. The gaze is the act of looking at something that is restricted, like the health record of a patient, to which someone should not have access. This in itself violates the individual's privacy. The gossip inflicts additional harm to the individual by affecting his or her reputation. This could lead to harms such as denial of insurance, loss of employment, or social stigma. The grab is when the peeping is done for financial gain.

There are many examples of peeping, also known as snooping, that have become known publicly. Some of these examples and their variety are summarized in this chapter. These illustrate that even trusted health care professionals and their staff are tempted to look at the medical information of other people that they know, famous people, or even people that they do not know. In the context of de-identification this is important because data recipients may also be tempted to peep. Even if the organization in which an individual works has strong security practices, an individual who has access to health information may still look at records that he or she is not supposed to. This kind of risk has also been referred to as spontaneous recognition or spontaneous re-identification in the literature, and considers the situation when an individual inadvertently recognizes someone in the data. A malicious version of an inadvertent recognition is an adversary who is attempting to find a record of a specific someone. De-identification can protect against these types of attempts by making it difficult for the culprit to determine the identity of the records.

Examples of Peeping

An example of this is the Lawanda Jackson case in which Ms. Jackson sold information about the health records of celebrities to the *National Enquirer* [1]. Lawanda Jackson was an administrative specialist at the UCLA Medical Center. Beginning in 2006, the *National Enquirer* paid her to provide them with medical information about celebrities. Ms. Jackson reportedly used her supervisor's password to gain access to medical records at the center. Among the records Jackson peeped at were those of Britney Spears, Farrah Fawcett, and Maria Shriver. She was convicted in 2008 and faced up to 10 years in prison and a $250,000 fine [2].

Similar cases of peeping into celebrity medical records have appeared in recent years. After George Clooney suffered a motorcycle accident in 2007, up to 40 health care workers at the Palisades Medical Center in North Bergen were suspended for inappropriately accessing and/or leaking confidential medical information about Clooney and his girlfriend [3]. At UCLA, not only Ms. Jackson, but up to 127 health care workers were caught accessing medical records without authorization between 2004 and 2006 [4]. Breached records include those of celebrities such as Farrah Fawcett.

At Kaiser Permanente, several employees accessed the medical information of Nadya Suleman, the famous mother who gave birth to octuplets in 2009 [5]. Ms. Suleman visited Kaiser's Bellflower facility to give birth; however, an investigation found that eight health care workers at other facilities and employees at the regional office had also accessed Ms. Suleman's record. Kaiser was found to have failed to put safeguards in place to adequately protect Ms. Suleman's privacy and was fined $250,000 by the Department of Public Health [5].

And it is not only celebrities who have had their records peeped into by health care workers. In 2010, six California hospitals were fined for security breaches relating to unauthorized access to medical records [6]. Pacific Hospital of Long Beach was fined $225,000 after an employee accessed the records of nine patients for the purposes of identity theft. Regulators fined the Children's Hospital of Orange County $25,000 after an employee accessed the medical record of a co-worker. Kern Medical Center was fined twice for a total of $310,000 for multiple breaches, including unauthorized access to and disclosure of medical record information. A $60,000 fine was issued to Delano Regional Medical Center for an employee's unauthorized access of a family member's medical record. In another case of attempted identity theft, an employee of Kaweah Manor Convalescent Hospital accessed the records of five patients without authorization. The hospital was fined $125,000. Biggs Gridley Memorial Hospital was fined $5,000 due to two employees' unauthorized access of a co-worker's medical records [6].

In Canada, similar cases have appeared in the media, like the case of the clerk in Calgary who was fined in 2007 for inappropriately accessing the medical records of the spouse of the man with whom she was having an affair [7]. The patient, who was diagnosed with cancer at the time, had her record accessed several times by her husband's mistress, who was working in the office of a plastic surgeon at the time.

The prosecutor argued that it "constituted a death watch over the victim" [7]. The mistress was fined $10,000 for her behavior. More recently, a report came out about a former employee of the Capital District Health Authority in Nova Scotia who inappropriately viewed the medical records of family members and friends between 2005 and 2011 [8]. The health authority initially flagged 15 cases of unauthorized access by this employee in an investigation started in October 2011, and have since found dozens of additional incidents. The employee, Katharine Zinck Lawrence, said that she is not the only employee of the health authority to access medical records without authorization. Friends and family of Lawrence whose files were accessed were at the time of this writing planning a lawsuit against the health authority for not adequately protecting the privacy of their health information.

Swire writes that there seems to be an increase in peeping cases in the last few years [1]. Why is this? He argues that the means to peep have increased; more information is being stored electronically, which allows more people to access the information. In 1995, Dr. Beverly Woodward published an article outlining her concerns about the confidentiality of emerging electronic health records [9]. Included in these concerns was unauthorized access to or "browsing" of medical records. As we saw in the Lawanda Jackson case, one of the main threats outlined by Dr. Woodward was the potential for health care workers to be influenced into providing medical record information to outside parties. "Insiders (employees and affiliated personnel), who may number in the thousands in some health care networks and hospitals, become a tempting target for the growing number of people outside the hospital who wish to have access to medical records. Among the many insiders with access, some will be willing to sell information, to share a password, or to subvert the system in some other manner" [9].

Woodward points to another peeping case in which the medical records of children were inappropriately accessed by a convicted child rapist who was employed at a Boston hospital [9]. This man used the information found to place obscene phone calls to the homes of these children.

Information and Privacy Commissioners' Orders

Below is a summary of some Canadian peeping examples that have been uncovered by privacy commissioners. While these examples are not comprehensive, they do provide a little more context for why and how peeping occurs, especially when it does not involve famous individuals.

Ontario

HO-002

A complaint was submitted by a patient of the Ottawa Hospital who claimed that her health record was improperly accessed by a nurse who worked at the hospital [10]. The nurse was the girlfriend of her estranged husband, who also worked at the hospital. Although this nurse did not provide care to the patient during her stay, the patient believed that this nurse had accessed her record and disclosed the information to her estranged husband. An audit of the logs by the hospital's privacy office revealed that the nurse did indeed access this patient's record without just cause. The Office of the Information and Privacy Commissioner (IPC) found that the nurse was in contravention of the Personal Health Information Protection Act (PHIPA) when she accessed the patient's record and disclosed this information to the patient's estranged husband. They also found that the hospital failed to comply with its obligation under PHIPA to adequately protect the privacy of the patient's health information, and also failed to effectively rectify the situation after the breach occurred. In fact, the nurse accessed the record on several more occasions after the hospital was initially informed of the breach. The nurse and the estranged husband were disciplined by the hospital and required to sign agreements stating that they "did not alter, destroy, copy or print any or all of the complainant's personal health information" [10].

HO-010

A complaint was received in 2010 from a patient of the Ottawa Hospital [11]. The patient claimed that a diagnostic imaging technologist at the hospital had accessed her medical records without authorization on six separate occasions. The technologist was the ex-wife of the patient's current spouse. The patient believed that her personal health information was used and disclosed by the technologist for purposes unrelated to her care. The patient reported the incident to the hospital, which conducted an audit and discovered that the technologist had in fact accessed the patient's records inappropriately. The patient was not satisfied with the resolution of the incident by the hospital and filed a complaint with the IPC. The IPC found that the measures taken to prevent the unauthorized use and disclosure of personal health information by employees were not effective and were also not in compliance with PHIPA. The hospital was again ordered to revise its policies and procedures around privacy and its process for investigating privacy complaints/breaches.

HR06-53

A report was received from a hospital that clerical staff within the hospital had inappropriately accessed the personal health information of a total of seventeen patients [12]. Three clerks were reported to have accessed the records of patients with which they had no clinical relationship. In many cases, the records belonged to family members or friends of the clerks. The hospital took disciplinary action against the clerks.

HI-050013-1

A hospital reported that a staff member had inappropriately accessed a patient's record [13]. The access was discovered during an audit of the clinical information system used in the mental health department. The employee did not work in the department, but the audit revealed that she had viewed the patient's chart on multiple occasions. The employee admitted to accessing the patient's information for purposes not related to the patient's care. Evidence of other unauthorized access to health information by this employee was later found. The hospital dismissed the employee for her conduct.

Alberta

Investigation Report H2011-IR-004

A complaint was received that the record of a patient had been accessed by nine physicians through Alberta Netcare who were not his personal physician [14]. The patient's partner and mother also found suspicious activity on their Netcare accounts around the same time. He suspected that his ex-wife, a nurse, and her partner, a doctor, may be responsible, although their names did not appear in the audit logs. The patient and his wife were going through divorce proceedings at the time. Although his ex-wife was found not to be responsible, her partner, a doctor with Covenant Health, admitted to using colleagues' accounts to access the records of the patient and his family members. The doctor claimed that she did not disclose any of the information to the patient's ex-wife. The doctor was at the time of writing under investigation by Alberta's College of Physicians and Surgeons.

IPC Investigation (Report Not Available)

A news release from the IPC of Alberta dated December 6, 2011, describes an investigation of a pharmacist who was charged under the Health Information Act and pleaded guilty in December 2011 [15]. The pharmacist, Marianne Songgadan, pleaded guilty to knowingly obtaining health information in contravention of the HIA and was fined $15,000.

A complaint was received by the IPC office in 2010 that the pharmacist had inappropriately accessed the record of a patient through Alberta Netcare, and had posted the information about the patient's prescription medication on Facebook. The audit logs showed that Songgadan had accessed the patient's record on four occasions. Records of eight of the patient's friends were also accessed by Songgadan around the same time, as shown by the Netcare audit logs. Songgadan's motive seems to have stemmed from a conflict that she was having with the patient and others who attended her church, centered around the romantic interests of one of the male church members. Songgadan posted disparaging comments about one woman on Facebook, and after a complaint was made to the church, Songgadan accessed the previously mentioned patient's records and posted her prescription information on Facebook. While at the time of writing there was only a news release about the incident, the investigation report is expected to be released by the commissioner's office shortly [15].

Saskatchewan

H-2010-001

The IPC received a complaint in regards to the unauthorized access by a pharmacist to the drug profiles of three individuals with whom the pharmacist was acquainted [16]. This incident took place at a time when none of the individuals were patients of that pharmacy, and had severed their relations with the pharmacist in question. The pharmacist had access to the drug profiles through his involvement in the Pharmaceutical Information Program. He indicated that he had accessed the records because he was concerned about the quality of care that the individuals were receiving since they had ceased being patients of the pharmacy. The IPC found that the pharmacy should be held responsible for the actions of the pharmacist, and that they were in violation of the provincial Health Information Protection Act (HIPA) because they did not have adequate policies and procedures in place to protect personal health information.

References

1. Swire P. Peeping. *Berkeley Technology Law Journal*, 2009; 24(3):1165–1194.
2. Mohajer S. Ex-UCLA worker pleads guilty to selling celebrity medical records. *The Huffington Post*, December 2, 2008.
3. Standora L. Staff suspended for leaking George Clooney medical records. *NY Daily News*, October 10, 2007.
4. Ornstein C. UCLA hospital scandal grows. *Los Angeles Times*, August 5, 2008.
5. Ornstein C. Breaches in privacy cost Kaiser. *Los Angeles Times*, May 15, 2009.
6. Hennessy-Fiske M. Six California hospitals fined for medical record security breaches. *Los Angeles Times*, November 19, 2010.
7. Slade D. Clerk fined for "death watch." *Calgary Herald*, April 14, 2007.
8. Former Capital Health worker sorry for privacy breach. CBC News, February 14, 2012.
9. Woodward B. The computer-based patient record and confidentiality. *New England Journal of Medicine*, 1995; 333(21): 1419–1422.
10. Cavoukian A. Order HO-002. Information and Privacy Commissioner of Ontario, July 2006.
11. Cavoukian A. PHIPA Order HO-010. Information and Privacy Commissioner of Ontario, December 31, 2010.
12. Beamish B. Personal Health Information Protection Act report, file no. HR06-53. Information and Privacy Commissioner of Ontario.
13. Cavoukian A. Personal Health Information Protection Act report, file no. HI-050013-1. Information and Privacy Commissioner of Ontario, August 9, 2005.
14. Hamilton B. Investigation Report H2011-IR-004. Information and Privacy Commissioner of Alberta, November 30, 2011.
15. Wood W. News release. Information and Privacy Commissioner of Alberta, December 6, 2011.
16. Investigation Report H-2010-001. Information and Privacy Commissioner of Saskatchewan, March 23, 2010.

Chapter 7

Unplanned but Legitimate Uses and Disclosures

The pressure to realize value from existing data sets is rising. This pressure exists in public health and the research community, as well as the commercial world and government. Realizing value means that the data collected for one purpose may be used or disclosed for other, often unplanned, purposes. Because it is unplanned at the outset, these uses and disclosures would also be unexpected by the patients. The patients may be unpleasantly surprised if they find out about these unexpected uses and disclosures. This has an impact on public trust in data custodians.

Data custodians may be reluctant to restrict themselves up front from realizing value from the data that they have collected. Therefore it will most likely fall upon the patients to insist on constraints on such unplanned uses and disclosures.

One way to allow the data custodians to realize value but still protect the interests of the patients is to de-identify these data at the earliest opportunity. In such a case any unplanned uses and disclosures would be of less concern to the patients (unless there are contracts prohibiting such secondary uses and disclosures).

Unplanned Uses by Governments

It will not be possible to discuss all known or possible unplanned uses of data collected by governments. Our objective is only to provide illustrative examples to make the point that some of these uses and disclosures may be unsettling to the public.

Data collected by governments is of particular interest because it can be compelled. A good example of this is the Canadian census, where criminal penalties apply for noncompliance with providing data. According to the assistant chief statistician, if explanation and persuasion do not work, then prosecution is considered [1]. Furthermore, he stated that there were 45 cases considered for prosecution after the 1986 census [1], and recently an individual has been found guilty of not completing her census form [2].

One does not have to go far into history to find unexpected uses of census data. In 1972 the British government considered the forcible expulsion of hundreds of thousands of Catholics in the Republic of Ireland as a solution to the Northern Ireland problem [3]. Evacuated areas would be repopulated by Protestants. Census records were used to identify areas with Catholic and Protestant majorities.* Of course this did not occur, but it was considered at a senior cabinet level as an option.

More recently in 2004, the U.S. Bureau of the Census was asked by the Department of Homeland Security to provide detailed tabulations of ZIP codes from the 2000 census with majorities of individuals with Arab ancestry [4].

In these examples the use or disclosure may be legitimate. However, from the individual citizen's perspective, the reason for the disclosure may be surprising, and perhaps more importantly, may play a role in eroding trust in institutions that collect information. Trust is an issue that we will return to in the next section.

For research purposes, the National Institutes of Health (NIH) can issue certificates of confidentiality to protect identifiable participant information from compelled disclosure, and allows researchers to refuse to disclose identifying information in any civil, criminal, administrative, legislative, or other proceeding, whether at the federal, state, or local level [5]. However, these would not be applicable to non-research projects or to projects that are not approved by an institutional review board (IRB). Furthermore, such certificates do not exist outside of the United States.

Data Sharing for Research Purposes

In January 2004 Canada was a signatory to the Organization for Economic Cooperation and Development (OECD) Declaration on Access to Research Data from Public Funding [6]. This is intended to ensure that data generated through public funds are publicly accessible for researchers as much as possible [7]. To the extent that this is implemented, potentially more personal health data about Canadians will be made available to researchers worldwide. The European Commission has passed a regulation facilitating the sharing with external researchers of data collected by community government agencies [8]. There is interest by the pharmaceutical industry and academia to share raw data from clinical trials [9, 10].

---

* Copies of the declassified report can be found at http://cain.ulst.ac.uk/publicrecords/1972/ prem15-1010-X.jpg, where X changed from 1 to 8 for images of each page.

Researchers in the future may have to disclose their data. The *Canadian Medical Association Journal* has recently contemplated requiring authors to make the full data sets from their published studies available publicly online [11]. Similar calls for depositing raw data with published manuscripts have been made recently [9, 12–16]. The Canadian Institutes of Health Research (CIHR) has a policy, effective on January 1, 2008, that requires making some data available with publications [17].* The UK Medical Research Council (MRC) policy on data sharing sets the expectation that data from its funded projects will be made publicly available [18]. The UK Economic and Social Research Council requires its funded projects to deposit data sets in the UK Data Archive (such projects generate health and lifestyle data on, for example, diet, reproduction, pain, and mental health) [19]. The European Research Council considers it essential that raw data be made available preferably immediately after publication, but not later than six months after publication [20]. The NIH in the United States expects investigators seeking more than $500,000 per year in funding to include a data sharing plan (or explain why that is not possible) [21]. If researchers do not make their data available, courts, in criminal and civil cases, may compel disclosure of research data [22, 23].

Open Government

U.S. president Barack Obama has recently brought into the spotlight the concept of open government, but this is certainly not a new concept, and the United States is one among many countries that are moving toward more transparency in government. Governments around the world have been working for some time now toward opening up their operations to the public and providing government information in a proactive fashion. There are several reasons for this movement toward more transparency. First, openness of government policy and procedures allows for public observation and scrutiny and ensures accountability. Accountability, in turn, helps to develop and maintain the trust of the people. "All government power in a modern democracy must be exercised, and be seen to be exercised, constitutionally and responsibly" [24]. Transparency and accountability form the basis for public trust in modern government [25]. This can be demonstrated by looking at governments on the other end of the spectrum: totalitarian governments. The Nazi and Stalinist governments of the last century are vivid examples of how secrecy and control of information can lead to widespread public distrust and fear of government [26].

An example within the Canadian government of such a move toward more transparency is the mandated disclosure of financial and human resource information to

---

* Since the initial writing of this chapter, CIHR has rescinded the policy for making data available, which was met with much criticisim: A. Silversides. Withdrawal of clinical trials policy by Canadian research institute is a "lost opportunity for increased transparency." *BMJ* 2011;342:d2570.

ensure accountability for government spending. This proactive disclosure involves mandatory publication of travel and hospitality expenses, the reclassification of positions, as well as any government contracts over $10,000 on departmental websites [27]. Similar moves are taking place in the UK, Australia, New Zealand, and the United States, while places like Mexico, Finland, and India have had proactive disclosure in their legislation for some time [28].

Beyond accountability, openness in government is "intended to provide the opportunity for individuals to participate in the policy process and to utilize information for that purpose" [29]. Democracy is defined by participation of the people—the power of rule in a democracy is supposed to lie with its people. In modern democracy, we have elected representatives to exercise power on our behalf because populations are too large for each individual to be involved. However, the intention remains for the will of the people to reign through these representatives. Opening up government to public participation harkens back to a more classic form of democracy where the voice of the people is heard directly. This intention can be found in Obama's 2009 Memorandum on Transparency and Open Government: "Executive departments and agencies should offer Americans increased opportunities to participate in policymaking and to provide their Government with the benefits of their collective expertise and information" [30]. Similarly, the UK plan for open government, "Putting the Frontline First: Smarter Government," stresses making raw data publically available as well as the tools that will facilitate interaction between citizens and government to engage the public in the policy and decision-making process [28, 31]. A model of this type of direct interaction between the public and government is currently being developed in British Columbia. The BC provincial government is working toward the goal of allowing affected citizens to participate in policy making by providing the relevant data, policy documents, and interactive tools for citizens to collaborate directly with public service departments [32].

Governments, particularly on the local level, have been opening up their data to other organizations and, in some instances, the public, in order to facilitate data analysis, applications development, and possibly even seed commerce [28, 32]. This is of benefit to all groups involved, as organizations, researchers, and others can gain from having access to these types of data for research, development, and commercial purposes, while the government is able to utilize the products of this external R&D, resulting in a decrease in its own internal costs. In Canada, as well as internationally, such open data sets are already being used to facilitate mash-ups, which merge information from multiple sources into one integrated web application. For example, a Research Funding Explorer application has been developed in the UK using data available through the government's open data portal, data.gov.uk [28]. In Canada, Edmonton is one of several municipalities across the country that has piloted data portals to make municipal government data sets available online. These portals contain data sets of information such as detailed election results, public transit information, geospatial information, and service requests. Edmonton held a contest, "Apps4Edmonton," in 2010 to encourage the development of applications using data from its portal, data.edmonton.ca [28, 33]. The winner was an application called "DinerInspect," which used government inspection data to compile restaurant inspections by location [33]. Other municipal data portals include Toronto,* Ottawa,† and Vancouver.‡

The federal government of Canada has also shown some interest in opening up government and sharing information with the public, particularly in regards to financial spending. Of course, there is also an obligation under the Access to Information Act for government to provide information to individuals when requested [34]. However, the Information and Privacy Commissioners across Canada have recently indicated that more needs to be done. They have called for more openness and transparency from government by way of a move from reactive disclosure to proactive disclosure of information [35]. This move toward open government is intended to ensure that government is accountable, to encourage public participation, and to make information "open, accessible and reusable" [35]. Some departments have moved significantly in this direction already. Statistics Canada has a historical mandate under the Statistics Act to provide data on the Canadian population to the public, through its publications and now online [36]. Along with this, it provides more detailed information for research purposes to academic institutions via the Data Liberation Initiative subscription service [37]. Natural Resources Canada has more recently endeavored to provide open data online via three web portals that they have established: Geobase [38], Geogratis [39], and GeoConnections Discovery Portal [28, 40]. However, as the information commissioner pointed out recently, a large number of federal government departments are falling behind in their obligation to respond to access to information requests [41]. Therefore it appears that much work still needs to be done to facilitate a transition from a reactive to a proactive disclosure model.

Open Data for Research

Open data have been an issue in the research community for many years now, and this debate shares some of the same arguments as those for open government. Open data are said to ensure accountability in research by allowing others access to researchers' data and methodologies [42–45]. Having research data available to peers and the public helps to ensure that reported study results are valid and protects against faulty data [9, 42–48]. Another asset of open data in research is that it allows researchers to build on the work of others more efficiently and helps to speed the progress of science [43, 44, 46]. In order to build on previous discoveries, there must be trust in the validity of prior research. Openness of research methods

---

* http://www.toronto.ca/open/.

† http://www.ottawa.ca/online_services/opendata/index_en.html.

‡ http://data.vancouver.ca/.

as well as raw data facilitates trust between researchers as well as with the public [43]. And having research data available to other researchers allows for secondary analyses that expand the usefulness of data sets and the resulting knowledge gained [42, 44–46]. Connected to this is the decrease in the burden on research subjects through the reuse of existing research data [42, 44, 46]. Also, reuse of data can help to decrease the cost of data collection; however, there may be costs associated with the preparation of data for redistribution [42, 44–46].

More and more pressure is being put on researchers to make not only their research results but also their raw data publically available. The "Panton Principles" were created by academics in conjunction with the Open Knowledge Foundation Working Group on Open Data in Science, as an ideal of openness toward which the research community should strive. The principles call for scientific data to be "freely available on the public internet permitting any user to download, copy, analyze, re-process, pass them to software or use them for any other purpose without financial, legal, or technical barriers other than those inseparable from gaining access to the internet itself" [49]. Research journals that aspire toward this ideal encourage researchers who publish in their journals to make their raw data available, typically by depositing it into an institutional data repository or publishing it as supplementary material [48, 50, 51]. Some public funding agencies, for example, the NIH in the United States and the Social Sciences and Humanities Research Council of Canada (SSHRC), have placed conditions on awards requiring that researchers submit a data sharing plan at the time of application and make the results of their work openly available via open access journals [21, 51–53]. To facilitate sharing, many academic institutions now have archives for researchers to deposit and obtain research data. A list of Canadian institutions can be found on the SSHRC website and includes the University of Alberta data library, the University of British Columbia data library, and the Carleton University Social Science data archive, to name a few [52].

Although there is some evidence that sharing raw research data increases the citation rate of research papers [54], researchers do have concerns about open data and how it will affect them. Such concerns could prevent them from sharing data, and include the privacy of research subjects, ownership of data and copyrights, as well as concerns about future use of data [42, 44, 45, 47, 48, 51, 53, 55]. Research subjects put their trust in the research team to protect their privacy and keep their information confidential [44, 45, 48, 53, 56]. If this information is shared with a third party without prior consent, researchers worry that this could be considered a breach of trust, if not a violation of their ethical and legal obligations [45, 53]. In terms of use of data, researchers who have spent their time and funding collecting data may wish to maintain control over the use of their data in order to publish subsequent analyses once the initial study results are made public [9, 47, 51]. Considering that academic institutions take the quantity of publications into account when determining tenure, protecting one's own interests in regard to research data is understandably a concern for, if not a deterrent to, data sharing

[9, 51, 53]. There have also been concerns expressed about the quality of reanalysis of original research data and the impact on the original researchers; however, it is assumed that the peer review process would weed out any poorly performed reanalyses [9, 47].

There do seem to be legitimate concerns about sharing information in both the research and government realms, but the benefits of opening up information, and the trust that is developed as a result, provide strong motivations to address these concerns and to find ways to continue the progress of these movements.

Unplanned Uses and Disclosures by Commercial Players

There is increasing interest by data custodians to package data, de-identify them in some way, and sell them. Here are a few examples.

Some vendors are providing electronic medical records (EMRs) for free to practitioners, but then selling the data to generate revenue.* Some providers have seriously considered, are planning to, or are already selling data about their patients. This is done directly or by creating subsidiary companies responsible for the commercialization of data, for example, Partners Healthcare in Boston,† the Joint Commission on Accreditation for Healthcare Organizations,‡ the Cleveland Clinic,§ and the Geisinger Health System [57].

Competitions

The public disclosure of health data for the purposes of attracting data analysts to solve complex problems or to bring rapid advances to a field is not new. In such a case, the data are released as part of a competition whereby the best solution to an analytical or practical problem is rewarded with prestige, cash, or both. Table 7.1 summarizes four recent competitions. The public disclosure of large health data sets accessible by individuals globally raises privacy concerns, especially around the identifiability of patients. In those competitions, even if the terms of the competition restrict entrants from a re-identification attempt, the entrants are often global and the enforcement of these restrictions would be a practical challenge. Therefore a strong case must be made that the competition data have a low probability of re-identification under a broad set of plausible attacks.

---

* See these articles about EMR vendors: http://www.modernhealthcare.com/article/20071008/ FREE/310080003# and http://www.bmj.com/cgi/content/full/331/7509/128-c.
† See http://www.boston.com/business/healthcare/articles/2006/03/24/your_data_for_sale/.
‡ See http://www.allbusiness.com/health-care/health-care-facilities-hospitals/10579564-1.html.
§ See http://www.ama-assn.org/amednews/2009/11/30/biscl130.htm.

Table 7.1   Recent Examples of Public Releases of Health Data for the Purpose of Competitions

Competition Objective	Description
Predicting HIV progression [58]	Find markers in the HIV sequence that predict a change in the severity of the infection
INFORMS data mining contest [59]	Predicting hospitalization outcomes: transfer and death
Practice Fusion medical research data [60, 61]	Develop an application to manage patients' chronic disease
Heritage Health Prize [62]	Develop a model to predict patient hospitalization in a future year

References

1. Statistics Sweden. *Statistics and privacy: Future access to data for official statistics—Cooperation or distrust?* 1987.
2. Winsa P. Woman could go to jail for not filling out census. *The Star*, 2011. http://www.thestar.com/news/canada/article/921600—woman-faces-jail-time-for-refusing-to-fill-out-census. Archived at http://www.webcitation.org/5vmxl3Rek.
3. Cahill K. When Catholics were "to be removed." *Washington Post*, 2003.
4. Electronic Privacy Information Center. Department of Homeland Security obtained data on Arab Americans from the Census Bureau. 2001.
5. Department of Health and Human Services. Certificates of confidentiality kiosk. http://grants.nih.gov/grants/policy/coc/.
6. Organization for Economic Cooperation and Development. Science, technology and innovation for the 21st century. 2004.
7. Organization for Economic Cooperation and Development. Promoting access to public research data for scientific, economic, and social development: OECD follow up group on issues of access to publicly funded research data. 2003.
8. Commission regulation (EC) no 831/2002 of 17 May 2002 on implementing council regulation (EC) no 322/97 on community statistics, concerning access to confidential data for scientific purposes. *Official Journal of the European Communities*, 133, 18.5.2002, p. 7–9. 2002.
9. Kirwan J. Making original data from clinical studies available for alternative analysis. *Journal of Rheumatology*, 1997; 24(5):822–825.
10. Wager L, Krieza-Jeric K. Report of public reporting of clinical trial outcomes and results (PROCTOR) meeting. Canadian Institutes of Health Research, 2008.
11. Are journals doing enough to prevent fraudulent publication? *Canadian Medical Association Journal*, 2006; 174(4):431.
12. Vickers A. Whose data set is it anyway? Sharing raw data from randomized trials. *Trials*, 2006; 7(15).
13. Chalmers I, Altman D. How can medical journals help prevent poor medical research? Some opportunities presented by electronic publishing. *Lancet*, 1999; 353:490–493.

14. Eysenbach G, Sa E-R. Code of conduct is needed for publishing raw data. *British Medical Journal*, 2001; 323:166.
15. Delamothe T. Whose data are they anyway? *British Medical Journal*, 1996; 312: 1241–1242.
16. Hutchon D. Publishing raw data and real time statistical analysis on e-journals. *British Medical Journal*, 2001; 322(3):530.
17. Canadian Institutes of Health Research. Policy on access to research outputs. 2007. http://www.cihr-irsc.gc.ca/e/34846.html. Archived at http://www.webcitation.org/5XgxgoBzj.
18. Medical Research Council. *MRC policy on data sharing and preservation.* 2006.
19. Economic and Social Research Council. *ESRC research funding guide.* 2008.
20. *ERC Scientific Council guidelines for open access.* European Research Council, 2007.
21. National Institutes of Health. Final NIH statement on sharing research data. http://grants.nih.gov/grants/guide/notice-files/not-od-03-032.html.
22. Yolles B, Connors J, Grufferman S. Obtaining access to data from government-sponsored medical research. *New England Journal of Medicine*, 1986; 315(26):1669–1672.
23. Cecil J, Boruch R. Compelled disclosure of research data: An early warning and suggestions for psychologists. *Law and Human Behavior*, 1988; 12(2):181–189.
24. Chapman RA, Hunt M. Open government in a theoretical and practical context. In *Open government in a theoretical and practical context*, ed. RA Chapman and M Hunt, 139–147. Aldershot: Ashgate, 2006.
25. Barberis P. The morality of open government. In *Freedom of information: Local government and accountability*, ed. RA Chapman and M Hunt, 121–134. Surrey: Ashgate, 2010.
26. Adie K, Platten S. *Open government: What should we really know?* Norwich: Canterbury Press, 2003.
27. Treasury Board of Canada Secretariat. Proactive disclosure. http://www.tbs-sct.gc.ca/pd-dp/index-eng.asp (accessed December 31, 2010).
28. Davies A, Lithwick D. *Government 2.0 and access to information. 2. Recent developments in proactive disclosure and open data in the United States and other countries.* Ottawa: Parliamentary Information and Research Service, Library of Parliament.
29. Chapman RA, Hunt M. Open government and freedom of information. In *Open government in a theoretical and practical context*, ed. RA Chapman and M Hunt, 1–10. Aldershot: Ashgate, 2006.
30. Obama B. Memorandum on transparency and open government, ed. E Branch. *Federal Register*, 2009.
31. Great Britain. Treasury. *Putting the frontline first: Smarter government.* Cm. 2009. Norwich: Stationery Office, 2009.
32. Davies A, Lithwick D. *Government 2.0 and access to information. 1. Recent developments in proactive disclosure and open data in Canada.* Ottawa: Parliamentary Information and Research Service, Library of Parliament.
33. Apps4Edmonton contest. http://contest.apps4edmonton.ca/ (accessed December 31, 2010).
34. Access to Information Act. 1985.
35. Access to Information and Privacy Commissioners of Canada. Open Government: Resolution of Canada's access to Information and Privacy Commissioners. 2010. Whitehorse: Office of the Access to Information Commissioner of Canada.
36. Statistics Act. Government of Canada, 1985.

37. Statistics Canada. Data liberation initiative. http://www.statcan.gc.ca/dli-ild/dli-idd-eng.htm (accessed January 1, 2011).

38. Natural Resources Canada. Geobase. http://www.geobase.ca/ (accessed January 1, 2011).

39. Natural Resources Canada. Geogratis. http://geogratis.cgdi.gc.ca/ (accessed January 1, 2011).

40. Natural Resources Canada. GeoConnections Discovery Portal. http://geodiscover.cgdi.ca/web/guest/home (accessed January 1, 2011).

41. Boisclair T. Information commissioner issues a dire diagnosis for access to information in Canada. Ottawa: Office of the Information Commissioner, 2009.

42. Fienberg S. Sharing statistical data in the biomedical and health sciences: Ethical, institutional, legal, and professional dimensions. *Annual Review of Public Health*, 1994; 15:1–18.

43. Sztompka P. Trust in science. *Journal of Classical Sociology*, 2007; 7(2):211–220. 10.1177/1468795x07078038.

44. Fienberg S, Martin M, Straf M. Sharing research data. Committee on National Statistics, National Research Council, 1985.

45. Sieber JE. Data sharing: Defining problems and seeking solutions. *Law and Human Behavior*, 1988; 12(2):199–206.

46. Hedrick T. Justifications for the sharing of social science data. *Law and Human Behavior*, 1988; 12(2):163–171.

47. Stanley B, Stanley M. Data sharing: The primary researcher's perspective. *Law and Human Behavior*, 1988; 12(2):173–180.

48. Hrynaszkiewicz I, Altman DG. Towards agreement on best practice for publishing raw clinical trial data. *Trials*, 2009; 10:17.

49. Murray-Rust P, Neylon C, Pollock R, Wilbanks J. Panton principles. http://pantonprinciples.org/ (accessed December 20, 2010).

50. Hrynaszkiewicz I. BioMed Central's position statement on open data. http://blogs.openaccesscentral.com/blogs/bmcblog/resource/opendatastatementdraft.pdf (accessed December 20, 2010).

51. Tananbaum G. Adventures in open data. *Learned Publishing*, 2008; 21:154–156. 10.1087/095315108x254485.

52. Social Sciences and Humanities Research Council. Research data archiving policy. http://www.sshrc-crsh.gc.ca/funding-financement/policies-politiques/edata-donnees_electroniques-eng.aspx (accessed December 31, 2010).

53. Perry CM. Archiving of publicly funded research data: A survey of Canadian researchers. *Government Information Quarterly*, 2008; 25(1):133–148. 10.1016/j.giq.2007.04.008.

54. Piwowar HA, Day RS, Fridsma DB. Sharing detailed research data is associated with increased citation rate. *PLoS ONE*, 2007; 2(3):e308.

55. Murray-Rust P. Open data in science. *Serials Review*, 2008; 34(1):52–64. 10.1016/j.serrev.2008.01.001.

56. Duncan G, Jabine T, de Wolf S. *Private lives and public policies: Confidentiality and accessibility of government statistics*. Washington, DC: National Academies Press, 1993.

57. PWC Healthcare. *Transforming healthcare through secondary use of health data*. Dallas, TX: PriceWaterhouseCoopers, 2009.

58. Kaggle. Predict HIV progression. 2010. http://www.kaggle.com/c/hivprogression.

59. INFORMS. INFORMS data mining contest. 2009. http://pages.stern.nyu.edu/~cperlich/INFORMS/.

60. Practice Fusion. Disease control app for doctors wins health 2.0 data challenge; analyze this! 2010. http://www.practicefusion.com/pages/pr/disease-control-application-for-doctors-ins-health-2.0-data-challenge.html.
61. Practice Fusion. Practice Fusion medical research data. 2010. https://datamarket.azure.com/dataset/8c30d4d3-0846-4b08-9991-104958f24ca7.
62. Kaggle. Heritage Health Prize. 2011. http://www.heritagehealthprize.com/.

Chapter 8

Public Perception and Privacy Protective Behaviors

With the growing use of information technology in the provision of health care [1–8], patients and physicians are worried about unauthorized disclosure and use of PHI [9–16]. In addition, a considerable amount of PHI is also disclosed with patient consent through compelled authorizations (e.g., to obtain insurance, make an insurance claim, or seek employment) [17].

The public is uncomfortable providing personal information, or having their personal information used for secondary purposes, if they do not trust the organization collecting and using the data. For example, individuals often cite privacy and confidentiality concerns and lack of trust in researchers as reasons for not wanting their health information used for research [18]. One study found that the greatest predictor of patients' willingness to share information with researchers was the level of trust they placed in the researchers themselves [19]. A number of U.S. studies have shown that attitudes toward privacy and confidentiality of the census are predictive of people's participation [20, 21], and also that there is a positive association between belief in the confidentiality of census records and the level of trust one has in the government [22]. These trust effects are amplified when the information collected is of a sensitive nature [22, 23].

Between 15% and 17% of U.S. adults have changed their behavior to protect the privacy of their PHI, doing things such as going to another doctor, paying out-of-pocket when insured to avoid disclosure, not seeking care to avoid disclosure to an employer, giving inaccurate or incomplete information on medical history, self-treating or self-medicating rather than seeing a provider, or asking a doctor not to write down the health problem or record a less serious or embarrassing condition [9, 24, 25]. Privacy concerns have sometimes caused individuals not to be totally honest with their health care provider [13]. In a survey of physicians in the United States, nearly 87% reported that a patient had asked that information be kept out of their record, and nearly 78% of physicians said that they had withheld information from a patient's record due to privacy concerns [26].

Public opinion surveys in Canada found that, over the prior year, between 3% and 5% of Canadians withheld information from their provider because of privacy concerns, and 1% to 3% decided not to seek care for the same reasons [27]. Furthermore, between 11% and 13% of Canadians have at some point withheld information from a health care provider because of concerns over with whom the information might be shared, or how it might be used [28–30], with the highest regional percentage in Alberta at 20% [28]. Similar results have been reported by the Canadian Medical Association [31]. An estimated 735,000 Canadians decided not to see a health care provider because of concerns about the privacy of their information [32].

Specific vulnerable populations have reported similar privacy protective behaviors, such as adolescents, people with HIV or at high risk for HIV, women undergoing genetic testing, mental health patients, and battered women [33–39]. A survey of California residents found that discussing depression with their primary care physician because of privacy concerns was a barrier to 15% of the respondents [40].

Arguably, as individuals adjust their current behaviors to more privacy protective ones, this behavior change will be hard to reverse. Once trust in data custodians has been eroded, it will be difficult to regain. Studies in risk management demonstrate how trust in organizations is hard to gain but easy to lose [41]. This asymmetry of trust can be explained by several interrelated factors, including a negativity bias on the part of the public where negative information (such as news about data breaches) carries more weight and is more diagnostic than positive information [41–43], a strong aversion to loss that causes people to weigh negative information more greatly in an effort to avoid loss [42, 43], and the perception that sources of negative information are more credible and less self-serving than sources of positive information [41, 43]. Furthermore, people have a tendency toward avoiding the negative, and consequently often avoid organizations or people that are deemed untrustworthy. This avoidance helps to sustain distrust by eliminating opportunities to witness events or gather information that would counter currently held beliefs and increase trust in the individual or organization [41]. People also tend to interpret events and information in accordance with their current beliefs, a confirmatory bias, which causes us to be more likely to accept negative information about people or organizations we distrust and to reject positive information [44, 45]. This bias also contributes to the self-perpetuating nature of distrust. On the other hand, it has been observed that those who have a high level of trust in a person or organization can feel a deeper sense of betrayal once this trust is breached [46]. Due to the fact that a breach would be contrary to their strongly held trust beliefs, such an event would cause great stress and anxiety, exacerbating their sense of betrayal and leading to greater distrust in the end [46].

One of the factors that can help to make the public more comfortable with their health information being used for research purposes is its de-identification at the earliest opportunity [18, 47–53]. As many as 86% of respondents in one study were comfortable with the creation and use of a health database of de-identified information for research purposes, whereas only 35% were comfortable with such a database that included identifiable information [51].

References

1. Irving R. 2002 *Report on information technology in Canadian hospitals.* Thornhill: Canadian Healthcare Technology, 2003.
2. HIMSS. *Healthcare CIO results.* Healthcare Information and Management Systems Society Foundation, 2004.
3. Andrews J, Pearce K, Sydney C, Ireson C, Love M. Current state of information technology use in a US primary care practice-based research network. *Informatics in Primary Care,* 2004; 12:11–18. PMID: 15140348.
4. Bower A. *The diffusion and value of healthcare information technology.* Santa Monica, CA: RAND Health, 2005.
5. Fonkych K, Taylor R. *The state and pattern of health information technology adoption.* Santa Monica, CA: RAND Health, 2005.
6. Jha A, Ferris T, Donelan K, DesRoches C, Shields A, Rosenbaum S, Blumenthal D. How common are electronic health records in the United States? A summary of the evidence. *Health Affairs,* 2006; 25(6):w496–w507.
7. Shields A, Shin P, Leu M, Levy D, Betancourt R-M, Hawkins D, Proser M. Adoption of health information technology in community health centers: Results of a national survey. *Health Affairs,* 2007; 26(5):1373–1383.
8. Gans D, Kralewski J, Hammons T, Dowd B. Medical groups' adoption of electronic health records and information systems. *Health Affairs,* 2005; 24(5):1323–1333.
9. California Health Care Foundation. Medical privacy and confidentiality survey. 1999. http://www.chcf.org/publications/1999/01/medical-privacy-and-confidentiality-survey. Archived at http://www.webcitation.org/5Q2YtO8yH.
10. HarrisInterractive. Health information privacy (HIPAA) notices have improved public's confidence that their medical information is being handled properly. 2005. http://www.harrisinteractive.com/news/allnewsbydate.asp?NewsID=894. Archived at http://www.webcitation.org/5Q2YQkeWM.
11. Grimes-Gruczka T, Gratzer C, the Institute for the Future. Ethics survey of consumer attitudes about health web sites. 2000. California Health Care Foundation.
12. Willison D, Kashavjee K, Nair K, Goldsmith C, Holbrook A. Patients' consent preferences for research uses of information in electronic medical records: Interview and survey data. *British Medical Journal,* 2003; 326:373.

13. Mitchell E, Sullivan F. A descriptive feast but an evaluative famine: Systematic review of published articles on primary care computing during 1980–97. *British Medical Journal*, 2001; 322:279–282.

14. Medix UK plc survey of doctors' views about the National Programme for IT (NPfIT). Medix UK, 2006.

15. 8th Medix Survey re the NHS National Programme for IT (NPfIT). Medix UK, 2007.

16. BMA News press release: Doctors have no confidence in NHS database, says BMA News poll. BMA, 2008. http://www.bma.org.uk/pressrel.nsf/wlu/SGOY-7BELTV? OpenDocument&vw=wfmms. Archived at http://www.webcitation.org/5VOJUSTaJ.

17. Rothstein M, Talbott M. Compelled authorizations for disclosure of health records: Magnitude and implications. *American Journal of Bioethics*, 2007; 7(3):38–45.

18. Nass S, Levit L, Gostin L, eds. *Beyond the HIPAA Privacy Rule: Enhancing privacy, improving health through research*. Washington, DC: National Academies Press, 2009.

19. Damschroder L, Pritts J, Neblo M, Kalarickal R, Creswell J, Hayward R. Patients, privacy and trust: Patients' willingness to allow researchers to access their medical records. *Social Science and Medicine*, 2007; 64:223–235.

20. Mayer TS. *Privacy and confidentiality research and the US Census Bureau: Recommendations based on a review of the literature*. Washington, DC: U.S. Bureau of the Census, 2002.

21. Singer E, van Hoewyk J, Neugebauer RJ. Attitudes and behaviour: The impact of privacy and confidentiality concerns on participation in the 2000 census. *Public Opinion Quarterly*, 2003; 67:368–384.

22. National Research Council. *Privacy and confidentiality as factors in survey response*. Washington, DC: National Academy of Sciences: 1979.

23. Martin E. *Privacy concerns and the census long form: Some evidence from census 2000*. Washington, DC: Annual Meeting of the American Statistical Association, 2001.

24. HarrisInteractive. Many US adults are satisfied with use of their personal health information. 2007. http://www.harrisinteractive.com/harris_poll/index.asp?PID=743.

25. Lee J, Buckley C. For privacy's sake, taking risks to end pregnancy. *New York Times*, 2009. http://www.nytimes.com/2009/01/05/nyregion/05abortion.html?_r=1.

26. Association of American Physicians and Surgeons. New poll: Doctors lie to protect patient privacy. 2001. http://www.aapsonline.org/press/nrnewpoll.htm. Archived at http://www.webcitation.org/5NzvR0MX2.

27. EKOS Research Associates. *Wave 2 graphical summary report: Part of the information highway study*. 2007.

28. Canadian Medical Association, Angus Reid Group, Inc. *Canadians' perceptions on the privacy of their health information*. 1998.

29. Canadian Medical Association, Angus Reid Group, Inc. *Canadians' perceptions of health information confidentiality*. 1999.

30. *Rethinking the information highway*. EKOS, 2003.

31. Day B. Why are doctors so concerned about protecting the confidentiality of patients records? *Healthcare: Information Management and Communications Canada*, 2008; 22(2):36–37.

32. Saravamuttoo M. Privacy: Changing attitudes in a tumultuous time. Sixth Annual Privacy and Security Workshop, Toronto, 2005.

33. Sankar P, Moran S, Merz J, Jones N. Patient perspectives on medical confidentiality: A review of the literature. *Journal of General Internal Medicine*, 2003; 18:659–669.

34. Britto MT, Tivorsak TL, Slap GB. Adolescents' needs for health care privacy. *Pediatrics*, 2010; 126(6):e1469–1476.

35. Thrall JS, McCloskey L, Ettner SL, Rothman E, Tighe JE, Emans SJ. Confidentiality and adolescents' use of providers for health information and for pelvic examinations. *Archives of Pediatrics and Adolescent Medicine*, 2000; 154(9):885–92.

36. Reddy DM, Fleming R, Swain C. Effect of mandatory parental notification on adolescent girls' use of sexual health care services. *Journal of the American Medical Association*, 2002; 288(6):710–714. joc11794 [pii].

37. Lothen-Kline C, Howard DE, Hamburger EK, Worrell KD, Boekeloo BO. Truth and consequences: Ethics, confidentiality, and disclosure in adolescent longitudinal prevention research. *Journal of Adolescent Health*, 2003; 33(5):385–394.

38. Ginsburg KR, Menapace AS, Slap GB. Factors affecting the decision to seek health care: The voice of adolescents. *Pediatrics*, 1997; 100(6):922–930.

39. Cheng T, Savageau J, Sattler J, DeWitt A, Thomas G. Confidentiality in health care: A survey of knowledge, perceptions, and attitudes among high school students. *Journal of the American Medical Association*, 1993; 269(11):1404–1408.

40. Bell RA, Franks P, Duberstein PR, Epstein RM, Feldman MD, Garcia EF, Kravitz RL. Suffering in silence: Reasons for not disclosing depression in primary care. *Annals of Family Medicine*, 2011; 9(5):439–446.

41. Slovic P. Perceived risk, trust, and democracy. *Risk Analysis*, 1993; 13(6):675–682.

42. Baumeister RF, Bratslavsky E, Finkenauner C, Vohs KD. Bad is stronger than good. *Review of General Psychology*, 2001; 5(4):323–370.

43. Siegrist M, Cvetkovich G. Better negative than positive? Evidence of bias for negative information about possible health dangers. *Risk Analysis*, 2001; 21(1):199–206.

44. White MP, Pahl S, Buehner M, Haye A. Trust in risky messages: The role of prior attitudes. *Risk Analysis*, 2003; 23(4):717–726.

45. Poortinga W, Pidgeon NF. Trust, the asymmetry principle, and the role of prior beliefs. *Risk Analysis*, 2004; 24(6):1475–1485.

46. Robinson SL, Dirks KT, Ozcelik H. Untangling the knot of trust and betrayal. In *Trust and distrust in organizations: Dilemmas and approaches*, ed. RM Kramer and KS Cook, 327–341. New York: Russell Sage Foundation, 2004.

47. Pullman D. Sorry, you can't have that information: Stakeholder awareness, perceptions and concerns regarding the disclosure and use of personal health information. *e-Health 2006*, 2006.

48. *OIPC stakeholder survey, 2003: Highlights report*. GPC Research, 2003.

49. Willison D, Schwartz L, Abelson J, Charles C, Swinton M, Northrup D, Thabane L. Alternatives to project-specific consent for access to personal information for health research: What is the opinion of the Canadian public? *Journal of the American Medical Informatics Association*, 2007; 14:706–712.

50. Nair K, Willison D, Holbrook A, Keshavjee K. Patients' consent preferences regarding the use of their health information for research purposes: A qualitative study. *Journal of Health Services Research and Policy*, 2004; 9(1):22–27.

51. Kass N, Natowicz M, Hull S, et al. The use of medical records in research: What do patients want? *Journal of Law, Medicine and Ethics*, 2003; 31:429–433.

52. Whiddett R, Hunter I, Engelbrecht J, Handy J. Patients' attitudes towards sharing their health information. *International Journal of Medical Informatics*, 2006; 75:530–541.

53. Pritts J. The importance and value of protecting the privacy of health information: Roles of HIPAA Privacy Rule and the common rule in health research. 2008. http://iom.edu/Object.File/Master/53/160/Pritts%20Privacy%20Final%20Draft%20web.pdf (accessed July 15, 2009).

Chapter 9

Alternative Methods for Data Access

There are five alternative methods to de-identification that can provide access to health information that are in common use today or are expected to increase in use in the near future. These are (1) remote access to data, (2) on-site access to data, (3) remote execution, (4) remote query, and (5) secure computation. They have a number of advantages and disadvantages compared to de-identification, which will be summarized below. On balance, we argue that in practice de-identification remains an attractive method in many situations compared to the alternatives.

Remote Access

With remote access, the data custodian provides the data analysts electronic access to the data through a secure communications channel. The data custodian may assign or sub-contract the task to a trusted third party who would manage the data holdings and provide the remote access to analysts.

Under this setting, the analysts would not be able to download any data. Even though in principle the analyst would not be able to directly print any of those data, it is always easy to "print screen" and then page through data files to print a large data set. In principle, this "read only" access model allows the data recipient to perform the analysis.

The primary advantage of this method is that there is no loss in the precision of the data, as would be the case with de-identification. Since the analyst works on the original data or a data set that still has a high probability of re-identification, there would be no loss in data utility that often accompanies de-identification.

There are variants of the remote access model. In one approach remote access is provided from certain trusted locations only. For example, a data custodian may only allow remote access to the raw data from a certain machine at the local university [1]. Any data user who wishes to access the data must physically go to the local university. Another approach is to allow remote access to anyone who has an account irrespective of where he or she may be located.

A key disadvantage of the remote access mechanism is that if the credentials of data users are compromised, then the adversary would be able to access the data as well. It is not difficult to compromise user account credentials using social engineering techniques. Many social engineering techniques exist [2–4], and have been used to obtain very personal information from individuals and organizations (as well as to commit more dramatic crimes, such as bank robberies) [5, 6]. A recent review of data breaches indicated that 12% of data breach incidents involved deceit and social engineering techniques [7]. It has been argued that the main threat to medical privacy is social engineering, and such techniques have been used by private investigators to surreptitiously obtain health information [8, 9].

The data custodian can impose more stringent credential checking to access the data. For example, users may need to answer a secret question or enter a temporary time-limited password. These additional steps will increase the inconvenience of remote access, but reduce the security risks.

Another consideration is that making the databases containing the identifiable health information available on the Internet does, in principle, expose the database to attacks. Adversaries may be able to find weaknesses in the network defenses and penetrate them to access the database. There are many ways that such attacks can occur, and it is difficult to provide guarantees that such attacks are not possible.

By constraining the remote access to be from certain locations or by using the on-site access model, a visual check of an individual's identity through his or her physical presence greatly reduces the risks. This, however, limits access to only those data users who can travel to the designated locations. In practice, an analysis of a data set requires many days or even months of effort, and therefore proximity to the location where the analysis will be performed is important. This disadvantage can be mitigated by hiring local analysts who perform the analysis from the designated locations (through remote access or on-site) on behalf of the data user.

Remote access methods assume that the data user or analyst can be completely trusted. Since the data have a high probability of re-identification, an unscrupulous data user would have direct access to personal health information. To justify that trust, such individuals would normally go through some form of background screening (e.g., a criminal background check). This additional process step increases the barriers to data access, and can also delay data access.

Even if the data users are deemed trustworthy, an inadvertent disclosure could occur if the user notices a record of someone that he or she knows. Such disclosures are often referred to as spontaneous recognition [10], and need to be protected against. The data user would not need to exert any effort or have any special skills or resources for such an inadvertent disclosure to occur.

Perhaps the biggest challenge with remote access is the cost of setting up the infrastructure and sustaining it over time. Creating a highly secure environment that is continuously monitored is not cheap and requires significant up-front investment.

On-Site Access

With on-site access the data recipient has to physically go to the data custodian site and access the data from there [11]. The data user would then access the raw data and analyze it locally. While on-site the data user would not be able to take any printouts off-site, and any data transfers off-site would have to be screened to ensure that no identifiable information is included in that transfer (for example, if the data user wishes to take the results of the analysis off-site). This methods also addresses risks from providing data over the Internet.

On-site access has mostly the same advantages and disadvantages as remote access. However, it is even more costly to set up than remote access because a physical space needs to be created for data users and continuously monitored.

Remote Execution

Another solution is remote execution [11]. Using this method, data users, by using metadata of data sets, prepare Statistical Analysis Software (SAS) or Statistical Package for the Social Sciences (SPSS) scripts and send them to the data custodian. Then, the data custodian will check every received script to ensure that any possible inference of personal information from the final results is not possible alone or in combination with the previous results sent to researchers.

Then he or she executes the safe scripts and sends back the results to the researchers. This method has some advantages for the data users: They do not need to physically be at the data center, and they can send their queries whenever they want. However, this can be more time-consuming for the data user because he or she is not directly running the analysis, and is not able to correct any possible errors in the request immediately. The data custodian would have to return a description of errors and outputs to the data user for modification, and several such attempts may have to be made before the problem is corrected. The data custodian will likely disallow certain SAS or SPSS commands because these would generate logs or results that disclose individual level information. This means that the set of analytical tools would be limited. Also, the response time could be long because of program checking by the data custodian. Finally, this method is very time-consuming for the data custodian, who has to check every program and its result.

A potential shortcut is to provide the data user with synthetic data that have similar characteristics to the real data. The data user would then prepare the analysis programs and test them on the synthetic data. Once the data user is content that the scripts are working, they would be sent in for remote execution. The challenge in this case is to create a synthetic data set that has a covariance and distributional structure similar to the original data.

Instead of synthetic data, the data custodian may create a public use file that is based on the real data. A public use file is one that has been de-identified using the techniques described in this book. The data user can then create his or her analysis programs on that. The public use file would be based on the original data, and therefore would have a similar structure as the original data.

A more fundamental risk with remote execution is that it can leak personal information. One concern is that a remotely constructed model on the original data that fits data very well can lead to accurate, possibly even perfect, predictions (which could be used to match to an external data set). Assume, for example, a model with a sensitive outcome, such as the presence of a rare or stigmatized disease (e.g., alcoholism). The parameter estimates could be used with known covariate values to predict outcomes. For observations with the same combination of covariate values (which is common with categorical data) and the same outcomes, the predictions on that same combination of values will be exact [12, 13]. Very small standard errors could also be used to directly or indirectly identify a sensitive population, potentially revealing information about them.

Often one will build several models before deciding which provides the best fit for the purposes of explaining or predicting outcomes. For example, interactions may be included but then found not to be practically or statistically significant, and therefore dropped. The process of fitting multiple models can in itself lead to disclosures. This is a common subject of consideration in the study of remote analysis methods [12–15].

Remote Queries

Remote queries are similar to remote execution except that the data user only executes database queries and gets the tabular results. They can be run against a single remote database or multiple databases (i.e., in a distributed fashion). In a distributed query architecture each site executes the query and sends the results back to the central user [16–19]. Such networks retain the data at the sites and only send summary information back to the central user in response to specific queries.

It has been well established for some time that it is possible to leak sensitive information by running multiple overlapping queries on a database—this is known as the problem of inference from statistical databases [20]. The ability to extract

Table 9.1 Example Table to Illustrate Tracker Queries

	Name	Age	Gender	Postal Code	Language	Diagnosis Code
1	N1	72	F	K1K	En	305
2	N2	63	F	K1N	En	294
3	N3	58	M	K1K	Fr	153
4	N4	56	F	K2K	En	231
5	N5	51	M	K1P	Fr	294
6	N6	48	M	K1R	It	282
7	N7	39	M	K2K	Fr	745
8	N8	38	F	K1P	En	523
9	N9	31	F	K1M	En	310
10	N10	29	M	K1K	En	312
11	N11	29	F	K1L	En	300
12	N12	23	M	K1J	It	482

sensitive information when multiple tables are available about the same population has been demonstrated on student data released by educational departments in the United States [21] and on the re-identification of federal capital cases by combining information from multiple tables released by the Department of Justice [22].

The major problem in inference from statistical databases comes from queries that return a subset of data [23, 24]. The two main inference attacks are queries with very small or very large outputs, and query overlapping (inference chaining) [25, 26]. An attribute in a statistical database could be compromised exactly or partially. If there is no restriction on the user's queries, the exact value of a specific attribute could be deduced, especially if the user has some initial knowledge of the contents in the underlying table. Consider Table 9.1. Suppose that an adversary already knows that N11 is one of the patients in this data set. An adversary can run the following query:

```
SELECT COUNT(*)
FROM Diagnosis
WHERE Name = 'N11' AND DiagnosisCode BETWEEN 290 AND 319
```

This query would return a result set of size one, revealing the patient's diagnosis. If the adversary does not know the patient's name but the postal code instead, then the following query will return the diagnosis:

```
SELECT COUNT(*)
FROM Diagnosis
WHERE PostalCode = 'K1L' AND DiagnosisCode BETWEEN 290 AND 319
```

These types of queries can be prevented by setting a restriction on the size of the result returned by the query. However, there are some inference methods, such as tracker queries [25], which are able to bypass this restriction by sending some related and overlapping queries and combining the results to infer some individual data. Different types of trackers, general, double, and union, have been discussed with examples in articles to show how a query can be applied even if the eligible queries are those with half of the whole data records as the result. More importantly, the examples show that sometimes the number of queries needed for trackers could be small.

Attempts to protect against such inferences by restricting the size of the query result (query set) would not be effective. Query set size control will block any query that produces a query set larger than some threshold, say k records. It also blocks any query set with $N - k$ records, where N is the total number of records in the table. This is because the complement of the query will have less than k records, which violates the inference control limit. Now, suppose instead of the complement of a query with the query set of k records, we create a query that is the complement of another query, or more than one query, which in this case is not prohibited.

Even with restrictions on the result set size, the adversary can run the following two queries:

```
SELECT COUNT (*)
FROM Diagnosis
WHERE Gender = 'F' AND Language = 'En' AND DiagnosisCode
BETWEEN 290 AND 319
```

and

```
SELECT COUNT (*)
FROM Diagnosis
WHERE Name < > 'N11' AND
Gender = 'F' AND Language = 'En' AND DiagnosisCode BETWEEN 290
AND 319
```

If we assume that $k = 2$, both of the above queries have query sets with more than k and $N - k$ records, and therefore would not be blocked. However, by subtracting the results of the above two queries, the adversary will obtain the singleton query set equal to the result of the prohibited query, and can figure out the range of N11's diagnosis code. This and other examples will lead us to set another, stricter condition on the query set size. For instance, the allowable size for a query set has to be between $2k$ and $N - 2k$. However, consider the following two queries, which are both allowed because of the size of the query sets, nine and eight records, respectively:

```
SELECT COUNT (*)
FROM Diagnosis
WHERE Gender = 'M' OR Language = 'Fr' OR DiagnosisCode BETWEEN
290 AND 319
```

and

```
SELECT COUNT (*)
FROM Diagnosis
WHERE Gender < > 'M' AND Language < > 'Fr' OR DiagnosisCode
BETWEEN 290 AND 319
```

The adversary can pad a condition to each of the above queries as follows:

```
SELECT COUNT (*)
FROM Diagnosis
WHERE (Name < > 'N11' AND DiagnosisCode
BETWEEN 290 AND 319)
OR (Gender = 'M' OR Language = 'Fr')
```

and

```
SELECT COUNT (*)
FROM Diagnosis
WHERE (Name < > 'N11' AND DiagnosisCode
BETWEEN 290 AND 319)
OR (Gender < > 'M' AND Language < > 'Fr')
```

The first query set has nine records and the second one has seven. Now by adding up these two and subtracting from the total of the previous two queries, N11's diagnosis code will be confirmed.

Queries that reveal information are not limited to 'count' queries. Suppose we also know that N11's age is 72, then we can construct the following 'max' query:

```
SELECT MAX (Age)
FROM Diagnosis
WHERE DiagnosisCode BETWEEN 290 AND 319
```

By returning 72, the adversary can conclude that N11's diagnosis code is in a specific range. Similar conclusions are possible using 'min' queries. Also, 'sum' queries can be used. As a simple example, suppose S is a sensitive numeric field and we want to have the result from the following query:

```
SELECT SUM(S)
FROM Diagnosis
WHERE Name = 'N11'
```

This query has the query set size problem and is not allowed to be replied to. However, the following two eligible queries could be applied to get the sensitive value:

```
SELECT SUM(S)
FROM Diagnosis
WHERE Name<>'N11' and Language = 'En'
```

and

```
SELECT SUM(S)
FROM Diagnosis
WHERE Language = 'En'
```

By subtracting the results from the two above queries, the value of S for N11 will be disclosed.

These examples illustrate the ineffectiveness of the inference control using query set size. The experimental results show that an adversary who has some prior information about the distribution of attribute values in the underlying data sets is able to find a general tracker with as few as one or two queries.

Alternatives to query set size restrictions have been proposed, but these require the perturbation of the data [27, 28]. Such perturbative techniques will reduce the accuracy of analyses based on the data. More importantly, we are not aware of many real-world uses of perturbation on health data and its empirical impact on health data utility.

Secure Computation

Secure computation has only been recently applied in practical health care contexts [29, 30]. The basic concept is that encrypted data are shared and computations are performed on the encrypted data. Specialized cryptosystems, such as the Paillier cryptosystem [31], are used in those circumstances.

Secure computation is suitable when the analysis is known in advance. This would be the case in public health surveillance contexts where specific models or tests are performed on incoming data feeds or registries on a regular basis. Keeping the analysis open presents practical challenges in that it is possible to leak personal information from the results of the analysis (as in remote execution and remote queries).

Summary

Therefore, in summary, these alternative approaches have some important weaknesses that need to be considered when making the decision on how to provide

Table 9.2 Summary of Advantages and Disadvantages of Alternative Data Access Methods

Method	Advantages	Disadvantages
Remote access	No loss in data utility	Infrastructure setup and maintenance can be costly
		Databases with PHI are exposed on the Internet
		Screening of users is generally required
		Risk of spontaneous recognition of patients
		Risk of credential theft
On-site access	No loss in data utility	Infrastructure setup and maintenance can be costly
		Screening of users is generally required
		Risk of spontaneous recognition of patients
		Risk of credential theft
Remote execution	No loss in data utility	Costly, labor-intensive, and has long turnaround times
Remote queries	No loss in data utility	These are not secure and can leak personal information
Secure computation	No loss in data utility	Requires knowledge of analytics in advance

access to health data. These are summarized in Table 9.2. By examining these, it would be challenging not to prefer de-identification on balance. The primary caveat is to ensure that de-identification methods maximize data utility.

References

1. El Emam K. *Practices for the review of data requests and the disclosure of health information by health ministries and large data custodians.* Health Information Privacy Group, Canada Health Infoway, 2010. http://www.ehealthinformation.ca/documents/Practices_for_the_review_of_data_requests_June_2010_EN_FINAL.pdf.
2. Dolan A. *Social engineering.* SANS Institute, 2004.
3. National Infrastructure Security Coordination Center. *Social engineering against information systems: What is it and how do you protect yourself?* 2006.

4. Winkler I, Dealy B. Information security technology? Don't rely on it: A case study in social engineering. Proceedings of the Fifth USENIX UNIX Security Symposium, 1995.

5. Mitnick K, Simon W. *The art of deception: Controlling the human element of security*. Indianapolis, IN: Wiley, 2002.

6. Long J. *No tech hacking: A guide to social engineering, dumpster diving, and shoulder surfing*. Burlington, MA: Syngress Publishing, 2008.

7. Verizon Business Risk Team. *2009 data breach investigations report*. 2009.

8. Anderson R. *Security engineering: A guide to building dependable distributed systems*. Indianapolis, IN: Wiley, 2008.

9. Anderson R. Clinical system security: Interim guidelines. *British Medical Journal*, 1996; 312(7023):109–111.

10. Willenborg L, de Waal T. *Elements of statistical disclosure control*. New York: Springer-Verlag, 2001.

11. Hundepool A. *Handbook on statistical disclosure control*. The Hague: Netherlands: ESSNet SDC, 2010.

12. Reiter J. New approaches to data dissemination: A glimpse into the future. *Chance*, 2004; 17(3):12–16.

13. Reiter J, Kohnen C. Categorical data regression diagnostics for remote access servers. *Journal of Statistical Computation and Simulation*, 2005; 75(11):889–903.

14. Sparks R, Carter C, Donnelly J, O'Keefe C, Duncan J, Keighley T, McAullay D. Remote access methods for exploratory data analysis and statistical modelling: Privacy-preserving analytics. *Computer Methods and Programs in Biomedicine*, 2008; 91(3):208–222.

15. O'Keefe C, Good N. Regression output from a remote server. *Data and Knowledge Engineering*, 2009; 68(11):1175–1186.

16. Brown J, Holmes J, Shah K, Hall K, Lazarus R, Platt R. Distributed health networks: A practical and preferred approach to multi-institutional evaluations of comparative effectiveness, safety, and quality of care. *Medical Care* 2010; 48(6 Suppl. 1):S45–S51.

17. Behrman R, Benner J, Brown J, McClellan M, Woodcock J, Platt R. Developing the sentinel system—A national resource for evidence development. *New England Journal of Medicine*, 2011; 364(6):498–499.

18. Platt R, Wilson M, Chan K, Benner J, Marchibroda J, McClellan M. The new sentinel network—Improving the evidence of medical-product safety. *New England Journal of Medicine*, 2009; 361(7):645–647.

19. Platt R, Davis R, Finkelstein J, Go A, Gurwitz J, Roblin D, Soumerai S, Ross-Degnan D, Andrade S, Goodman M, Martinson B, Raebel M, Smith D, Ulcickas-Yood M, Chan K. Multicenter epidemiologic and health services research on therapeutics in the HMO Research Network Center for Education and Research on Therapeutics. *Pharmacoepidemiology and Drug Safety*, 2001; 10(5):373–377.

20. Adam N, Wortman J. Security-control methods for statistical databases: A comparative study. *ACM Computing Surveys*, 1989; 21(4):515–556.

21. Muralidhar K, Sarathy R. *Privacy violations in accountability data released to the public by state educational agencies*. Federal Committee on Statistical Methodology Research Conference, 2009.

22. Algranati D, Kadane J. Extracting confidential information from public documents: The 2000 Department of Justice report on the federal use of the death penalty in the United States. *Journal of Official Statistics*, 2004; 20(1):97–113.

23. Chin F. Security problems on inference control for SUM, MAX, and MIN queries. *Journal of the ACM*, 1986; 33(3):451–464.
24. Chin FY, Gzsoyo LG. Auditing and inference control in statistical databases. *IEEE Transactions on Software Engineering*, 1982; 8(6):574–582.
25. Denning DE, Denning PJ, Schwartz MD. The tracker: A threat to statistical database security. *ACM Transactions on Database Systems (TODS)*, 1979; 4(1):76–96.
26. Domingo-Ferrer J. Inference control in statistical databases: From theory to practice. *Lecture Notes in Computer Science*, 2002; 2316.
27. Schatz JM. Survey of techniques for securing statistical databases. University of California at Davis, 1998.
28. Gopal R, Garfinkel R, Goes P. Confidentiality via camouflage: The CVC approach to disclosure limitation when answering queries to databases. *Operational Research*, 2002; 50(3):501–516.
29. El Emam K, Hu J, Mercer J, Peyton L, Kantarcioglu M, Malin B, Buckeridge D, Samet S, Earle C. A secure protocol for protecting the identity of providers when disclosing data for disease surveillance. *Journal of the American Medical Informatics Association*, 2011; 18:212–217.
30. El Emam K, Samet S, Hu J, Peyton L, Earle C, Jayaraman G, Wong T, Kantarcioglu M, Dankar F, Essex A. A protocol for the secure linking of registries for HPV surveillance. *PLoS ONE*, 2012.
31. Paillier P. Public-key cryptosystems based on composite degree residuosity classes. In *International Conference on the Theory and Application of Cryptographic Techniques (EUROCRYPT)*, Prague, Czech Republic, 1999, pp. 223–238.

UNDERSTANDING DISCLOSURE RISKS

Chapter 10

Scope, Terminology, and Definitions

The scope of this book is limited to the de-identification of structured data. Therefore we do not consider free-form text as a type of data, nor do we consider images and video. We refer to data using multiple terms, just to avoid being repetitious and dense. Therefore terms like *data set*, *database*, and *file* will mean the same thing.

Perspective on De-Identification

The perspective we take here is that of the data custodian. Therefore the measurement of the probability of re-identification and the assessment of re-identification risks will be framed from what a data custodian is expected to know and do. The reasoning for this is that it is the data custodian who needs to make the decisions about de-identification. Any discussion of metrics and methods that does not take account of the data custodian's perspective would not be very useful in practice.

Original Data and DFs

We denote the original data set that is being prepared for disclosure as the "original data set." When the original data set is transformed into a de-identified data set it becomes a de-identified file (DF). The DF may be a sample of the records in the original data set, or it may include all of the records in the original data set.

Furthermore, the DF may contain all of the variables in the original data set or only a subset of the variables.

It is not our intention to create new terminology, but we needed a short acronym to refer to all of the types of data that can be used or disclosed to avoid having long and repetitive sentences. Therefore a DF will be a generic type of data file that is being used or disclosed.

No assumptions are made about the kind of data that are being represented in the original data set. These can be data that have been collected previously for a different purpose, and the creation of a DF is a secondary purpose. Alternatively, there may be a prospective data collection of this original data set, with the explicit intention of making it a DF at some later point.

In practice, more than one DF may be created from a single original data set. Therefore we may sometimes talk about the DFs (plural) that have been disclosed. When we refer to a single DF, that does not exclude the possibility that there may be multiple DFs.

During the process of creating a DF, intermediate DFs will be created and evaluated. When it is important to make the distinction, we refer to these as "candidate DFs" to distinguish them from the final DFs that are actually used or disclosed.

Unit of Analysis

An original data set may be at many units of analysis, such as individuals, businesses, or countries. In this book we limit ourselves to individual-level data.

The data set is assumed to have multiple "rows" or "records" and a set of "attributes" or "variables" as columns. The unit of analysis when evaluating the identifiability of individuals will depend on the type of data.

The original data set is assumed to be about individuals. The records in the data set, however, may pertain to individuals or other units of analysis. Other units of analysis can be events related to individuals, for example, patient visits or claims.

If the unit of analysis is an individual, we sometimes use the term *data subject*. Because the individuals may be healthy members of the public (e.g., if the data set is about controls in a clinical research study) or health care providers (e.g., if the data set pertains to their insurance or performance), we will refrain from using the term *patient* exclusively to refer to these individuals.

Types of Data

There are a number of ways to characterize the data. The methods used for evaluating the probability of re-identification, as well as the methods for de-identification, will depend on the characterization of the data. We can characterize the data by the number of levels and the type of data.

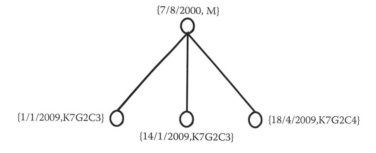

{7/8/2000, M}

{1/1/2009,K7G2C3}   {14/1/2009,K7G2C3}   {18/4/2009,K7G2C4}

Figure 10.1   An example of a two-level data set.

For multilevel data, level 1 of a data set characterizes intrinsic characteristics of individuals, such as individual date of birth and gender. Level 2 of a data set would characterize an event that occurs multiple times to that individual. An example of a two-level data set for a patient is shown in Figure 10.1. Level 1 consists of the patient's date of birth and gender. Level 2 contains information about that patient's visits, with the date of the visit and the residence postal code of that patient at that date. This two-level representation is for a longitudinal data set characterizing patient visits.

Another example of a two-level data set would be a birth registry. The level 1 component would characterize the mother's information, and level 2 would be the infant information. There would be multiple nodes at level 2 if there were multiple births (e.g., twins or babies at different points in time).

A three-level data set example from Figure 10.1 would be diagnosis codes: Each patient would have multiple diagnosis codes during each visit. The patient may also have multiple drug prescriptions and multiple procedures at level 3.

A one-level data set is essentially a cross-sectional data set. For example, a data set with age, gender, race, language spoken at home, as well as some sensitive financial or health information would be a single-level data set. Our primary focus in this book will be on one-level data.

There are five different types of data that can make up the original data set, as discussed in the sections below.

Relational Data

This is the most common type of data and consists of a fixed number of variables (fields or columns) and a fixed number of rows. All records have the same number of fields. Each record pertains to a single individual, and an individual would appear only once in the original data set. For example, clinical data in a disease or population registry would typically look like that, with a fixed number of fields collected from each individual. An example of a relational data set is illustrated in Table 10.1.

Table 10.1 Example of a Relational Data Set (based on example in [1])

PID	Race	Date of Birth	Sex	ZIP	Marital Status	Disease
1	Asian	64/04/12	F	94142	Divorced	Hypertension
2	Asian	64/09/13	F	94141	Divorced	Obesity
3	Asian	64/04/15	F	94139	Married	Diabetes
4	Asian	63/03/13	M	94139	Married	Obesity
5	Asian	63/03/18	M	94139	Married	Diabetes
6	Black	64/09/27	F	94138	Single	Depression
7	Black	64/09/27	F	94139	Single	Obesity
8	White	64/09/27	F	94139	Single	Diabetes
9	White	64/09/27	F	94141	Widow	Depression

Relational data are almost always level 1 data. Sometimes a two-level data set can be flattened into a single-level relational data set. In such cases an individual may appear more than once. For example, if a mother has twins, then there may be two records in a birth registry with information about that mother. Note that this is still cross-sectional data, but a record can appear multiple times. In that case the record pertains to the birth event rather than to the individual. An event can occur only once in the original data set.

Transactional Data

This kind of data has a variable number of columns. For example, purchases from a store would consist of a set of items that were purchased. Different individuals may have a different number of transactions and items in each transaction.

Items may be simple, consisting of a single attribute. For example, the transactions may be the names of the purchased products. Table 10.2 shows a transaction data set of a hospital in which each transaction consists of a set of diagnoses corresponding to a patient. In a binary representation of transactional data, the data set would have a fixed number of columns, and each item is a binary attribute, and for each transaction the attribute gets a value of 1 if the transaction contains that item. Otherwise, it gets a value of 0.

The attributes can also be discrete or continuous, for instance, the number of each item purchased or the price of each item. Each item may be a composite of fields as well; for example, it could be the item name, its price, and quantity bought.

Transactional data are often at level 2 or level 3 in a multilevel data set. In such a case the transactional data have some fixed fields that all of the records have values

Table 10.2 Example of a Transactional Data Set

PID	Diagnosis Codes
1	a, c, f, h
2	b, c, h, j, k
3	a, b, f, k
4	c, d, g, i, j
5	b, g, h, i
6	a, b, c, f, g, h

for. For example, if a record pertains to an individual consumer, then the first few fields in the record would be for the consumer's age, gender, and postal code (level 1), followed by a series of purchased items (level 2).

It is possible to have quite complex transactional data, with level 1 being the individual information, level 2 the visits to the store, and level 3 the items that were purchased. Also note that in transactional data no assumption is made about the order of the transactions (e.g., time or location order): It is just a set of unordered items.

Sequential Data

Sequential data often look like transactional data, but there is an order to the items in each record. For example, data sets that contain time stamps or visit dates would be considered sequential data because certain items appear before others. Web server log data can be considered sequential data. Examples of sequential data are provided in Tables 10.3 and 10.4.

Table 10.3 Time Stamps Assigned to Transactions

Time	Customer	Items purchased
t1	C1	A, B
t2	C3	A, C
t2	C1	C, D
t3	C2	A, D
t4	C2	E
t5	C1	A, E

Table 10.4   Time Stamps Assigned to Attributes

Customer	Time and Items Purchased
C1	(t1:A,B) (t2:C,D) (t5:A,E)
C2	(t3:A,D) (t4:E)
C3	(t2:A,C)

There is another type of data set that is very similar to a sequential data set and is referred to as a sequence data set. A sequence data set contains a collection of ordered sequences. Instead of time stamps, the positions of items in each sequence are important. An example of sequence data is genomic data.

Trajectory Data

Trajectory data are sequential as well as having location information. For example, data on the movement of individuals would have the location as well as a time stamp.

A trajectory data set can be seen as a collection of sequences of spatiotemporal data points belonging to a moving object such as GPS devices, cell phones, and radio frequency identification (RFID) tags. One example of trajectory data is shown in Table 10.5. Each record in this data set contains a path, which is a sequence of pairs (loc_i, t_i) specifying that an individual visited location loc_i at time t_i [2].

If trajectory data are not transactional by nature (i.e., a variable number of fields), then we can treat them as relational data for the purposes of re-identification and de-identification. For example, if the number of hops in the trajectory is pre-determined for all records, then the number of fields is fixed.

Table 10.5   Example of a Trajectory Data Set

ID	Path
1	((b, 2) → (d, 3) → (c, 4) → (f, 6) → (c, 7))
2	((f, 6) → (c, 7) → (e, 8))
3	((d, 3) → (c, 4) → (f, 6) → (e, 8))
4	((b, 2) → (c, 5) → (c, 7) → (e, 8))
5	((d, 3) → (c, 7) → (e, 8))
6	((c, 5) → (f, 6) → (e, 8))
7	((b, 2) → (f, 6) → (c, 7) → (e, 8))
8	((b, 2) → (c, 5) → (f, 6) → (c, 7))

Graph Data

These kind of data show relationships among objects. For example, data showing telephone calling, emailing, or instant messaging patterns among individuals would be represented as a graph. Also, social network data can be represented as a graph (e.g., people are connected to each other because they are friends).

While the metrics and methods we present here are relevant to all types of data, our main focus in this chapter is on single-level relational data, and all of the examples use single-level relational data.

The Notion of an Adversary

In discussions about re-identification we refer to the "adversary" who is trying to re-identify the records in the DF. Sometimes the term *intruder* is also used. This is the individual or organization that we are trying to protect against. The term *adversary* is not intended to imply that someone who re-identifies records is somehow bad or evil. Many of the individuals who are known to have successfully re-identified databases were researchers and journalists. Therefore do not read too much into the negative connotations of the term.

Examples of adversaries that we assume are neighbors, co-workers, ex-spouses, employers of the individuals in the DF, journalists, researchers, lawyers, or expert witnesses in court cases.

We assume that the adversary (1) has access to the DF and (2) has some background knowledge that he or she will use during the re-identification attack. The nature of that background knowledge will depend on the assumptions one is willing to make.

Also note that in this text we often refer to the adversary in the neutral term "it" because we did not want to assign a gender to someone who would launch a re-identification attack on the data set.

Types of Variables

It is useful to differentiate among the different types of variables in a data set. The way the variables are handled during the de-identification process will depend on how they are categorized. We make a distinction among four types of variables [3, 4], as shown in the following sections.

Directly Identifying Variables

One or more direct identifiers can be used to uniquely identify an individual, either by themselves or in combination with other readily available information. For example, there are more than 200 people named John Smith in Ontario; therefore the name by itself would not be directly identifying, but in combination with the address it would be directly identifying information. A telephone number is not directly identifying by itself, but in combination with the readily available White Pages it becomes so. Other examples of directly identifying variables include email address, health insurance card number, credit card number, and social insurance number. These numbers are identifying because there exist public and/or private databases that an adversary can plausibly get access to where these numbers can lead directly, and uniquely, to an identity. For example, Table 10.6 shows the names and telephone numbers of individuals. In that case the name and number would be considered identifying variables.

Indirectly Identifying Variables (Quasi-Identifiers)

The quasi-identifiers are the background knowledge variables about individuals in the DF that an adversary can use, individually or in combination, to re-identify a record with a high probability. If an adversary does not have background knowledge of a variable, then it cannot be a quasi-identifier. The manner in which an adversary can obtain such background knowledge will determine which attacks on a data set are plausible. For example, the background knowledge may be available because the adversary knows a particular target individual in the disclosed data set, an individual in the data set has a visible characteristic that is also described in the data set, or the background knowledge exists in a public or semi-public registry.

Another important criterion for a variable to be considered a quasi-identifier is that it must have analytical utility. This means that if a variable will be used for data analysis, and meets the criterion above, then it should be considered a quasi-identifier.

Examples of quasi-identifiers include sex, date of birth or age, locations (such as postal codes, census geography, information about proximity to known or unique landmarks), language spoken at home, ethnic origin, aboriginal identity, total years of schooling, marital status, criminal history, total income, visible minority status, activity difficulties/reductions, profession, event dates (such as admission, discharge, procedure, death, specimen collection, visit/encounter), codes (such as diagnosis codes, procedure codes, adverse event codes), country of birth, birth weight, and birth plurality. For example, Table 10.6 shows the patient sex and year of birth (from which an age can be derived) as quasi-identifiers.

Sensitive Variables

These are the variables that are not really useful for determining an individual's identity but contain sensitive health information about the individuals. Examples of sensitive variables are laboratory test results and drug dosage information. In Table 10.6 the lab test that was ordered and the test results are the sensitive variables.

Other Variables

Any variable in the data set that does not fall into one of the above categories falls into this catchall category. For example, in Table 10.6 we see the variable PayDelay, which indicates how long (in days) it took the insurer to pay the provider. In general, this information is not considered sensitive and would be quite difficult for an adversary to use for re-identification attack purposes.

Individuals can be re-identified because of the directly identifying variables and the quasi-identifiers. A good example illustrating this is the HIPAA Safe Harbor de-identification standard. This specifies 18 elements that must be removed from a data set to claim that it is de-identified. The dates and geographic information are quasi-identifiers, whereas the remaining 16 elements would be considered direct identifiers. De-identification methods are classified as those that work on direct identifiers and those that work on quasi-identifiers. We often refer to the methods that operate on direct identifiers as masking methods. We use this term for historical reasons in that there has been a masking industry for a number of years focusing on the needs of the software and financial services industries to help them prepare data sets for software testing.

Sidebar 10.1: *Rules to Determine if a Variable Is a Direct Identifier or a Quasi-Identifier*

1. If a variable can be known by an adversary (i.e., it can plausibly be considered as adversary background knowledge), then it can be either a direct identifier or a quasi-identifier.
2. If the variable is useful for data analysis, then it must be treated as a quasi-identifier. If it is not useful for analytic purposes, then treat it as a direct identifier.
3. If the variable can uniquely identify an individual, then it should be considered a direct identifier.

In Sidebar 10.1 we highlight the general rules to determine whether a variable should be treated as a direct identifier or a quasi-identifier. We illustrate these through some examples.

A variable classified as a quasi-identifier in one context may be classified as a sensitive variable in another context. For example, diagnosis codes in health data sets can be treated as a quasi-identifier or as a sensitive variable. The distinction in this case will depend on whether the adversary can gain background knowledge on diagnosis codes. If the adversary can get background knowledge on diagnosis

Table 10.6 Hypothetical Example Illustrating a Number of Concepts Used Throughout the Analysis

	Identifying Variable		Quasi-identifiers		Sensitive Variables		Other Variables
ID	Name	Telephone Number	Sex	Year of Birth	Lab Test	Lab Result	Pay Delay
1	John Smith	(412) 688-5468	Male	1959	Albumin, serum	4.8	37
2	Alan Smith	(413) 822-5074	Male	1969	Creatine kinase	86	36
3	Alice Brown	(416) 886-5314	Female	1955	Alkaline phosphatase	66	52
4	Hercules Green	(613) 763-5254	Male	1959	Bilirubin	Negative	36
5	Alicia Freds	(613) 586-6222	Female	1942	BUN/creatinine ratio	17	82
6	Gill Stringer	(954) 699-5423	Female	1975	Calcium, serum	9.2	34
7	Marie Kirkpatrick	(416) 786-6212	Female	1966	Free thyroxine index	2.7	23
8	Leslie Hall	(905) 668-6581	Female	1987	Globulin, total	3.5	9
9	Douglas Henry	(416) 423-5965	Male	1959	B-Type natriuretic peptide	134.1	38
10	Fred Thompson	(416) 421-7719	Male	1967	Creatine kinase	80	21
11	Joe Doe	(705) 727-7808	Male	1968	Alanine aminotransferase	24	33
12	Lillian Barley	(416) 695-4669	Female	1955	Cancer antigen 125	86	28

13	Deitmar Plank	(416) 603-5526	Male	1967	Creatine kinase	327	37
14	Anderson Hoyt	(905) 388-2851	Male	1967	Creatine kinase	82	16
15	Alexandra Knight	(416) 539-4200	Female	1966	Creatinine	0.78	44
16	Helene Arnold	(519) 631-0587	Female	1955	Triglycerides	147	59
17	Almond Zipf	(519) 515-8500	Male	1967	Creatine kinase	73	20
18	Britney Goldman	(613) 737-7870	Female	1956	Monocytes	12	34
19	Lisa Marie	(902) 473-2383	Female	1956	HDL cholesterol	68	141
20	William Cooper	(905) 763-6852	Male	1978	Neutrophils	83	21
21	Kathy Last	(705) 424-1266	Female	1966	Prothrombin time	16.9	23
22	Deitmar Plank	(519) 831-2330	Male	1967	Creatine kinase	68	16
23	Anderson Hoyt	(705) 652-6215	Male	1971	White blood cell count	13.0	151
24	Alexandra Knight	(416) 813-5873	Female	1954	Hemoglobin	14.8	34
25	Helene Arnold	(705) 663-1801	Female	1977	Lipase, serum	37	27
26	Anderson Heft	(416) 813-6498	Male	1944	Cholesterol, total	147	18
27	Almond Zipf	(617) 667-9540	Male	1965	Hematocrit	45.3	53

codes, then it would be considered a quasi-identifier. If the diagnosis codes in the data set are rare and make individuals unique in the population, then they may be considered direct identifiers. However, in practice, there is a broad distribution of diagnosis codes that they would not all be uniquely identifying. Therefore in this case the diagnosis code variable would be considered a quasi-identifier.

As another example, date of birth and six-character postal codes are often known to adversaries and are often used for data analysis. Therefore they would generally be considered quasi-identifiers.

Consider an individual's initials, which can be known by an adversary. Initials often do not make individuals unique by themselves and are rarely useful for data analysis. Therefore they are often considered direct identifiers.

Equivalence Classes

All the records that share the same values on a set of quasi-identifiers are called an equivalence class. For example, all the records in a data set about 17-year-old males admitted to a hospital on January 1, 2008, are an equivalence class. Equivalence class sizes for a data concept (such as age) potentially change during de-identification. For example, there may be three records for 17-year-old males admitted on January 1, 2008. When the age is recoded to a five-year interval, then there may be eight records for males between 16 and 20 years old admitted on January 1, 2008. In general, there is a tradeoff between the level of detail provided for a data concept and the size of the corresponding equivalence classes, with more detail associated with smaller equivalence classes.

Aggregate Tables

Some data custodians consider data sets that are represented in tabular form to be "aggregate data." As such they are no longer considered to be personal information, and therefore do not need to go through a process of de-identification. This is a dangerous assumption because certain types of tables can be converted to individual-level relational data.

Consider the table in Table 10.7. This is a table of counts. It can be converted into the data set in Table 10.8. Therefore simply representing a data set as a table does not reduce the re-identification risks in any meaningful way.

Table 10.7 Example of an Aggregate Data Table

	HPV Vaccinated	Not HPV Vaccinated
Religion A	1	3
Religion B	2	2

Table 10.8 Aggregate Table Converted to an Individual-Level Data Set

HPV Vaccination Status	Religion
N	A
N	A
N	A
N	B
N	B
Y	A
Y	B
Y	B

References

1. Ciriani V, De Capitani di Vimercati S, Foresti S, Samarati P. k-Anonymity. In *Secure data management in decentralized systems*. Springer, 2007.
2. Mohammed N, Fung B, Debbabi M. Walking in the crowd: Anonymizing trajectory data for pattern analysis. CIKM '09: Proceedings of the 18th ACM Conference on Information and Knowledge Management, 2009.
3. Samarati P. Protecting respondents identities in microdata release. *IEEE Transactions on Knowledge and Data Engineering*, 2001; 13(6):1010–1027. [10.1109/69.971193].
4. Sweeney L. k-Anonymity: A model for protecting privacy. *International Journal on Uncertainty, Fuzziness and Knowledge-Based Systems*, 2002; 10(5):557–570.

Chapter 11

Frequently Asked Questions about De-Identification

The following are commonly asked questions that have come up during our work. They need to be addressed up front, as otherwise they can create confusion and misunderstandings about re-identification risk metrics as well as how to interpret them, de-identification methods and when they should be applied, and also to set expectations appropriately.

Can We Have Zero Risk?

Some commentators, including data custodians, have required that the only acceptable probability of re-identification is zero. This is phrased as a "zero-risk" or "impossible to re-identify" requirement. The only way to meet this requirement is not to disclose any data at all. If any data are disclosed, then the probability of re-identification will not be zero. Even if one were to randomly match a DF with the telephone book's White Pages, the probability of re-identification will not be zero. It will be small, but it will not be zero.

Therefore the requirement for zero risk is not realistic if one wants to disclose data. Rather, the approach that needs to be taken is to define an acceptable probability of re-identification. If the actual probability of re-identification is below that acceptable value, then the data set can be disclosed.

The challenge with any de-identification initiative is to define this acceptable probability. A large part of this book focuses on that exact issue.

To be precise, we therefore do not talk about a data set being de-identified because that implies, at least to some observers, that the probability of re-identification has reached zero. Rather, we will talk about data sets whose probability of re-identification is "very small," "acceptably low," or just "low."

Will All DFs Be Re-Identified in the Future?

It is sometimes stated that re-identification technology is moving forward all the time, and that new databases useful for linking are being made increasingly available, and therefore that it is futile to apply de-identification to any data sets. Any advances in the future can pose heightened re-identification risk to the data.

While there is no question that more databases are being created all the time, the merits of this statement in terms of its implications on the ability to re-identify individuals is debatable, and will be addressed at some length later on in this chapter. Notwithstanding these doubts, there are pragmatic counterarguments to the logic behind this view.

If we adopted the "advances in technology will happen" argument, then there is no point in using encryption technology either. New ways are being devised to break existing encryption algorithms, either through faster computers, newly discovered weaknesses in current algorithms, or clever new algorithms that can optimize certain computations. We know this is likely to happen. When this happens, then material that was encrypted with the old technology may be compromised. We hope that this will happen far enough in the future that the compromised information has little value. A good example of this is the commentator who says "What about quantum computing?" which could make computation so fast that all assumption about bounded computation capability of an adversary would become irrelevant. Again, while this may happen, we cannot use that as an excuse not to encrypt sensitive data today. While the risk is not zero, we cannot stop doing sensible things because there is a small probability that there will be compromises at an undefined point in the future.

Another argument that has been made is that certain types of information have a limited life span, whereas other types of information would be relevant for a long time. For example, financial transaction information may convey details that are relevant in the short term that may not be as relevant in, say, five or ten years, whereas health information may be relevant for the rest of an individual's life (e.g., information about chronic conditions), or even into the life of an individual's siblings and children for genetic information. In the latter case the "future" we have to worry about is a long time.

However, the logical consequence of that argument then is not to bother using encryption for any data that will be disclosed because it is futile. For example, if encryption algorithms today may be broken in the future, and if the value lifetime of health information is very long, then one should not encrypt health information. A reasonable observer would see that this would not be a meaningful or desirable course of action. The key point here is that the future is a potential problem for all data protection technologies, some in wide use today, and is not a unique concern with de-identification.

Rather, we can do two things to manage risks that can happen in the future. First, we can use metrics so that we can estimate the probability of re-identification should future data sets become available and proceed on that basis. Second, we can impose restrictions on the availability of certain types of auxiliary data that would dramatically increase the probability of re-identification.

Is a Data Set Identifiable If a Person Can Find His or Her Record?

One question that sometimes comes up is whether a data set can be considered identifiable if a person can find his or her own record(s) in it. In this case the adversary is the targeted individual.

If we accept the above definition, then we are setting a high standard. A common way we model an adversary is to consider the kind of background knowledge the adversary would have about the target person (or persons) being re-identified. The more background information the adversary has, the greater the re-identification probability. In general, a person will have the maximum possible background information about himself or herself, possibly much more than any other adversary would know. It is true that many people tell their friends and family many things, but they do not tell them absolutely everything. Therefore the background knowledge of a person about himself or herself represents close to the maximum possible background information, and therefore close to the maximum possible risk. If one wants to be very conservative, then this is a good approach. But in many cases assuming that an adversary will know absolutely everything does not seem very plausible and sets quite a high standard. In fact, the standard would be so high that we would not be able to share any information at all.

The caveat here is that individuals may not know all detailed health information about themselves. A good example would be detailed diagnosis codes. Diagnosis codes are very specialized and an individual may not know which specific part of an organ or bone was affected. In that case the DF may contain more details than the individual would know.

A counterargument that can be made is that people are now voluntarily (and involuntarily through their friends and colleagues) revealing more and more about themselves on their blogs, Facebook pages, and tweets. This is certainly the case, and more and more is being revealed every day. Whether this type of self-exposure of personal information amounts to individuals revealing everything about themselves such that an intruder has the same background knowledge as the persons themselves remains an empirical question—although it is easy to argue that we have not quite reached that point yet.

Can De-Identified Data Be Linked to Other Data Sets?

Sometimes it is important to link the DF with other data sets to enhance it. A classic example would be to link a Canadian DF with the socioeconomic data available from Statistics Canada using the six-character postal codes. There are many instances where adding socioeconomic information would be very valuable.

The short answer to this question is "no." As will become apparent later in the book, a big part in applying de-identification techniques is to reduce the probability of successfully linking the DF with other data sets. Therefore an attempt to link the DF with other data sets should have a low probability of being successful.

In general, any linking that needs to be performed on a data set must be done before any de-identification is applied. If there are privacy concerns with the linking process itself, there are privacy preserving protocols and algorithms that have been developed to solve that problem. We do not address privacy preserving linking protocols here.

Doesn't Differential Privacy Already Provide the Answer?

Generally speaking, differential privacy requires that the answer to any query be "probabilistically indistinguishable" with or without a particular row in the database. In other words, given an arbitrary query f with domain $\wp$ and range P ($f:\wp \rightarrow P$), and two databases D and D', drawn from population $\wp$, that differ in exactly one record, if K_f is a randomized function used to respond to query f, then K_f gives ε differential privacy if for any $s \subseteq \text{Range}(K_f)$, $\Pr[K_f(D) \in s] \le e^\varepsilon \Pr[K_f(D') \in s]$.

One of the key mechanisms used within differential privacy to meet the above condition is to add Laplace noise centered at zero. This is a form of data perturbation. It is also suited to an interactive mechanism of data access, whereby a user runs queries against a database and gets answers. The user does not actually get the raw data under the interactive mechanism.

The disclosure of health data has a number of characteristics that need to be considered in any practical mechanism used to preserve privacy. These characteristics have to do with current practices and data sets, and the introduction of any new mechanism for privacy protective data disclosure or analysis would have to address these issues before it can be adopted widely. The considerations below are driven by our experiences creating health data sets for many different purposes over the last seven years, some of which have been documented, as well as empirical studies of health data sharing practices and challenges.

Health data contain categorical data (e.g., diagnosis codes, procedure codes, drugs dispensed, laboratory tests ordered, and geographical information about the patient and the provider) as well as numeric data (e.g., age in years, length of stay in hospital, and time since last visit). Therefore both types of variables need to be addressed. There is evidence that the addition of Laplace noise to numeric data can distort the values significantly.

Users of health data are accustomed to data publishing, which is where the data are disclosed to the end user. There are multiple reasons. Health data are often messy, with data errors and sometimes unexpected distributions. Analysts need to look at the data to determine the appropriate transformations to apply, compute appropriate indices from the original data, and extract the appropriate cohort of patients for the analysis. This is easiest to do when one has access to the data directly. Furthermore, biostatisticians and epidemiologists will often have a suite of analysis methods and tools that are commonly used, that they have used for many years, that they understand, for which they can interpret the results correctly, and for which they have code in languages such as SAS that they use. From a behavior change perspective, it would be challenging to convince data analysts to abandon their current methods and SAS code, which they may have been using for decades, in favor of an interactive system that is less understood. Therefore, at least in the short term, a non-interactive mechanism would be most suitable for this community.

Another important consideration is the law. The health care sector often has specific privacy laws in many jurisdictions. Current health privacy statutes in the United States, Canada, and Europe do not specify the acceptable risk and often use the "reasonableness" standard. In practice, one relies on precedent to justify the risk thresholds that are used. For currently used privacy models, such as k-anonymity, there is a significant amount of precedent for different values of k. Data custodians have been releasing data for more than two decades, including health data. During that period guidelines, policies, court cases, and regulatory orders have come out that define what can be considered acceptable levels of risk. A data custodian, if confronted in a court case or by a regulator, for example, can point to these precedents to justify its decisions. In the case of differential privacy, important parameters such as ε have no intrinsic meaning, and there are few existing precedents of actual health data releases to justify the choice of any value. A data custodian needs to consider how it would justify its choice in a dispute, and it is much easier to do so under current models, such as k-anonymity, and risky (financially and reputationally) under differential privacy.

Many fields in health data sets are correlated or have natural constraints. For example, one treatment would often precede another, or certain drugs given in combination. There are correlations among drugs, and diagnoses, and between lab results and diagnoses. Distortions to the data that produce results that do not make sense erode the trust of the data analysts in the data and act as barriers to the acceptability of the techniques used to protect the privacy of the data. For example, if the distorted data show two drugs that are known to interact in a way that can be damaging to a patient's health, a drug that would never be prescribed with a particular treatment appears for the same patient, or a dose that does not make sense for a patient, then the analysts will cease to trust the data. In practice, this has created challenges for introducing mechanisms that add noise to data because it is not possible to guarantee that nonsense data cannot be output.

Reference deployments of differential privacy in practice are also important. A powerful argument in convincing data analysts to use a data set that has been transformed in some way to deal with privacy concerns is to show them actual examples where such data have produced useful and valid results. To our knowledge, thus far there have been limited real-world disclosures of differentially private health data, and consequently few examples of useful and valid analytical results.

While not often explicitly considered when designing new mechanisms to protect data, convincing the public that stewardship of their data is being conducted in a responsible way is becoming a necessary objective. For instance, patients and providers have expressed concerns about the disclosure and use of health information, and as noted earlier, there is evidence that patients adopt privacy protective behaviors when they have concerns about how their own information is being used or disclosed, especially among vulnerable patient groups. In practice this means there is an ongoing need to explain in non-specialist terms the parameters of the privacy mechanisms used and how much protection they really provide. In the context of differential privacy, it is quite challenging to explain to a data subject the meaning of the ε value used to disclose his data or provide analytical access to his or her data, for example. It is necessary to relate these parameters to more common notions to allow easier communication to the public.

While the above observations are limited by our experiences, we believe they represent real challenges that the differential privacy model and mechanisms need to address to ensure wider acceptability and adoption within the health domain. As of today, these challenges remain, making differential privacy unsuitable as a general privacy model for the use and disclosure of health data.

Chapter 12

Definitions of Identifiability

To define and measure the probability of re-identification, it is first necessary to define the concept of identifiability. Most privacy laws treat the identifiability of information as a binary construct: information is either identifiable (personal) or not. The definitions of when information is on one side or the other vary and take into account multiple, and sometimes conflicting, criteria. In this chapter we review the different ways in which identifiability has been characterized and the different factors that have been proposed as important for determining if data is identifiable or not.

Definitions

Under the EU Data Protection Directive, an "individual shall not be regarded as identifiable if the identification requires an unreasonable amount of time and manpower," and the German Data Protection Act defines "rendering anonymous" as "the modification of personal data so that the information concerning personal or material circumstances can no longer or only with a disproportionate amount of time, expense and labour be attributed to an identified or identifiable individual" [2]. These two definitions refer to the amount of effort or resources required for re-identification as a criterion for deciding if a data set is de-identified.

The Article 29 Data Protection Working Party notes that the term *identifiable* should account for "all means likely reasonably to be used either by the controller or by any other person to identify the said person" [3], although the controller (the data custodian) would usually have access to more detailed information about the individuals in the data that they would not disclose. This gives the data custodian a re-identification advantage over anyone else. The inclusion of the custodian as also a possible adversary would exaggerate the re-identification risk considerably.

The reasonableness argument is also used often in Canadian health privacy legislation [1]. For example, Ontario's Personal Health Information Protection Act (PHIPA) states that "identifying information" means "information that identifies an individual or for which it is reasonably foreseeable in the circumstances that it could be utilized, either alone or with other information, to identify an individual." Other Canadian definitions from health privacy laws are summarized in Table 12.1, and Table 12.2 outlines the definitions found in Canadian public and private sector privacy legislation.

The Canadian Institutes of Health Research (CIHR) offered the following interpretation of "information about an identifiable individual" to include only information that can [4]: (1) identify, either directly or indirectly, a specific individual; (2) be manipulated by a reasonably foreseeable method to identify a specific individual; or (3) be linked with other accessible information by a reasonably foreseeable method to identify a specific individual. CIHR also noted that "information about an identifiable individual" shall not include [4]: (1) anonymized information that has been permanently stripped of all identifiers or aggregate information that has been grouped and averaged, such that the information has no reasonable potential for any organization to identify a specific individual, or (2) unlinked information that, to the actual knowledge of the disclosing organization, the receiving organization cannot link with other accessible information by any reasonably foreseeable method, to identify a specific individual. It notes that whether or not a method is reasonably foreseeable shall be assessed with regard to the circumstances prevailing at the time of the proposed collection, use, or disclosure of the information. Therefore, for example, the prospect of "quantum computing" making all forms of data protection futile would not be considered reasonably foreseeable. Using the reasonableness standard "identifiable" would encompass only those technical possibilities that are realistically, practically, and rationally foreseeable in the circumstances, while excluding those that are highly unlikely, immoderate, or unfeasible to expect [5].

Another EU regulation on data sharing defines *anonymized microdata* as "individual statistical records which have been modified in order to minimize, in accordance with current best practice, the risk of identification of the statistical units to which they relate" [6]. One of the standards specified in the U.S. HIPAA Privacy Rule is to get a qualified statistician to certify that a data set is de-identified. The Secretary of Health and Human Services has approved two federal documents as sources of guidance to what is generally accepted statistical and scientific principles for de-identification [7]. In these cases the definition of identifiability refers to what are considered current best practices.

Table 12.1 Examples of the Definition of Identifiability in Some Canadian Health Privacy Laws

Privacy Law	Definition
Personal Health Information Protection Act (PHIPA), S.O. 2004 c. 3 (Ontario)	"Identifying information" means information that identifies an individual or for which it is reasonably foreseeable in the circumstances that it could be utilized, either alone or with other information, to identify an individual.
Protection of Personal Health Information (PPHI), S.Nfld and Lab. 2008, c. P-7.01 (Newfoundland and Labrador)	"Identifying information" means information that identifies an individual or for which it is reasonably foreseeable in the circumstances that it could be utilized, either alone or with other information, to identify an individual.
The Health Information Protection Act (HIPA), S.S. 1999, c. H-0.021 (Saskatchewan)	"De-identified personal health information" means personal health information from which any information that may reasonably be expected to identify an individual has been removed.
Health Information Act (HIA), R.S.A. 2000, c. H-5 (Alberta)	"Individually identifying," when used to describe health information, means that the identity of the individual who is the subject of the information can be readily ascertained from the information; "nonidentifying," when used to describe health information, means that the identity of the individual who is the subject of the information cannot be readily ascertained from the information.
Protection of Personal Information Act, S.N.B. 1998, c. P-19.1 (New Brunswick)	"Identifiable individual" means an individual who can be identified by the contents of information because the information includes the individual's name, makes the individual's identity obvious, or is likely in the circumstances to be combined with other information that includes the individual's name or makes the individual's identity obvious.

The privacy commissioner of Canada has proposed the "serious possibility" test to determine whether information is about an identifiable individual: "Information will be about an identifiable individual where there is a serious possibility that an individual could be identified through the use of that information, alone or in combination with other available information" [8]. In Canadian common law, the concept of "serious possibility" means something more than a frivolous chance

Table 12.2 Examples of the Definition of Identifiability in Canadian Public and Private Sector Privacy Laws

Privacy Law	Definition
Privacy Act, R.S., 1985, c. P-21 (Federal)	"Personal information" is defined as "information about an identifiable individual that is recorded in any form."
Freedom of Information and Protection of Privacy Act (FOIPPA) [RSBC 1996], Chapter 165 (British Columbia)	"Personal information" is defined in part as "recorded information about an identifiable individual."
Freedom of Information and Protection of Privacy Act, R.S.A. 2000, c. F-25 (Alberta)	"Personal information" is defined in part as "recorded information about an identifiable individual."
Freedom of Information and Protection of Privacy Act, S.S. Chapter F-22.01 (Saskatchewan)	Defines "personal information" as "personal information about an identifiable individual that is recorded in any form."
The Freedom of Information and Protection of Privacy Act, C.C.S.M. c. F175 (Manitoba)	"If an individual is named in a record or it is possible to determine his or her identity from the contents of the record, the record is about an 'identifiable' individual. For example, if it is reasonable to expect that a requester will be able to identify particular individuals based on a combination of the information requested and information otherwise available to him or her, it is information about an 'identifiable individual'" (referencing Order P-316, Ontario Information and Privacy Commissioner (re Archives of Ontario, June 16, 1992)).
Protection of Personal Information Act, S.N.B. 1998, c-19.1 (New Brunswick)	"An individual is identifiable for the purposes of this Act if (a) information includes his or her name, (b) information makes his or her identity obvious, or (c) information does not itself include the name of the individual or make his or her identity obvious but is likely in the circumstances to be combined with other information that does."

Table 12.2 (continued)   Examples of the Definition of Identifiability in Canadian Public and Private Sector Privacy Laws

Privacy Law	Definition
An act respecting access to documents held by public bodies and the protection of personal information, R.S.Q., chapter A-2.1 (Quebec)	"Information concerning a natural person that allows the person to be identified."
An act respecting the protection of personal information in the private sector, R.S.Q., chapter P-39.1 (Quebec)	"Personal information" is defined in the same manner as in the public sector legislation—"information concerning a natural person that allows the person to be identified."
Personal Information Protection Act [SBC 2003], Chapter 63 (British Columbia)	Defines the relevant part of "personal information" in the same way as in FOIPPA, the public sector legislation; i.e., "information about an identifiable individual."
Personal Information Protection Act, Chapter P-6.5 (Alberta)	Defines "personal Information" as information about an identifiable individual.
Personal Information Protection and Electronic Documents Act S.C. 2000, c. 5 (federal)	"Personal information" means "information about an identifiable individual."

and something less than a balance of probabilities. This is a more stringent test than a "reasonable expectation" test, which is sometimes proposed, in that if it is expressed probabilistically, the probability of re-identification threshold is higher than for a "serious possibility."

Another test that has been proposed to determine whether information is identifiable is to ask: "Could this information ever be linked to the individual by the police for use as evidence?" [9]. It is argued that anything that is easy for the police to do is usually easy for hackers or insider adversaries to do.

The Supreme Court of the State of Illinois ruled that even if re-identification was shown empirically to be possible by an expert in the field, it was not reasonable to expect that non-experts, or even different experts in the art of re-identification, would be able achieve the same re-identification outcome [10]. By that interpretation, it must be demonstrated that non-experts and multiple different experts can correctly re-identify records in a DF before it can be considered personal information.

Under the U.S. HIPAA statistical standard considers information not to be identifiable if an expert applying generally accepted statistical and scientific principles and methods determines that the risk is very small that the information could be used, alone or in combination with other reasonably available information, by an anticipated recipient to identify an individual who is a subject of the information. A key phrase here is "anticipated recipient." This means that one should only be concerned about anticipated recipients of the information as potential adversaries.

Many definitions assume that an adversary would use some other information to re-identify a data set. Yakowitz argues that this information was intended to encompass only *public* information and not information that may be privately known by the adversary or in private databases [11]. She further makes the point that if an individual makes certain information about himself or herself or colleagues public, that should not mean any data set that contains that information would be considered identifiable. For example, if a single individual writes a blog detailing her blood pressure after a doctor's visit, does that mean blood pressure is now a quasi-identifier whose existence in any data set increases the risk of re-identification (because there is an example of blood pressure being public information that can be used for re-identification)? Stated another way, how many people need to have public information about them for information to be considered public for the purposes of re-identification risk assessment?

The most precise definition of de-identified information is provided in the Safe Harbor standard of the U.S. HIPAA Privacy Rule [12]. This lists 18 specific data elements whose absence deem a data set to have a low probability of re-identification.

An interesting observation about all of the above definitions is that they do not consider the probability that an adversary would discover something new about an individual; they only consider the probability of correctly assigning an identity to a record (i.e., they only consider identity disclosure and not attribute disclosure).

Common Framework for Assessing Identifiability

At first sight it would seem that these many definitions do not provide much guidance for how to ensure that the data set is not identifiable. However, the above definitions can be mostly accommodated within the risk-based methodology for creating DFs that we present here. In Table 12.3 we summarize the key criteria that have been used to define identifiability, and provide an explanation as to how the methodology described here can allow that.

Table 12.3 Definition of Identifiability (key criteria)

Identifiable Information Criteria	Our Assumptions
Records	
It must be recorded information Information can be recorded in any form	It is assumed in our methodology that the information is electronically recorded.
Who Can Re-Identify	
The data custodian/controller Anticipated data recipient Anyone else apart from the data custodian A non-expert in re/de-identification Multiple experts in re/de-identification	We only consider re-identification attacks from anyone else apart from the data custodian since the custodian would have inherent advantages for re-identification. Inclusion of the custodian as a potential adversary would set a difficult standard to meet.
Source of Background Information	
Public information Private information	We do not limit our assumptions to public background information only. However, the nature of the background information will depend on the assumptions about the adversary. These assumptions are driven by empirical evidence from actual attacks.
Specific Fields to Generalize or Suppress	
Name or information that makes identity obvious The HIPAA Privacy Rule Safe Harbor 18 elements	We do not make assumptions about a pre-defined set of identifiers or quasi-identifiers. The appropriate quasi-identifiers would be determined using our methodology on a case-by-case basis.
Specific Adversaries	
Law enforcement being able to re-identify the data	We do not specify adversaries upfront, but the adversaries that are of concern are decided upon as part of the methodology.

continued

Table 12.3 (continued) Definition of Identifiability (key criteria)

Identifiable Information Criteria	Our Assumptions
Probabilistic Interpretation	
Reasonableness standard: technical possibilities that are realistically, practically, and rationally foreseeable in the circumstances; foreseeable is assessed with regard to the circumstances prevailing at the time of the proposed disclosure Serious possibility test (which has a lower threshold than a reasonableness standard)	Our metric-based approach quantifies these statements which allows precise decisions on whether the risk is acceptable or not.
Effort and Resources Required to Re-Identify	
Re-identification requires an unreasonable or disproportionate amount of time, expense, and manpower	The methodology presented here allows the assumptions about the effort and resources the adversary will spend on re-identification to be made explicit.
Skill of Adversary	
Data is not identifiable if it does require an expert to determine the identity of individuals	The methodology presented here allows the assumptions about the skill of the adversary to be made explicit.
Best Practices	
Data is not identifiable if best practices have been used to de-identify it	This document presents what can be considered best practices in this area.

References

1. El Emam K, Kosseim P. Privacy interests in prescription records. Part 2. Patient privacy. *IEEE Security and Privacy*, 2009; 7(2):75–78. DOI: 10.1109/MSP.2009.47.
2. Federal Data Protection Act (Germany). 2006.
3. Article 29 Data Protection Working Party. Opinion 4/2007 on the concept of personal data: Adopted on 20th June. 2007. http://ec.europa.eu/justice_home/fsj/privacy/docs/wpdocs/2007/wp136_en.pdf. Archived at http://www.webcitation.org/5Q2YBu0CR.
4. Canadian Institutes of Health Research. Recommendations for the interpretation and application of the Personal Information Protection and Electronic Documents Act (S.C.2000, c.5) in the health research context. Canadian Institutes of Health Research, 2001. http://www.cihr-irsc.gc.ca/e/documents/recommendations_e.pdf.
5. Canadian Institutes of Health Research. Background legal research and analysis in support of CIHR's recommendations with respect to the Personal Information Protection and Electronic Documents Act (PIPEDA) (S.C. 2000, c. 5). 2001. http://www.cihr-irsc.gc.ca/e/documents/legal_analysis_e.pdf.
6. Commission regulation (EC) no. 831/2002 of 17 May 2002 on implementing council regulation (EC) no. 322/97 on community statistics, concerning access to confidential data for scientific purposes. *Official Journal of the European Communities*, 133, 18.5.2002, p. 7–9. 2002.
7. Brownlee C, Waleski B. *Privacy law*. New York: Law Journal Press, 2006.
8. Gordin M and the Minister of Health and the Privacy Commissioner of Canada. Memorandum of fact and law of the privacy commissioner of Canada. Federal Court, 2007.
9. Long M, Perrin S, Brands S, Dixon L, Fisher F, Gellman R. *Privacy enhancing tools and practices for an electronic health record (EHR) environment: Phase 2 of a research report for Health Canada's Office of Health and the Information Highway*. Health Canada, 2003.
10. Supreme Court of the State of Illinois. *Southern Illinoisan v. the Illinois Department of Public Health*. 2006.
11. Yakowitz J. *Tragedy of the commons*. Social Sciences Research Network, 2011. http://ssrn.com/abstract=1789749.
12. Pabrai U. *Getting started with HIPAA*. Norwood, MA: Premier Press, 2003.

Chapter 13

A Methodology for Managing Re-Identification Risk

This chapter provides the high-level principles behind our risk-based methodology to the creation of DFs with a low probability of re-identification.

A DF may be disclosed with different levels of access. One type of access may have no restrictions whatsoever, for example, when data are posted publicly. This means that the data custodians will not know who the data recipient may be, and how they will manage the DF. On the other hand, the data custodian may have significant access restrictions in place, requiring that the data recipient have strong security and privacy practices in place to ensure that the data are well protected and processed appropriately.

The methodology presented here allows the data custodian to disclose data along this full spectrum. Such a methodology ensures that the amount of de-identification that is applied to the data is proportionate to the amount of risk that the data custodian is taking when disclosing the DF (the transaction risk). Higher-risk disclosures will require more de-identification. As one can imagine, in the former situation where there are no access restrictions, the amount of de-identification that the data custodian would have to perform can be substantial. In the latter case, where many restrictions are in place, the data custodian can make the case that less de-identification is justified.

Re-Identification Risk versus Re-Identification Probability

It is important to make a distinction between *re-identification risk* and *re-identification probability*. Risk is a bigger concept and includes some subjectivity. It captures the overall risk that the custodian is taking by disclosing the DF. This may be legal, ethical, financial, and reputational risk.

To manage risk a custodian may impose restrictions on access to data, for example. Managing risk may also involve reducing the probability of re-identification, whereas managing the probability of re-identification strictly involves the application of de-identification techniques.

To be specific, we define re-identification risk to be affected by four factors, as illustrated in the conceptual diagram of Figure 13.1. Only one of them is the probability of re-identification. The higher the probability of re-identification, the greater the re-identification risk. The other three factors are defined as follows [1]:

- **Mitigating controls.** This is the set of security and privacy practices that the data recipient has in place. A recent review has identified a union of practices used by large data custodians, and recommended by funding agencies and research ethics boards for managing sensitive health information [2]. Although the mitigating controls were derived for health information, they can be useful for other types of information that individuals often consider as sensitive as well, such as financial and lifestyle information. The more mitigating controls that are in place, the less the re-identification risk. This is indicated with a negative relationship.

- **Invasion of privacy.** This characterizes the extent to which a particular disclosure would be an invasion of privacy to the individuals. There are three

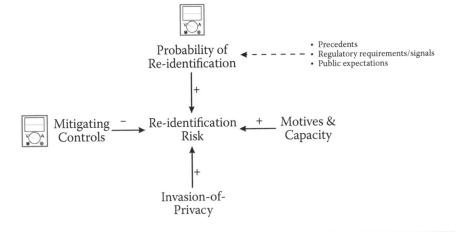

Figure 13.1   General factors that affect re-identification risk.

considerations: (a) the sensitivity of the data: the greater the sensitivity of the data the greater the invasion of privacy, (b) the potential injury to individuals from an inappropriate processing of the data: the greater the potential for injury the greater the invasion of privacy, and (c) the appropriateness of consent for disclosing the data: the less appropriate the consent the greater the invasion of privacy. The more there is an invasion of privacy, the greater the re-identification risk.

■ **Motives and capacity.** This considers the motives and capacity of the data recipient to re-identify the data, considering issues such as conflicts of interest, the potential for financial gain from a re-identification, and whether the data recipient has the skills and financial capacity to re-identify the data. The greater the motives and capacity of the data recipient to re-identify data, the greater the re-identification risk.

The tradeoffs among those four factors have been suggested previously [3–5] and have been in use informally by data custodians for at least the last decade and a half [6]. Section V of the book includes checklists that can be used to assess and score each of these three dimensions.

The invasion of privacy and motives and capacity constructs characterize the original data and the data recipient, respectively. Therefore, they are fixed once the basic parameters of the disclosure are known. However, mitigating controls and the probability of re-identification can be manipulated by the data custodian (that is why these two dimensions have the dials next to them in the figure). The former can be manipulated by requiring certain practices to be in place by the data recipient, and the latter by applying de-identification techniques to the original data set to create the DF. Because these two factors work in opposite directions in terms of their impact on re-identification risk, trade-offs will be necessary. A re-identification risk management methodology would explain how these trade-offs can be made by the data custodian. Such a methodology is described in the remainder of the book.

It should also be noted that the amount of de-identification that is applied is influenced by external factors that must be taken into account: precedents, regulatory requirements and signals, and the public's expectations. It is difficult in practice to ignore precedents, especially if there is no strong reasoning for a deviation from precedents. Regulators may indicate preferences for certain amounts of de-identification through regulations, orders, and guidance documents. Finally, it is important to consider the public's expectations. For example, if, in a particular case, a high probability of re-identification can be justified when disclosing a DF, the data custodian may still be wise to reduce that probability to retain the public's confidence and trust. On the other hand, if the public good that will come from disclosing a particular data set is so high (for example, prevention of a dangerous infection in the community), then the data custodian may choose to accept a greater than usual probability of re-identification.

Re-Identification Risk for Public Files

The conceptual model illustrated in Figure 13.1 would be suitable if there are access restrictions on a DF. In such a case the data custodian can demand that certain mitigating controls are put in place by the data recipient. Furthermore, because the data recipient will be known to the data custodian, it is possible for the data custodian to assess the motives and capacity dimension as well.

In the context of creating a DF with no access restrictions, the data custodian cannot impose any mitigating controls because, as noted earlier, the data custodian essentially loses control of the data once they are disclosed. Furthermore, it would be prudent for the data custodian to make the worst-case assumptions about the motives and capacity of the data recipient since anyone would be able to get hold of the data. Therefore, these two factors are not relevant in such a context.

For creating a DF without any access restrictions we end up with the conceptual model in Figure 13.2. This shows that only the invasion of privacy construct and the probability of re-identification are important.

Managing Re-Identification Risk

The process to follow for managing re-identification risk is shown in Figure 13.3. This involves the assessment of risk, measuring the probability of re-identification, and applying de-identification techniques to the data set to ensure that the risk in disclosing the DF is acceptable. Some of the steps in the process are technical and tool specific (e.g., importing and exporting data), and are therefore only discussed

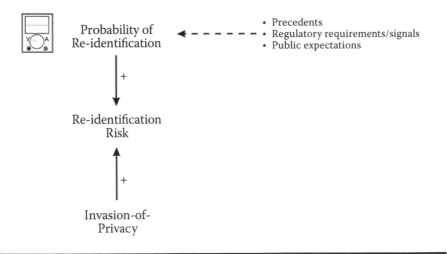

Figure 13.2   The factors that have an impact on re-identification risk in the case of creating a DF with no access restrictions.

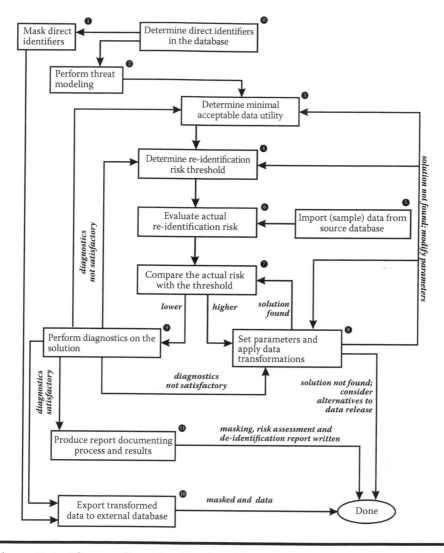

Figure 13.3   The overall re-identification risk management process.

minimally. They are nevertheless quite important, as they could consume significant resources during the process.

0. Determine which fields in the database are direct identifiers. These are fields that can individually or in combination uniquely identify individuals. For example, names and telephone numbers would be considered direct identifiers. If the database has already been stripped of direct identifiers, then this step may not be needed. But sometimes direct identifiers need to remain in the disclosed data set.

1. Once the direct identifiers have been determined, masking techniques must be applied to those direct identifiers. Masking techniques are discussed in Chapter 14. Once masking is completed there is virtually no risk of re-identification from direct identifiers. If the database has already been stripped of direct identifiers, then this step may not be needed.

2. Threat modeling consists of a number of activities: (a) identification of the plausible adversaries and what information they may be able to access, and (b) determination of the quasi-identifiers or the indirect identifiers in the database. Quasi-identifiers are generally considered to be fields like dates (birth, admission, discharge), geospatial information, demographics, socioeconomic fields, and some basic diagnosis information. There is accumulating evidence that the risk of re-identification from indirect identifiers can be high. Threat modeling is further discussed in Chapter 18.

3. It is important to determine in advance the minimal relevant data based on the indirect identifiers. This is essentially an examination of what fields are considered to be the most appropriate given the purpose of the use or disclosure. This step concludes with the imposition of practical limits on how some data may be de-identified. For example, suppose you need a data set to test a new or updated software program or to perform analysis for a research project. In this data set you need to retain temporal relationships between events, as well as track patients' diagnoses. However, in order to accomplish this goal, you may only need general information, such as a date within the same month of a patient's admission, but not the actual date. Or instead of a detailed diagnosis code, a higher-level code would be sufficient. This more general information would allow you to properly test the software program or do the research analysis, while at the same time minimize privacy risks to the patients.

4. What constitutes acceptable risk is based on the dimensions discussed earlier.

5. Importing the data from the source database may be a simple or complex exercise, depending on the data model of the source database. This step is included explicitly in the process because it can consume significant resources and must be accounted for in any planning of de-identification. For large data sets only a subsample is imported for analysis. The reason for subsampling is to speed up the data analysis, and there may also be practical limits to making a large data set available for analysis. A subsample is usually defined in terms of the percentage of patients. The exact parameters for the subsample would be project specific, but they must be defensibly representative of the full data set.

6. The actual risk is computed from the data set. Metrics are discussed at length in Section III.

7. Compare the actual risk with the threshold determined in step 4.

8. If the measured risk is higher than the threshold, then de-identification methods are applied to the data, such as generalization, suppression, and sub-sampling. Before these methods are run, some parameters need to be set, such as the maximum allowable suppression.

   Generalization means reducing the precision of the indirect identifiers. For example, the date of birth can be generalized to a five-year age interval. Suppression means removing a patient or a visit from the data set, or some details about the patient or the visit. Sub-sampling means taking a sample of patients rather than releasing the full set of patients.

   Sometimes a solution cannot be found within the specified parameters, and it is necessary to go back and reset the parameters. It may also be necessary to modify the threshold and adjust some of the assumptions behind the original risk assessment. Alternatively, some of the assumptions about acceptable data utility may need to be renegotiated.

   After a few iterations it may not be possible to produce a data set that meets the requirement. While this is rare, it is not impossible. Under these conditions, then, some of the alternative data access mechanisms discussed earlier should be considered.

9. If the measured risk is lower than the threshold, then diagnostics should be performed on the solution. Diagnostics may be objective or subjective. An objective diagnostic would evaluate the sensitivity of the solution to violations of assumptions that were made. For example, an assumption may be that an adversary might know the diagnosis code of a patient, or if there is uncertainty about the sampling fraction of the data set. A subjective diagnostic would determine whether the utility of the data is sufficiently high for the intended purposes of the use or disclosure.

   If the diagnostics are satisfactory, then the de-identified data are exported and a report is produced. On the other hand, if the diagnostics are not satisfactory, the re-identification parameters may need to be modified, the risk threshold may have to be adjusted, and the original assumptions about minimal, acceptable utility renegotiated with the data user.

10. Exporting the de-identified data to the destination database may be a simple or complex exercise, depending on the data model of the destination database. This step is included explicitly in the process because it can consume significant resources and must be accounted for in any planning of de-identification.

11. At the end of the re-identification risk assessment and de-identification, a report documenting the process and results is produced and provided to the data custodian.

References

1. El Emam K. Risk-based de-identification of health data. *IEEE Security and Privacy*, 2010; 8(3):64–67.
2. El Emam K, Dankar F, Vaillancourt R, Roffey T, Lysyk M. Evaluating patient re-identification risk from hospital prescription records. *Canadian Journal of Hospital Pharmacy*, 2009; 62(4):307–319.
3. El Emam K. *De-identifying health data for secondary use: A framework*. Ottawa: CHEO Research Institute, 2008.
4. Jabine T. Statistical disclosure limitation practices of United States statistical agencies. *Journal of Official Statistics*, 1993; 9(2):427–454.
5. Jabine T. Procedures for restricted data access. *Journal of Official Statistics*, 1993; 9(2):537–589.
6. El Emam K, Brown A, AbdelMalik P, Neisa A, Walker M, Bottomley J, Roffey T. A method for managing re-identification risk from small geographic areas in Canada. *BMC Medical Informatics and Decision Making*, 2010; 10(18).

Chapter 14

Data Masking Methods

In this chapter we provide a general overview of the most common data masking techniques that are defensible. Masking operates on the directly identifying variables in a data set only. If the original data set has directly identifying variables, then masking must be applied while creating the DF.

It should be noted that masking is often not sufficient for protecting against identity disclosure in the DF. In practice, de-identification techniques must be applied on the quasi-identifiers after the masking is complete.

Suppression

The simplest data masking method is suppression. This means the removal of a value from the data set or replacing a value with a NULL. One can suppress the whole field (or column) in a data set, or suppress rows, although in the context of masking, suppression almost always means field suppression. This approach is effective because it removes the whole variable that can potentially be used to re-identify records.

Suppression is used in situations where the directly identifying variables are not needed in the DF. For example, if a data set is being created for research purposes and there is no intention to contact the patients or data subjects to collect additional information, then there is no need to have any of the directly identifying variables in the DF.

Randomization

This technique keeps the identifying variables in the DF, but replaces the actual values with random values that look real. For example, the data custodian would replace the real names and addresses with fake names and addresses. The fake names and addresses would be taken from a large database of real Canadian/American names and addresses. This approach ensures that all of that information looks real (for example, if a masking tool replaces a male first name with a randomly selected name from its database, it will also be a male name) [1, 2].

A good randomization tool will select a name randomly with the same probability that it appears in the actual population of Canada/the United States. This ensures that very uncommon names do not appear disproportionally often in the masked data.

Various constraints can be placed on such value substitutions. Randomization tools can also replace the values of health insurance numbers with fake numbers that will pass validation checks (e.g., the Luhn algorithm). Similarly, social security numbers (SSN) and credit card numbers can be randomized. If a credit card number is substituted, it may be desirable to ensure that the replacement number is from the same financial institution or the same type of card.

More sophisticated randomization techniques will maintain the internal consistency within the data. For example, let there be two variables: "postal code" and "telephone number." If one of these is modified, say, "postal code," then a randomization system would also modify the area code for "telephone number" to make it consistent with the new "postal code" value. That way, if someone examines the masked data, the data will look realistic throughout.

For complex relational data sets, randomization needs to be performed carefully. For example, if there are two tables in a database that are related by a patient's health insurance number, then one would not want to randomize one table in one way and in the second table assign the same patient a different random health insurance number. Therefore referential integrity across tables must be ensured where appropriate.

Randomization should be irreversible, but there are instances where this would not be the case. For example, if an audit trail of all substitutions is maintained, then it would be possible for any person with access to the audit trail to check later on what the original values were. Therefore audit trails should be protected or disabled.

Irreversible Coding

One can irreversibly replace the identifying variables with a pseudonym [3, 4]. An irreversible pseudonym can be random or unique.

A random pseudonym will be different if it is generated multiple times for the same individual. For example, a random pseudonym would be used if a data custodian is disclosing two different DFs about overlapping individuals and does not wish to allow data recipients to link the two DFs. In such a case random pseud-onyms would be generated for each DF.

A unique pseudonym is the same when it is generated for the same individual. These are useful if the data custodian wants to allow the different DFs to be linked, for example, if DFs are being disclosed at intervals about the same individuals. Unique pseudonyms will allow data recipients to link the records about the same individuals in multiple DFs. These are also referred to as persistent pseudonyms.

Reversible Coding

When coding is reversible it allows individuals to be re-identified if necessary. This is also sometimes called reversible pseudonymization [3, 4]. Reversible coding is useful under certain situations. For example, in a research context it may be nec-essary to notify a study participant of important results that can affect his or his family's health. Normally this would be agreed to with the research ethics board. Rather than analyze identifiable information, the data may be coded with a revers-ible pseudonym, and only for the situations where notification is needed would that seal be broken.

Common reversible coding schemes that are used are single or double coding. Single-coded data means that direct identifiers are removed from the DF and each record is assigned a new code (a pseudonym). Identifiers are kept in a different data set with the pseudonym to allow linking back to the original data. This is illustrated in the clinical example of Figure 14.1. Note that the identity database must also be shuffled. Here the value "AF09XY" is the pseudonym. The identity database would normally be kept separate from the clinical database with different access control permissions where only specifically authorized individuals would have access.

If there is ever a need to re-identify a patient in the clinical database, then the party holding the identity database is contacted and asked to reveal the identity of

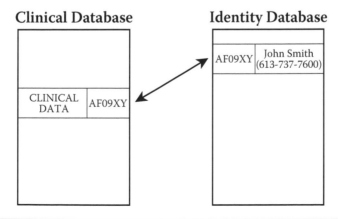

Figure 14.1   Re-identification by linking using single coding.

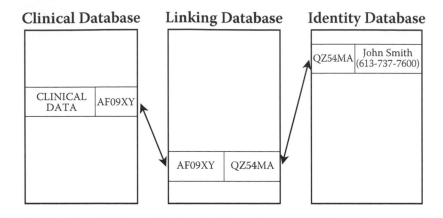

Figure 14.2　An example of double coding.

the individual with a particular pseudonym. The procedure for such re-identification would have to be decided upon in advance before data collection commences.

Double-coded data means that the pseudonyms associated with the original data and the identity database are different, and the information linking them is kept in a separate linking database. The linking database is maintained in a secure location by an authorized party (also referred to as a trusted third party), for example. This is illustrated in the clinical example of Figure 14.2.

Again, in this scenario if there is ever a need to re-identify a patient, both the authorized party and the party holding the identity database would be asked to facilitate the linking of the three tables. Double coding is useful where one wants to protect against collusion between the holder of the clinical database and the holder of the identity database. The same points on unique versus random pseudonyms apply to reversible coding as well.

Instead of using linking tables, one can also encrypt the values and only store the encryption key in a safe location. To ensure that the encrypted values have the same format as the original data, a specific type of encryption called Format Preserving Encryption can be used to retain the number and type of characters as the original variables.

Reversible Coding, HIPAA, and the Common Rule

A commonly used method for implementing reversible codes is a simple one-way hash function. Some of the older hash functions have been shown to be vulnerable, so we will assume that the data custodian is using one of the more recent hash functions. Nevertheless, a one-way hash could be reverse engineered using a dictionary attack in the context of creating pseudonyms for fields where a dictionary can be constructed (e.g., names, SSNs, health card numbers, and medical record numbers

(MRNs)). For example, if we are using an individual's SSN and that number is hashed, then an adversary would only need to hash all possible numbers of the same length and compare it to the targeted value until a match is found.

A special type of dictionary attack has also been proposed and utilized to reduce the computation time at the cost of more data storage capacity—the so-called rainbow tables [5]. In this method, a table of hash chains is precomputed for reversing the hash function by using a reduction function. The chains that create the items in the rainbow table are chains of one-way hash functions and reduction functions starting at a certain plaintext, and ending at a certain hashed value. However, only the starting plaintext and ending hashed value are stored in the rainbow table. By comparing against only the stored values, a significant reduction in computation can be gained during an attack.

In practice one always adds some randomness to the hash value. This random value is called a "salt" or a "key." This makes the range of possible values that would need to be checked in a dictionary attack, even with a rainbow table, computationally unattainable in any reasonable amount of time.

The HIPAA Privacy Rule does address the use of codes or pseudonyms directly, and it requires that "the code or other means of record identification is not derived from or related to information about the individual" and that the covered entity does not use or disclose the code for other purposes or disclose the mechanism for re-identification (45 CFR 164.514(c)). The second condition is relatively easy to meet by ensuring that the identification and linking are managed in a secure way. However, a hash value, with or without a salt, is derived from identifiable information and would therefore still be considered personal information under this definition.

The Privacy Rule allows the disclosure of information containing such coded information as a limited data set (45 CFR 164.514(e)). A limited data set would require a data sharing agreement with the data recipient, and the data can only be used for specific purposes: research, public health, or health care operations. Under this limited set of purposes, and if an appropriately constructed data sharing agreement is in place, this provision would allow the use of pseudonyms.

However, if a data set is disclosed for research purposes, then the Common Rule would also apply. Under the Common Rule, which guides IRBs, if the user of the information has no means of getting the key, for example, through an agreement with the other party prohibiting the sharing of keys under any circumstances or through organizational policies prohibiting such an exchange, then this would not be considered human subjects research and would not require an IRB review [6, 7] since the hash values would not be considered personally identifying information. This inconsistency between HIPAA and the Common Rule is well documented [8, 9].

However, the Privacy Rule does provide a mechanism for an expert with appropriate statistical knowledge to certify that the DF has a very small risk of re-identification (45 CFR 164.514(a)), at which point it would not be considered personal health information [10]. Therefore, coded date would not be considered identifiable if an expert deemed that the (salted) hashed value presents a very small risk of re-identification because it cannot be reversed and because adequate legal mechanisms exist prohibiting the inappropriate release of the salt.

In other jurisdictions, such precise prescriptions on the interpretability of coded information are absent, making it easier to argue that the use of hashed information (with a salt) as a pseudonym, with prohibitions on the sharing of that random value, would not constitute a disclosure of personal health information. This interpretation has recently been confirmed in the guidance issued by DHHS about the HIPAA de-identification standards.

Other Techniques That Do Not Work Well

There are a number of masking techniques that are sometimes used in practice. These techniques, discussed below, have known weaknesses and are generally not recommended.

Constraining Names

Some masking tools allow the user to put inappropriate constraints during randomization. For example, if a first name is substituted with a random one, a constraint can be imposed to ensure that the replacement name has the same ethnicity as the original name. This type of constraint can leak information about the data subject. For instance, if there is a single Asian name in the data set, then under certain conditions that could make it easier to re-identify that record. Ensuring that the replacement name is also Asian, then that individual still has a high risk of being re-identified.

Similarly, some tools ensure that the replacement names have the same number of characters as the original name. Figure 14.3 is the distribution of the number of characters in the first names of all doctors in Ontario (a data set of 19,433 distinct names obtained from the College of Physicians and Surgeons of Ontario). As can be seen, this distribution has a long tail. There is only one name with 23 characters, and only one name for all character lengths beyond that. There are only four names with 22 characters, 0.03% of the distinct names had 21 characters, and 0.06% of the distinct names had 19 or 20 characters. The key observation is that very few names have many characters. Therefore retaining the number of characters makes it easy to figure out the original name with a high probability using a dictionary (such as a phone book or a membership list).

Adding Noise

The challenge with noise addition (which is most often used with continuous variables) is problematic because there are many techniques that have been developed

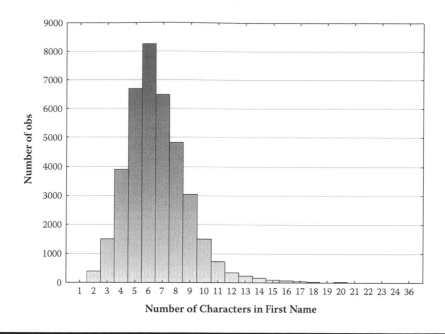

Figure 14.3 The distribution of the number of characters in the first names of doctors in Ontario.

to remove noise out of data. Therefore a sophisticated adversary can remove the noise from the data using various filters and recover the original values.

Additive noise is widely used as a tool for protecting privacy in statistical databases [11–13]. In this approach, a perturbed version of the data is created by adding random noise [14–16]. However, the privacy resulting from this technique is not always clear [17]. We examine different methods that have been used to remove noise from a data set and effectively reverse-engineer the privacy protective capabilities of this approach.

A privacy breach of the perturbed data is measured by how closely the original value can be estimated from the perturbed one [14, 16]. The authors in [18] questioned the privacy of the noise addition scheme. They presented a technique, random matrix-based spectral filtering, to estimate the original data from the perturbed one. They determined through a series of experimental results that the estimated data can be very close to the original data, and that "arbitrary randomization is not safe" [18]. Similarly, the authors in [19] showed that very accurate estimates can be constructed from the perturbed data. They found that the relationship among data attributes is important for reconstructing values. In [20], the authors present a noise removal technique; the technique reconstructs the distribution of the original data from the noisy one. The authors show that their technique can be used to attack "most practical noise addition methods" [20]. In [21, 22], the author presents an attack on the privacy of data that was sanitized using differential privacy. The author used several data mining algorithms from the Weka software package to obtain multiple predictions for each perturbed sensitive value, then these predictions were fused together to produce one estimate for each of the sensitive values. The author proved that up to 93% of the noise can be removed by using this attack. However, the author did not assume a limit on the number of queries per user; in fact, the author sets a budget per query (the values used are 0.5, 0.1, 0.05, and 0.01), but contrary to differential privacy theory, did not assume a limit on the total budget (and hence on the total number of queries).

Character Scrambling

Some masking tools will rearrange the order of the characters in a field. For example, "SMITH" may be scrambled to "TMHIS." This is quite easy to reverse. To illustrate, I took the surname table published by the U.S. Census Bureau from the 2000 census. It has 151,671 distinct surnames. Out of these, 113,242 of the names have distinct combinations of characters. There were 91,438 unique combinations of characters (i.e., they are the only name with that combination of characters). That means by just knowing the characters in a name, I can figure out the name 60% of the time because the characters that make up that name are unique. Another 13,721 have combinations of characters that appear in two names. As you can see, this is not a reliable way to protect information and leaves the data open to simple dictionary attacks (for example, using a phone book).

Character Masking

Character masking is when the last one or more characters of a string are replaced with an "*." An important decision is how many characters should be replaced in such a manner. In the surname example, we replaced the last character with an "*." In total, there were 102,312 (~67%) of the names that still had a unique combination of characters. If two characters are replaced, then 69,300 names are still unique (~46%). Without metrics to assess how many characters to replace, this type of masking may be giving a false sense of security when in fact the ability to accurately guess the name may be quite high.

Character masking only works well when accompanied by a way to measure the probability of re-identification. Only then is it possible to know how many characters to replace with "*." Without such metrics, too few or too many characters may be masked inadvertently.

Truncation

Truncation is a variant of character masking in that the last few characters are removed rather than replaced with an "*." This can also have the same risks as character masking. For example, the removal of the last character in a name still results in approximately 67% of the names being unique on the remaining characters.

Encoding

Encoding is when the value is replaced with another meaningless value. Hashing, even with a salt, would be an example of this kind of encoding. This process must be done with care because it is easy to perform a frequency analysis and figure out, say, the names by how often they appear. For example, in a multiracial data set, the most frequent name is likely to be "SMITH." Encoding should be performed only in the context of creating pseudonyms on unique values and not as a general masking function.

Summary

The above masking techniques that are not demonstrably protective should not be used in practice. The masking techniques that should be used (suppression, randomization, and coding) distort the data sufficiently that the affected direct identifiers cannot be used for data analysis. This is often not a problem because one rarely performs analytics on names, SSNs, medical record numbers, and so on. If analytics will be performed on a field, then the de-identification techniques described later on should be used, as they retain more utility in the data.

References

1. El Emam K, Sams S. Anonymization case study 1: Randomizing names and addresses. 2007. http://www.ehealthinformation.ca/documents/PACaseStudy-1.pdf. Archived at http://www.webcitation.org/5OT8Y1eKp.
2. El Emam K, Jonker E, Sams S, Neri E, Neisa A, Gao T, et al. *Pan-Canadian de-identification guidelines for personal health information*. 2007. http://www.ehealthinformation.ca/documents/OPCReportv11.pdf. Archived at http://www.webcitation.org/5Ow1Nko5C.
3. Numeir R, Lemay A, Lina J-M. Pseudonymization of radiology data for research purposes. *Journal of Digital Imaging* 2007; 20(3):284–295.
4. ISO/TS 25237. *Health informatics: Pseudonymization*. Geneva: International Organization for Standardization, 2008.
5. Oechslin P, ed. Making a faster cryptanalytic time-memory trade-off. Proceedings of 23rd Annual International Cryptology Conference, 2003.
6. Department of Health and Human Services. *Guidance on research involving coded private information or biological specimens*. 2004. http://www.hhs.gov/ohrp/archive/humansubjects/guidance/cdebiol04.htm.

7. Department of Health and Human Services. *OHRP—Guidance on research involving coded private information or biological specimens.* 2008. http://www.hhs.gov/ohrp/policy/cdebiol.html. Archived at http://www.webcitation.org/64zZAmJwa.

8. Rothstein M. Is deidentification sufficient to protect health privacy in research? *American Journal of Bioethics.* 2010; 10(9):3–11.

9. Rothstein M. Research privacy under HIPAA and the Common Rule. *Journal of Law, Medicine and Ethics.* 2005; 33:154–159.

10. National Institutes of Health. Health services research and the HIPAA Privacy Rule. 2005. http://privacyruleandresearch.nih.gov/healthservicesprivacy.asp. Archived at http://www.webcitation.org/650x1Wnx0.

11. Adam N, Wortman J. Security-control methods for statistical databases: A comparative study. *ACM Computing Surveys,* 1989; 21(4):515–556.

12. Brand R. Microdata protection through noise addition. In *Inference control in statistical databases,* ed. Domingo-Ferrer J, 97–116. Berlin: Springer, 2002.

13. Fung BCM, Wang K, Chen R, Yu PS. Privacy-preserving data publishing. *ACM Computing Surveys,* 2010; 42(4):1–53.

14. Du W, Zhan Z, eds. Using randomized response techniques for privacy-preserving data mining. New York: ACM, 2003.

15. Agrawal D, Aggarwal CC, eds. *On the design and quantification of privacy preserving data mining algorithms.* New York: ACM, 2001.

16. Agrawal R, Srikant R, eds. *Privacy-preserving data mining.* New York: ACM, 2000.

17. Chen B-C, Kifer D, LeFevre K, Machanavajjhala A. Privacy-preserving data publishing. *Foundations and Trends in Databases,* 2009; 2(1–2):1–167.

18. Kargupta H, Datta S, Wang Q, Sivakumar K, eds. *On the privacy preserving properties of random data perturbation techniques.* Proceedings of the Third IEEE International Conference on Data Mining (ICDM '03), 99 Washington, DC: IEEE Computer Society. 2003.

19. Huang Z, Du W, Chen B, ed. *Deriving private information from randomized data.* New York: ACM, 2005.

20. Domingo-Ferrer J, Sebé F, Castellà-Roca J. On the security of noise addition for privacy in statistical databases. In *Privacy in statistical databases,* ed. Domingo-Ferrer J, Torra V, 519. Lecture Notes in Computer Science, 3050. Berlin: Springer, 2004.

21. Sramka M. *A privacy attack that removes the majority of the noise from perturbed data.* The 2010 International Joint Conference on Neural Networks (IJCNN), Barcelona, 1–8, IEEE Computer Society. 2010.

22. Sramka M. Breaching privacy using data mining: Removing noise from perturbed data. *Computational Intelligence for Privacy and Security.* 2012; 135–157.

Chapter 15

Theoretical Re-Identification Attacks

There are a number of theoretical, but also very plausible, identity disclosure re-identification attacks. These are summarized in this chapter.

Background Knowledge of the Adversary

In an identity disclosure attack, the goal of the adversary can be to re-identify the record of an individual whose information is in the disclosed DF or try to re-identify as many records as possible in the DF by matching with a population registry [1]. In the former case, the adversary may know that the record of a specific individual is in the released data set, and she employs her background knowledge about that individual to re-identify that record. Alternatively, without targeting any specific individual, the adversary attacks the data set with the goal of re-identifying any record. In the latter case, the population registry may be complete in that it has information about all members of the population, or it may be incomplete but overlaps with the disclosed DF.

Identity disclosure is a potential privacy threat for any type of data being released, including relational data, transaction data, sequential data, and trajectory data. In a transaction data set, every subset of items can potentially act as a quasi-identifier to uniquely or nearly uniquely re-identify an individual's transaction. A sequential database is susceptible to identity disclosure if an adversary knows a subsequence of items about a specific individual, for instance, if the adversary knows a part of a sequence of events related to an individual whose data are found in the database. In a trajectory data set, a subset of spatiotemporal data points belonging to a moving object, such as a GPS device in an individual's car, may be known by an adversary and be employed by her to re-identify the record of that individual. In all these cases, the adversary can obtain such knowledge from various external sources. For instance, she may have access to a public database containing the record of the targeted data subject. The adversary may even use several scattered sources of information, and not just one external data source, to gain knowledge about an individual.

In the next sections, we present some key privacy attacks leading to identity disclosure and the methods to protect data against such attacks.

Re-Identification Attacks

Having some background knowledge about an individual, the adversary may be able to uniquely or nearly uniquely re-identify the individual's record in a released data set. For this purpose, the adversary employs her background knowledge to link an individual to a record in the data set. This kind of attack is called a linking attack [2] and was described by Sweeney [3] through the following example.*

Example of a Linking Attack on Relational Data [3]

The Group Insurance Commission (GIC) in Massachusetts, which is responsible for purchasing health insurance for all Massachusetts' employees, after removing all explicit identifiers, released a copy of its data set containing the medical information of all employees in Massachusetts as well as their demographic information, such as ZIP code, birth date, and gender. Besides having access to this data set, Sweeney purchased a copy of voter registration lists for Massachusetts, which is a public data set containing name, address, ZIP code, birth date, and gender of each voter. By linking these two data sets on the attributes ZIP code, birth date, and gender, Sweeney identified the medical record of former governor of Massachusetts, William Weld, including all diagnoses, procedures, and medications. In Figure 15.1, such re-identification through linkage is shown.

In addition to relational data, the other types of data, like transaction data, sequential data, trajectory data, etc., are also vulnerable to linking attacks. In the following paragraphs, through a set of examples, we illustrate linking attacks on different types of data.

---

* Recently a critical analysis of this attack suggested that the attack would be more difficult to replicate on someone who was not a famous personality, and that the success rate of such attacks is lower than one imagines because identification databases, such as the voter registration list, are incomplete. See Barth-Jones, Daniel C., The "Re-Identification" of Governor William Weld's Medical Information: A Critical Re-Examination of Health Data Identification Risks and Privacy Protections, Then and Now (June 4, 2012). Available at SSRN: http://ssrn.com/abstract=2076397 or http://dx.doi.org/10.2139/ssrn.2076397

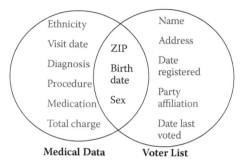

Figure 15.1   Re-identification by linking. (From Sweeney L, *International Journal on Uncertainty, Fuzziness and Knowledge-Based Systems,* **2002; 10(5):557–570. With permission.)**

Example of a Linking Attack on Transactional Data

Assume that a hospital wants to publish a data set containing the transactions of the patients who visited the hospital during the last year. Each transaction consists of a set of diagnoses corresponding to each patient. The hospital removes all directly identifying information, like names and social security numbers, prior to releasing the data set. An example of such a data set is shown in Table 15.1. Assume that Alice knows that her neighbor, Bob, was in this hospital two months ago because of toxoplasmosis (diagnosis code 130). If Alice obtains access to the released data set from the hospital, she will be able to infer that record 4 belongs to Bob, since this is the only record in this database that contains diagnosis code 130.

In the case of sequential data, if the adversary knows a subsequence of actions related to an individual, she may be able to re-identify that individual's record and, consequently, infer the individual's whole sequence. Pensa et al. [4] showed how this is possible using the following example.

Table 15.1   Example of Patient Data

PID[a]	Diagnosis Codes
1	208, 530, 727, 730
2	281, 530, 730, 264, 266
3	208, 281, 727, 266
4	530, 130, 288, 003, 264
5	281, 288, 730, 003
6	208, 281, 530, 727, 288, 730

[a] PID = Patent ID

Example of a Linking Attack on Sequential Data [4]

Assume that Alice has access to the city traffic data. If she knows that Bob often goes from commercial zone A to general hospital B, and the sequence A–B occurs a few times in the data set, then she will be able to easily identify Bob's sequence record in the released city traffic data.

Publication of a trajectory data set may also threaten the privacy of individuals if an adversary knows a specific path of spatiotemporal data points related to an individual. To illustrate this, we consider the following example.

Example of a Linking Attack on Trajectory Data [5]

Assume that a hospital needs to release the patient-specific trajectory and health data set, as shown in Table 15.2. Each record in this table contains a path, which is a sequence of pairs (loc_i, t_i) specifying that the patient visited location loc_i at time t_i. In addition, each record contains the sensitive attribute "Diagnosis." A linking attack can occur when there is a specific path that is not shared with many other patients. Assume that Alice knows that Bob visited locations b and d at times 2 and 3, respectively. Since there is only one record, ID = 1, that contains (b, 2) and (d, 3), Alice can uniquely re-identify Bob's record.

Table 15.2 Trajectory and Health Data

ID	Path	Diagnosis	...
1	((b, 2) → (d, 3) → (c, 4) → (f, 6) → (c, 7))	AIDS	...
2	((f, 6) → (c, 7) → (e, 8))	Flu	...
3	((d, 3) → (c, 4) → (f, 6) → (e, 8))	Fever	...
4	((b, 2) → (c, 5) → (c, 7) → (e, 8))	Flu	...
5	((d, 3) → (c, 7) → (e, 8))	Fever	...
6	((c, 5) → (f, 6) → (e, 8))	Diabetes	...
7	((b, 2) → (f, 6) → (c, 7) → (e, 8))	Diabetes	...
8	((b, 2) → (c, 5) → (f, 6) → (c, 7))	AIDS	...

Source: Mohammed N, Fung B, Debbabi M, Walking in the Crowd: Anonymizing Trajectory Data for Pattern Analysis, CIKM '09: Proceedings of the 18th ACM Conference on Information and Knowledge Management, 2009. With permission.

In all of the above examples, a linking attack occurred due to an exact match between the background knowledge that the adversary had about an individual and a part of that individual's record in the released data set. However, a linking attack may also happen based on the semantic information contained in the record of an individual, for instance, in her search queries [2]. To illustrate this kind of linking attack, we consider the case of AOL.

Example of a Linking Attack Based on Semantic Information [2, 6, 7]

On August 6, 2006, AOL released a data set containing 20 million web queries from 650,000 of its users collected over a period of three months. The data set also contained the URLs selected from each search result and their ranking. To anonymize the data before release, AOL replaced each user ID with a randomly generated number (i.e., a pseudonym). After the release, two *New York Times* reporters analyzed this data set based on the semantic content of users' search queries, such as the name of a town, age-related queries, several searches with a particular last name, etc. After three days of analysis, they were able to identify user number 4417749 as Thelma Arnold, a 62-year-old woman living in Lilburn, Georgia. In her search query logs, Thelma had hundreds of searches over a period of three months on topics like "60 single men," "dog that urinates on everything," and "numb fingers," which revealed personal information about her and her friends and family.

In addition to these examples, linking attacks can lead to privacy breaches in other domains, including social networks [8–10] and genomic records [11–13].

References

1. Elliot M, Dale A. Scenarios of attack: The data intruder's perspective on statistical disclosure risk. *Netherlands Official Statistics*, 1999; 14(Spring):6–10.
2. Chen B-C, Kifer D, LeFevre K, Machanavajjhala A. Privacy-preserving data publishing. *Foundations and Trends in Databases*, 2009; 2(1–2):1–167. DOI: 10.1561/1900000008.
3. Sweeney L. k-Anonymity: A model for protecting privacy. *International Journal on Uncertainty, Fuzziness and Knowledge-Based Systems*, 2002; 10(5):557–570.
4. Pensa R, Monreale A, Pinelli F, Pedreschi D. *Pattern-preserving k-anonymization of sequences and its application to mobility data mining*. PiLBA, 2008.
5. Mohammed N, Fung B, Debbabi M. Walking in the crowd: Anonymizing trajectory data for pattern analysis. CIKM '09: Proceedings of the 18th ACM Conference on Information and Knowledge Management, 2009.
6. Arrington M. AOL proudly releases massive amounts of private data. TechCrunch, 2006. http://techcrunch.com/2006/08/06/aol-proudly-releases-massive-amounts-of-user-search-data/ (accessed January 1, 2011).
7. Barbaro M, Zeller Jr. T. A face is exposed for AOL searcher no. 4417749. *New York Times*, August 9, 2006.

8. Backstrom L, Dwork C, Kleinberg J. *Wherefore art thou R3579X? Anonymized social networks, hidden patterns, and structural steganography.* WWW 2007. Banff: ACM, 2007.

9. Hay M, Miklau G, Jensen D, Towsley D, Weis P. Resisting structural re-identification in anonymized social networks. *Proceedings of the VLDB Endowment*, 2008; 1(1):102–114. DOI: 10.1145/1453856.1453873.

10. Narayanan A, Shmatikov V. De-anonymizing social networks. *Proceedings of the 30th IEEE Symposium on Security and Privacy*, 2009; 173–187.

11. Malin B. Re-identification of familial database records. Proceedings of the American Medical Informatics Association Annual Symposium, 2006.

12. Malin B, Sweeney L. How (not) to protect genomic data privacy in a distributed network: Using trails re-identification to evaluate and design anonymity protection systems. *Journal of Biomedical Informatics*, 2004; 37(3):179–192.

13. Malin B. An evaluation of the current state of genomic data privacy protection technology and a roadmap for the future. *Journal of the American Medical Informatics Association*, 2005; 12(1):28–34.

MEASURING RE-IDENTIFICATION RISK

Chapter 16

Measuring the Probability of Re-Identification

The application of de-identification algorithms in practice requires the data custodian to be able to measure the probability of re-identification. Such measurement will inform the custodian whether the probability of re-identification is high or not. If the probability is high, then de-identification methods need to be applied. This means that specific metrics for the measurement of the probability of re-identification are needed, as well as guidelines for interpreting their values. In this chapter we present a set of metrics and decision rules for measuring and interpreting the probability of re-identification for identity disclosure.

Simple and Derived Metrics

When we assess re-identification risk for a data set, we assign a probability of successful re-identification to each record in that data set. For identity disclosure, the probability of re-identification means the probability of that record being assigned a correct identity. We will denote the probability of a record i being correctly re-identified by θ_i where $\theta_i = 1, \ldots, n$, and n is the total number of records in the data set. Based on that, a number of derived metrics can be developed.

Let J be the set of equivalence classes in the disclosed data set, and $|J|$ be the number of equivalence classes in the data set. In practice, all of the records in the same equivalence class will have the same probability value, θ_i. Therefore we refer to the probability θ_j for an equivalence class where $j \in J$.

All of the derived metrics apply this simple individual equivalence class metric to the whole data set. For the sake of consistency we will scale all of the derived metrics to have a value between 0 and 1.

Derived metrics need to be converted to a binary value to reflect whether the probability is considered too high or not. The decision that needs to be made at the end of the measurement is a binary one after all. This is the *decision rule* for interpreting the metric value.

The decision rule converts measurements on a derived metric into a re-identification risk. Hence if the decision rule determines that the risk is high, then de-identification methods would be necessary to bring it to a low value. If the decision rule determines that the risk is low, then no de-identification is necessary.

This is achieved by the use of thresholds. The thresholds determine whether the derived metric is acceptable or not. Deciding on the threshold is the subjective component in risk management. We will defer a detailed discussion of exactly how to decide on a threshold to subsequent chapters, but will provide some general principles here.

If there are access restrictions on the DF, then the data custodian needs to consider our three risk constructs: mitigating controls, invasion of privacy, and motives and capacity. This is illustrated in Figure 16.1. Also, as noted earlier, other factors need to be considered when deciding on the threshold, such as (1) precedents of thresholds for the same kind of DF, (2) regulatory requirements and signals in terms of acceptable thresholds, and (3) public expectations about reasonable thresholds.

If there are no access restrictions, then only the invasion of privacy construct needs to be considered, as shown in Figure 16.2.

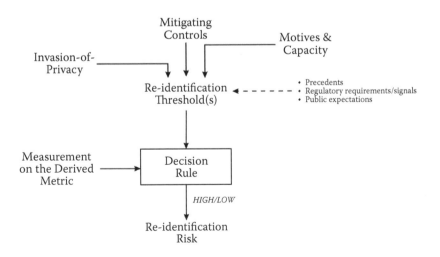

Figure 16.1 Schematics showing how the derived metrics and the decision rules determine re-identification risk: DF with access restrictions.

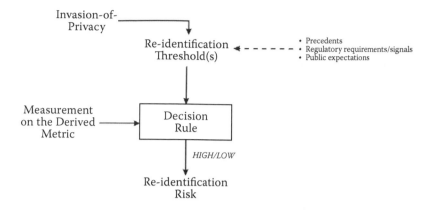

Figure 16.2 **Schematics showing how the derived metrics and the decision rules determine re-identification risk: DF without access restrictions.**

The first derived metric assesses the proportion of records that have a re-identification probability higher than a threshold. The threshold is denoted by τ:

$$R_a = \frac{1}{n} \sum_{j \in J} f_j \times I\left(\theta_j > \tau\right) \tag{16.1}$$

where $I(\cdot)$ is the indicator function (this returns 1 if the parameters are true and 0 otherwise) and f_j is the size of equivalence class j in the database. We will discuss how to set the value of τ below. If the value of R_a is too high, then the data set is considered to have a risk of re-identification that is not acceptable.

We will denote the threshold for the maximum proportion of records that have a high probability of re-identification by α. Therefore the decision rule for R_a is

$$D_a = \begin{cases} HIGH, \ R_a > \alpha \\ LOW, \ R_a \leq \alpha \end{cases} \tag{16.2}$$

If the R_a value is higher than the threshold, the re-identification risk is considered high. As will be noted, the D_a decision rule requires more than one threshold to be operationalized, τ and α.

Another kind of derived metric takes the worst-case scenario and assumes that the equivalence class with the highest re-identification probability represents the whole data set.

$$R_b = \max_{j \in J}\left(\theta_j\right) \tag{16.3}$$

This is quite a stringent standard because even records with a low probability of re-identification are penalized as much as the records with a high probability of re-identification. For instance, even if there is a single record in a million-record data set with a high value for θ_j, the value of R_b will take on that value. The situations where this metric will be appropriate are (1) when the data custodian wants to err on the quite conservative side, and (2) if we assume that the adversary is smart and will focus her attention on the records that have the highest re-identification probability. There are situations where the latter situation is the most reasonable one to make, and therefore R_b would be clearly appropriate to use. However, when it does not make sense to assume that an adversary can target the highest risk records, then it is up for debate whether R_b is suitable or not. The decision rule for R_b is

$$D_b = \begin{cases} HIGH, \ R_b > \tau \\ LOW, \ R_b \leq \tau \end{cases} \tag{16.4}$$

Note that the threshold for this decision rule is the same as for Equation (16.1) because that threshold has the same meaning: the maximum probability of a record being re-identified.

Another derived metric takes the average probability across all of the records in the data set. It is essentially the expected value. This expected value is

$$R_c = \frac{1}{n} \sum_{j \in J} f_j \theta_j \tag{16.5}$$

The decision rule for this type of derived metric is given by

$$D_c = \begin{cases} HIGH, \ R_c > \lambda \\ LOW, \ R_c \leq \lambda \end{cases} \tag{16.6}$$

where λ represents the maximum proportion of records that can be re-identified.

The R_c metric gives the proportion of records that would be re-identified by an adversary (on average). On the surface this would seem to be similar to the R_a metric, which measures the proportion of records that have a high probability of re-identification. However, the records accounted for in R_a are not necessarily those that will be re-identified.

For example, if we say that a data set has 100 records, $\tau = 0.2$, $\alpha = 0$, $\lambda = 0.2$, and only two records have a probability of re-identification $\theta_j = 0.3$, with the rest having $\theta_j = 0.1$. When we use the R_a metric we are assuming that the adversary will try to re-identify a single record and that the adversary may select one of those two records with $\theta_j > \tau$ to re-identify. In such a case the risk would be unacceptable because two records would have a high probability of re-identification if they were selected. On the other hand, when we use the R_c metric we are assuming that the adversary will try to re-identify *all* of the records in the data set by matching them against some registry and that he will likely get ten correct matches. Because that is a smaller proportion than λ, it would be considered acceptable risk.

When discussing re-identification risk metrics it is therefore important to be clear about what kind of metric we are talking about and the decision rule that is being used. Equally important, we need to be clear about the thresholds being used because these are instrumental for interpreting the results. There will be a great difference in interpreting the results, say, using $\tau = 0.2$ versus $\tau = 0.05$.

A summary of the derived metrics is provided in Table 16.1, of the decision rules in Table 16.2, and a summary of the thresholds and their interpretation is provided in Table 16.3.

Table 16.1 Summary of Derived Re-Identification Metrics

Derived Risk Metric	Interpretation
$R_a = \dfrac{1}{n}\displaystyle\sum_{j \in J} f_j \times I\left(\theta_j > \tau\right)$	The proportion of records that have a re-identification probability higher than a threshold
$R_b = \max_{j \in J}\left(\theta_j\right)$	The maximum probability of re-identification in the data set among all records
$R_c = \dfrac{1}{n}\displaystyle\sum_{j \in J} f_j \theta_j$	The proportion of records that can be correctly re-identified on average

Table 16.2 Summary of the Decision Rules

Decision Rule	Interpretation of High/Low Risk
$D_a = \begin{cases} HIGH,\ R_a > \alpha \\ LOW,\ R_a \le \alpha \end{cases}$	The proportion of records with a high probability of re-identification is not acceptable/acceptable.
$D_b = \begin{cases} HIGH,\ R_b > \tau \\ LOW,\ R_b \le \tau \end{cases}$	The highest probability of re-identification among all records is not acceptable/acceptable.
$D_c = \begin{cases} HIGH,\ R_c > \lambda \\ LOW,\ R_c \le \lambda \end{cases}$	The average proportion of records that can be re-identified is not acceptable/acceptable.

Table 16.3 Summary of Thresholds

Threshold	Interpretation
τ	The highest allowable probability of correctly re-identifying a single record
α	The proportion of records that have a high probability of re-identification that would be acceptable to the data custodian
λ	The average proportion of records that can be correctly re-identified that would be acceptable to the data custodian

Simple Risk Metrics: Prosecutor and Journalist Risk

There are two simple re-identification metrics, or rather, there are two instantiations of θ_j. The main criterion that differentiates them is whether the adversary can know whether a particular individual is in the DF [1]. This individual is the one that is being re-identified, and we will call that individual the *target*. The target may be a specific individual that the adversary already has background information about. For example, this may be the adversary's neighbor, co-worker, ex-spouse, relative, or a famous person. We will refer to this individual as the adversary's acquaintance. Or the target may be an individual selected at random from a population list such as a voter registry. For example, if the adversary is a journalist who wishes to embarrass or expose a data custodian, then the journalist may select a target at random because the re-identification of any record will achieve the purpose.

If the adversary can know whether the target is in the DF, then this is called *prosecutor risk*. If the target does not or cannot know whether the target is in the DF, then this is called *journalist risk*.

How can the adversary know if the target is in the DF? If any of the three following conditions are true, then the data custodian needs to care about prosecutor risk [1]:

- ▪ The DF represents the whole population (e.g., a population registry) or has a large sampling fraction from that population. If the whole population is being disclosed, then the adversary would have certainty that the target is in the DF. This would be true whether the adversary was trying to re-identify an acquaintance or a random person from a population registry. Also, a large sampling fraction means that the target is very likely to be in the DF. Examples of population registries are provincial or state disease registries, or registries that capture information about certain events, such as births or hospital discharges.
- ▪ The DF is not a population registry but is a sample from a population, and it can be easily determined who is in the DF. For example, if the DF is the data set from a sample drug use survey of teenagers, then a parent would likely

know that his or her teenager participated because he or she had to consent for the teen to participate.

■ The DF is a sample and the individuals in the DF self-reveal that they are part of the sample. For example, consider the public release of a clinical trials data set. Subjects in clinical trials do generally inform their family, friends, and even acquaintances that they are participating in a trial. An acquaintance may attempt to re-identify one of these self-revealing participants' data in the DF. Individuals may also disclose information about themselves on their blogs and social networking site pages, which may self-reveal that they are part of a study or a disease registry. However, it is not always the case that individuals do know that their record is in a data set. For example, for studies using existing data where consent has been waived or where individuals provide broad authorization for their data or tissue samples to be used in future research, the individuals may not know that their record is in a specific DF, providing them no opportunity for self-revealing their inclusion.

If a data set does not meet the above criteria, then the data custodian should be concerned about journalist risk and not prosecutor risk (i.e., it is either one or the other, not both). The distinction between the two types of risk is quite important because the way risk is measured or estimated does differ between them. Examples illustrating the choice between prosecutor and journalist risk are provided in Sidebar 16.1.

It is often the case that custodians hold a certain type of data, and therefore once they have decided that their data fall under prosecutor or journalist risk, they can apply that type of measurement moving forward.

Note that the term *population* is used loosely here. It does not necessarily mean the whole population of a geographic area, but the group of people who have defined characteristics. For example, a data set of all patients with renal cancer for a province would be in a renal cancer population registry since everyone with renal cancer would be in that registry. A data set of all patients with a particular disease within a geographic boundary, or that have a particular demographic (e.g., ethnicity, language spoken at home, or age group), would be considered a population, and therefore the data set would meet the first criterion above.

Sidebar 16.1: Examples of Prosecutor and Journalist Risk

The following are real examples to illustrate when each type of risk applies:

■ The Ontario birth registry, known as BORN, discloses data sets about the health of new mothers and infants for specific purposes, including research and public health investigations. Normally, the whole population data set is disclosed, or everyone who meets specific criteria (e.g., location or period of birth). Because the registry effectively includes the whole population (i.e., all births in the province), an adversary would know with certainty that any mother would be in the disclosed data set from the registry. In this case prosecutor risk would apply. However, if a random sample from the registry is disclosed, then journalist risk is applied. The reason is that an adversary would not know if any particular mother/infant is included in that sample.

- A study is performed at an office and employees volunteer to participate. Participation, however, cannot be hidden. For example, participating employees may have to skip a day of work to take a few tests or to take part in a focus group or training session. Or, participating employees need to have a device placed in their office/cubicle. In these situations only a sample of the employees would have data in the data set. However, it would be known among other employees (and potential adversaries) who has participated, and therefore who has data in the data set. In this case prosecutor risk would apply even though this is a sample.

- Data about patients who come to a hospital's emergency department are being disclosed. If the data on all patients are being disclosed, then prosecutor risk applies. The reason is that if an adversary knew that a particular individual went to the emergency room, then the adversary would also know that the patient's data are in that disclosed data set. However, if data only on patients who came in with complaints of an influenza-like illness were being disclosed, then this would be journalist risk if the adversary did not know that the target individual had influenza. In such a case, the adversary would not know if the target individual is in the data set or not.

- A government health insurer decides to make health information publicly available as a DF. Data on a random sample of 10% of the patients are included in the DF. In this case journalist risk applies because an adversary would not know who was in that random sample, and the patients themselves would not know if they were in that sample.

Measuring Prosecutor Risk

Let us assume that the adversary is attempting to re-identify a specific target, Alice. The adversary also knows that Alice is in the DF, and therefore the prosecutor risk criterion is met.

In the example shown in Figure 16.3 there is an original data set that contains patient information and some prescription information (DIN—the drug identification number). The directly identifying variable, the patient name, is suppressed. De-identification is applied by generalizing the year of birth. We now have a DF. The adversary has some background information about Alice, namely, her year of birth and gender. The adversary also knows that Alice is in the DF.

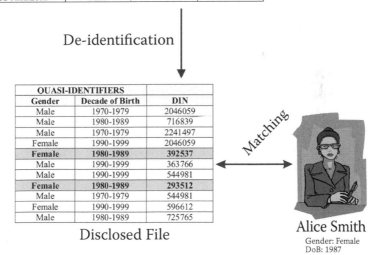

Original Database

IDENTIFYING VARIABLE	QUASI-IDENTIFIERS		
Name	Gender	Year of Birth	DIN
John Smith	Male	1979	2046059
Alan Patel	Male	1982	716839
Hercules Green	Male	1979	2241497
Gill Stringer	Female	1995	2046059
Alice Smith	Female	1987	392537
Bill Nash	Male	1995	363766
Albert Blackwell	Male	1998	544981
Beverly McCulsky	Female	1984	293512
Douglas Henry	Male	1979	544981
Freda Shields	Female	1995	596612
Fred Thompson	Male	1987	725765

De-identification

QUASI-IDENTIFIERS		
Gender	Decade of Birth	DIN
Male	1970-1979	2046059
Male	1980-1989	716839
Male	1970-1979	2241497
Female	1990-1999	2046059
Female	1980-1989	392537
Male	1990-1999	363766
Male	1990-1999	544981
Female	1980-1989	293512
Male	1970-1979	544981
Female	1990-1999	596612
Male	1980-1989	725765

Matching

Disclosed File

Alice Smith
Gender: Female
DoB: 1987

Figure 16.3 Illustration of prosecutor risk whereby the adversary is attempting to re-identify a record belonging to a specific target individual, Alice, about whom he or she has background information.

Because the adversary knows that Alice is in the DF, he or she can match on the year of birth and gender. There are two records that match. Therefore the matching equivalence class size is equal to 2. Since the adversary does not know which one of these two records pertains to Alice, the adversary will select one at random. Therefore her probability of re-identification is 0.5.

More generally, the probability of correct re-identification is given by

$$_p\theta_j = 1/f_j \tag{16.7}$$

where f_j is the size of the matching equivalence class in the DF. We use the notation p here to indicate that this is prosecutor risk.

In practice the data custodian will not know in advance that the adversary will be targeting Alice. The adversary may target any of the individuals in the DF. Therefore the custodian needs to compute the value of $_p\theta_j$ for all of the equivalence classes, as shown in Table 16.4.

The custodian must then choose a type of derived metric to compute from the individual $_p\theta_j$ values. The final equations and risk values based on the example in Figure 16.3 are shown in Table 16.5 assuming $\tau = 0.33$.

As can be seen, the risk values can be dramatically different, which makes it important to decide carefully in advance which types of derived risk metrics we will use for the assessment of prosecutor risk.

If the adversary has a population registry that has information about people who are known to be in the DF, then the adversary can select individuals from the registry in small equivalence classes as targets. In this case the adversary can target the smallest equivalence classes and the $_pR_b$ metric would make the most sense. However, if there is no known registry of individuals who are known to be in the DF, then either the maximum risk or the average risk would be appropriate, depending on the comfort level of the data custodian.

Table 16.4 Prosecutor Risk of Re-Identification for Every Equivalence Class in the Example Data Set

Gender	Year of Birth	$_p\theta_j$
Male	1970–1979	0.33
Male	1980–1989	0.5
Male	1990–1999	0.5
Female	1990–1999	0.5
Female	1980–1989	0.5

Table 16.5   Computation of All Three Types of Derived Prosecutor Risk Metrics for Our Example

Derived Risk Metric	Equation	Risk Value
$_pR_a$	$\dfrac{1}{n}\sum_{j \in J} f_j \times I\left(\dfrac{1}{f_j} > \tau\right)$	0.73
$_pR_b$	$\max_{j \in J}\left(\dfrac{1}{f_j}\right) = \dfrac{1}{\min_{j \in J}(f_j)}$	0.5
$_pR_c$	$\dfrac{1}{n}\sum_{j \in J} f_j \times \dfrac{1}{f_j} = \dfrac{|J|}{n}$	0.45

Measuring Journalist Risk

For journalist risk to apply the data set has to be a sample of some sort. The reasoning is that if the disclosed data set is a population registry, then the adversary will likely know for sure that the target is in the population (because everyone is). Note that the reverse is not necessarily true: If a data set is a sample, that does not mean that journalist risk applies.

There are two general types of re-identification attacks under journalist risk: (1) The adversary is targeting a specific individual, and (2) the adversary is targeting any individual. With the former the adversary has background knowledge about a specific individual (e.g., a neighbor or a famous person), whereas with the latter, the adversary does not care which individual is being targeted.

For journalist risk we assume that the adversary will match the disclosed data set with another *identification database*. For now we also assume that there is an identification database that is known to be a superset of the disclosed data set. The voter registration list in the United States is often taken to represent the whole population [2]—although approximately only two-thirds of eligible citizens actually register to vote [3]. For our illustrative purposes we will carry on with the common assumption that the voter list covers the whole population.

Under this scenario let K be the set of equivalence classes in the identification database, $|K|$ and the number of equivalence classes in the identification database. We also have that $J \subseteq K$, where $J = \{x | \forall x : x \in K \wedge f_x > 0\}$. Let the number of records in an equivalence class j in the identification database be denoted by F_j, where $F_j > 0$ for $j \in K$, and the total number of records in the identification database is given by

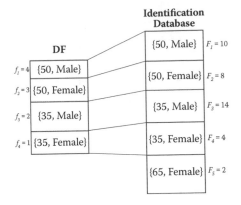

Figure 16.4   An example of a sample DF drawn from an identification database.

$$N = \sum_{j \in K} F_j$$

The equivalence class size in the disclosed database is given by f_j, and the total number of records in this sample is

$$n = \sum_{j \in J} f_j$$

We assume that the disclosed database is a simple random sample from the identification database.

Take the example in Figure 16.4. Let's say that the adversary wishes to re-identify a specific individual, his neighbor, who is a 50-year-old male. The adversary knows that the neighbor is in the identification database. Then we need to consider the probability that the selected 50-year-old male is in the DF and the probability of a correct match with the background information given that the target is in the DF. If we assume that this target individual is in equivalence class j, this gives us a probability

$$\frac{f_j}{F_j} \cdot \frac{1}{f_j} = \frac{1}{F_j}$$

More generally, the probability of a correct match is

$$_j\theta_j = 1/F_j$$

for any equivalence class where $f_j > 0$. We use the J subscript to indicate that this is journalist risk. If the adversary focuses on the smallest equivalence classes, then the appropriate risk metric is

$$_j R_b = \max_{j \in J}\left(1/F_j\right)$$

We provide proofs for this in Chapter 23 in the case where the adversary selects a record from the DF and attempts to match with an identification database, and also under the attack where the adversary selects a record from the identification database and attempts to match against the DF.

If we know that the adversary will not focus on the smallest equivalence classes, then we can measure the average risk. Consider that the DF consists of data on cancer patients. An adversary who is trying to re-identify a record belonging to an acquaintance will not target the smallest equivalence classes, but will match against the equivalence classes that belong to the acquaintance. In such a case the average risk is relevant.

For a randomly selected record from the DF that is matched against an identification database, the average probability of re-identification is

$$_j R_{c_1} = \frac{1}{n} \sum_{j \in J} \frac{f_j}{F_j} \tag{16.8}$$

On the other hand, for a randomly selected record from the identification database that is matched against the DF, the average probability of re-identification is

$$_j R_{c_2} = \frac{|J|}{\displaystyle\sum_{j \in J} F_j} \tag{16.9}$$

Given that it is not possible to know in advance which method of attack an adversary will use, the overall average risk needs to be formulated as the maximum of Equations (16.8) and (16.9):

$$_j R_c = \max\left(\frac{|J|}{\displaystyle\sum_{j \in J} F_j}, \frac{1}{n} \sum_{j \in J} \frac{f_j}{F_j} \right) \tag{16.10}$$

In practice the data custodian will often not have access to the identification database to compute the journalist risk. Therefore the value of $_j \theta_j$ must be estimated using only the information in the disclosed database. Various methods for doing so have been developed [1, 4].

There are good reasons why the data custodian would not have an identification database. Often, a population database is expensive to obtain. Plus, it is likely that the data custodian will have to protect multiple populations, hence multiplying the effort and expense to obtain such a population database. For example, the construction of a single profession-specific database using semipublic registries that can be used for re-identification attacks in Canada costs between \$150,000 and \$188,000 [5]. Commercial databases can be comparatively costly. In the United States, the cost for the voter registration list from Alabama is more than \$28,000, \$5,000 for Louisiana, more than \$8,000 for New Hampshire, \$12,000 for Wisconsin, and \$17,000 for West Virginia [2]. Commercial databases would likely be more costly than the semipublic ones. Furthermore, an adversary may misrepresent itself or commit illegal acts to get access to population registries. For example, privacy legislation and the Elections Act in Canada restrict the use of voter lists to running and supporting election activities [5]. There is at least one known case where a charity allegedly supporting a terrorist group has been able to obtain Canadian voter lists for fund-raising [6–8]. A legitimate data custodian would not engage in such acts and therefore may not even be able to get hold of an appropriate identification database. In the United States voter lists in some states are only available for purposes related to elections [2], and an adversary may misrepresent itself to get access to these lists. Under those conditions, the data custodian's ability to estimate $_j\theta_j$ is important.

The data custodian must then choose a type of derived risk to compute from the individual $_j\theta_j$ values. The final equations and risk values for the example in Figure 16.4 are shown in Table 16.6 assuming $\tau = 0.33$.

Table 16.6 Computation of All Three Types of Derived Journalist Risk Metrics for Our Example under the Scenario of the DF Being a Proper Subset of the Identification Database

Derived Risk Metric	Equation	Risk Value
$_jR_a$	$\dfrac{1}{n}\sum_{j\in J} f_j \times I\left(\dfrac{1}{F_j} > \tau\right)$	0
$_jR_b$	$\max_{j\in J}\left(\dfrac{1}{F_j}\right) = \dfrac{1}{\min_{j\in J}(F_j)}$	0.25
$_jR_c$	$\max\left(\dfrac{|J|}{\sum_{j\in J} F_j},\ \dfrac{1}{n}\sum_{j\in J}\dfrac{f_j}{F_j}\right)$	0.12

Thus far we have been assuming that the DF is a sample from the identification database. However, there will be many instances where this assumption will not hold, and there will not be a complete overlap of individuals between the DF and the identification database. This is illustrated as scenario (b) in Figure 16.5. The case where the DF is a subset of the identification database is illustrated by scenario (a) in the figure.

Under scenario (b), some of the individuals in the DF also exist in the identification database. This is illustrated in Figure 16.6. We assume that there is some complete population database, say, the census. Then individuals are sampled from the census with equal probability to create the DF, and individuals are sampled

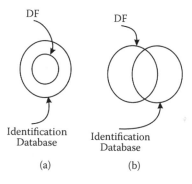

Figure 16.5   Two scenarios for journalist risk.

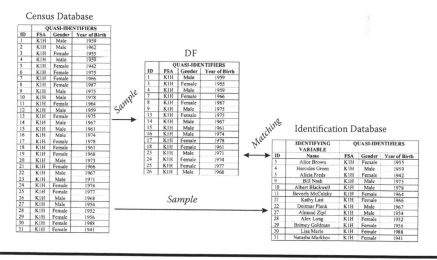

Figure 16.6   An example of matching when the DF and identification database overlap.

from the census, independently of the DF, to create the identification database. The concern is then about the probability of re-identifying an individual.

Let an equivalence class in the census database be denoted by C_j. Then the probability of a random individual in the identification database being correctly matched with the DF is given by $_j\theta_j = 1/C_j$ [9]. The best way to get information about C_j is to count it from published census data or tables, or to use census samples to estimate the value for C_j. If there is another source of information that is more precise than the census for a particular DF, then that can be used as well. Note that with the assumptions of simple random samples, the probability of a correct match is independent of the sampling fraction of the DF or the identification database.

Applying the Derived Metrics and Decision Rules

In the context of de-identification, we often set α to zero; therefore the $_.R_a$ type derived metrics inform us of how many (or what proportion) of records need to be suppressed. For example, if the value of $_.R_a = 0.053$, then it means just over 5% of the records would have to be suppressed to ensure that there are no records with a risk higher than τ.

The $_.R_a$ type metrics are complementary to the others. For example, if we have $_.R_b = 0.4$, which is higher than our τ threshold of 0.33, then the $_.R_a = 0.053$ the value tells us that only 5% of the records are leading to this high risk for the whole file.

The $_.R_c$ type derived metrics also have a special interpretation: the average proportion of records in the DF that would be correctly re-identified if the adversary tried to match *all of the records in the DF* with an identification database. With that interpretation these derived metrics give us a measure of how many records, on average, would be re-identified, and we therefore label it as *marketer risk* [4, 10]. There are two marketer risk metrics, $_mR_1$ and $_mR_2$, depending on whether the identification database has exactly the same records and data subjects as the DF.

The full set of metrics is now summarized in Table 16.7.

The appropriate decision rule from Equations (16.2), (16.4), and (16.6) would then be used to decide whether the risk of re-identification is too high. If it is determined that the risk is high, then de-identification methods can be applied to reduce that risk.

Relationship among Metrics

One other point to consider is the relationship among the risk metrics. For the same data sets and thresholds, numerically we have a number of inequalities holding. These inequalities can be useful in practice for deciding which metrics to use.

Because for all $j, f_j \leq F_j$, for $j \in J$ we have $_pR_b \geq {}_jR_b$. And if $I(1/F_j > \tau)$ is true for some fixed j, then $I(1/f_j > \tau)$ must also be true, but not vice versa, which means $_pR_a \geq {}_jR_a$.

Table 16.7   Summary of the Re-Identification Risk Metrics

Risk Type	Equation	Notes and Conditions
Prosecutor	$$_pR_a = \frac{1}{n}\sum_{j\in J} f_j \times I\left(\frac{1}{f_j} > \tau\right)$$ $$_pR_b = \frac{1}{\min_{j\in J}(f_j)}$$ $$_pR_c = \frac{|J|}{n}$$	Where f_j is the size of the equivalence class in the DF. If the DF is the same as the whole population, then $f_j = F_j$, where F_j is the equivalence class size in the population.
Journalist	$$_jR_a = \frac{1}{n}\sum_{j\in J} f_j \times I\left(\frac{1}{F_j} > \tau\right)$$ $$_jR_b = \frac{1}{\min_{j\in J}(F_j)}$$ $$_jR_c = \max\left(\frac{|J|}{\sum_{j\in J} F_j}, \frac{1}{n}\sum_{j\in J}\frac{f_j}{F_j}\right)$$	These metrics are suitable for the situation where the DF is a proper subset of the identification database. The value of which would have to be estimated by the data custodian unless the whole population registry is readily available, in which case can just be counted.
Marketer	$$_mR_1 = \frac{|J|}{N}$$	This metric is suitable when matching all records in two databases; then $n = N$ (i.e., the adversary has access to an identification database with records on exactly the same individuals as in the DF).
	$$_mR_2 = \frac{1}{n}\sum_{j\in J}\frac{f_j}{F_j}$$	This metric is suitable for the situation where $n < N$ and the disclosed data set is a proper subset of the identification database ($J \subseteq K$). The value of $1/F_j$ would have to be estimated by the data custodian unless the whole population registry is readily available, in which case F_j can just be counted. This gives the (average) proportion of records in the DF that would be correctly matched.

Also, we have [4]

$$\frac{1}{n}\sum_j \frac{f_j}{F_j} \leq \left(\frac{1}{\min_j(F_j)}, \frac{\sum_j f_j}{n} \right) = \frac{1}{\min_j(F_j)} \tag{16.11}$$

which means that $_jR_b \geq {}_jR_c$.
When $n = N$, we have

$$|J| \times \min_{j \in J}(f_j) \leq N$$

which means that $_pR_b \geq {}_mR_1$. Also,

$$|J| \times \min_{j \in J}(F_j) \leq N$$

which means $_jR_b \geq {}_mR_1$, and

$$|J| \times \min_{j \in J}(f_j) \leq n$$

which means $_pR_b \geq {}_pR_c$. Finally,

$$\frac{|J|}{\sum_{j \in J} F_j} \geq \frac{|J|}{N} \quad \text{and} \quad \frac{|J|}{n} \geq \frac{|J|}{N}$$

which leads us to $_jR_c \geq {}_mR_1$ and $_pR_c \geq {}_mR_1$. Because

$$\sum_{j \in J} F_j \geq n, \text{ then } \frac{|J|}{\sum_{j \in J} F_j} \geq \frac{|J|}{n}$$

and $_pR_c \geq {}_jR_c$.

Therefore by comparing the possible values, in summary we have

$$_pR_b \geq {_pR_c} \geq {_jR_c} \geq {_mR_1} \geq {_mR_2}$$

$$_pR_b \geq {_jR_b} \geq {_jR_c} \tag{16.12}$$

$$_pR_a \geq {_jR_a}$$

The primary importance of these relationships is that if the custodian determines that more than one type of risk needs to be managed, then these relationships can help decide which metrics to actually compute and which risks to manage.

References

1. El Emam K, Dankar F. Protecting privacy using k-anonymity. *Journal of the American Medical Informatics Association*, 2008; 15:627–637.
2. Benitez K, Malin B. Evaluating re-identification risks with respect to the HIPAA Privacy Rule. *Journal of the American Medical Informatics Association*, 2010; 17(2):169–177.
3. File T. *Voting and registration in the election of November 2006*. U.S. Census Bureau, 2008.
4. Dankar F, El Emam K. A method for evaluating marketer re-identification risk. Proceedings of the 3rd International Workshop on Privacy and Anonymity in the Information Society, 2010.
5. El Emam K, Jabbouri S, Sams S, Drouet Y, Power M. Evaluating common de-identification heuristics for personal health information. *Journal of Medical Internet Research*, 2006; 8(4):e28. PMID: 17213047.
6. Bell S. Alleged LTTE front had voter lists. *National Post*, July 22, 2006.
7. Bell S. Privacy chief probes how group got voter lists. *National Post*, July 25, 2006.
8. Freeze C, Clark C. Voters lists "most disturbing" items seized in Tamil raids, documents say. *Globe and Mail*, May 7, 2008. http://www.theglobeandmail.com/servlet/story/RTGAM.20080507.wxtamilssb07/BNStory/National/home. Archived at http://www.webcitation.org/5Xe4UWJKP.
9. El Emam K, Paton D, Dankar F, Koru G. De-identifying a public use microdata file from the Canadian National Discharge Abstract Database. *BMC Medical Informatics and Decision Making* 2011; 11(53).
10. El Emam K. Risk-based de-identification of health data. *IEEE Security and Privacy*, 2010; 8(3):64–67.

Chapter 17

Measures of Uniqueness

The uniqueness of individuals means that they are in an equivalence class of size one, and is often used as a measure of re-identification risk [1–6]. For example, if a woman is the only 92-year-old in her ZIP code, because she lives in a college town, then she would be considered unique in the population.

We first describe common uniqueness metrics and then explain the differences between uniqueness and the metrics that we have described in the previous chapter.

Uniqueness under Prosecutor Risk

In situations where prosecutor risk applies, uniqueness is measured as the proportion of records in the disclosed data set that are unique. For example, consider Table 17.1, which shows an adversary with some background information about Alice Smith. The adversary is attempting to find her record in a disclosed prescription records database. Alice is female and was born in 1987. In this case there is a single record that matches Alice's information. If the adversary knew that Alice was in the DF (as you may recall, this is a condition for prosecutor risk to apply), then the adversary would know with certainty that Alice's record was found. The metric that is often used is the proportion of records in the disclosed data set that are unique:

$$U_1 = \frac{1}{n} \sum_{j \in J} I\left(f_j = 1\right) \tag{17.1}$$

Table 17.1 Prescription Records DF where Alice is Unique, Example 1

Quasi-Identifiers		
Gender	*Year of Birth*	*Drug Identification Number (DIN)*
Male	1959	02172100
Male	1962	00015547
Female	1955	02239607
Male	1959	02239766
Female	1942	02236974
Female	1975	02357593
Female	1966	02238282
Female	1987	02298538
Male	1975	01989944
Male	1978	02017849
Female	1964	02043394
Male	1959	02248088
Female	1975	02091879
Male	1967	02184478

The decision rule for this metric is based on how large this proportion can be

$$D_1 = \begin{cases} HIGH, & U_1 > \chi \\ LOW, & U_1 \le \chi \end{cases} \tag{17.2}$$

Often the value of χ is set to zero or close to zero such that no or few uniques are acceptable in the disclosed data set.

The first difference between uniqueness metrics and our metrics is that the former only consider situations where re-identification is certain, whereas even if the probability of re-identification is uncertain (i.e., below 1), it can still be unacceptably high.

Consider a different DF in Table 17.2. In this case there are two females who were born in 1987. Now the record that matches Alice is not unique, and would therefore not be considered a high-risk record, and would not be counted at all

Table 17.2   Prescription Records DF where Alice is Not Unique, Example 2

Quasi-Identifiers		
Gender	*Year of Birth*	*Drug Identification Number (DIN)*
Male	1959	02172100
Male	1962	00015547
Female	1955	02239607
Male	1959	02239766
Female	1942	02236974
Female	1975	02357593
Female	1966	02238282
Female	1987	02298538
Male	1975	01989944
Male	1978	02017849
Female	1964	02043394
Male	1959	02248088
Female	1987	02091879
Male	1967	02184478

under Equation (17.1). But Alice has a 0.5 probability of being correctly matched to her record, which would be considered a high risk by most standards.

Therefore if a data set fails on the uniqueness criterion (i.e., the risk is high), then by definition the risk on our prosecutor risk metrics will also be high. However, if the uniqueness risk is low, that does not necessarily mean that it will also be low on our prosecutor risk metrics.

Uniqueness under Journalist Risk

A number of different uniqueness metrics have been proposed under the journalist risk assumptions [7]. Under journalist risk, a record that is unique in the disclosed data set is not necessarily unique in the population data set (as represented by an identification database). Therefore one metric considers the probability that a sample unique is also unique in the identification database:

$$U_2 = \frac{\sum_{j \in J} I\left(f_j = 1, F_j = 1\right)}{\sum_{j \in J} I\left(f_j = 1\right)} \tag{17.3}$$

In this case the numerator is the number of records that are both unique in the DF and unique in the population. The decision rule for this metric is based on how large this probability can be

$$D_2 = \begin{cases} HIGH, & U_1 > \omega \\ LOW, & U_1 \leq \omega \end{cases} \tag{17.4}$$

Note that the values for χ and ω have different interpretations. The former is the maximum acceptable proportion of uniques in the DF, while the latter pertains to the maximum proportion of uniques in the data set (sample uniques) that are also unique in the population (identification database).

However, the denominator for this risk metric considers only the number of records that are unique in the disclosed data set, which ignores the risk from the remaining records in the data set. For example, consider a 1,000-record data set where there are only two unique records, and they are both also unique in the identification database. In this case $U_2 = 1$, indicating that all records are at risk, when in fact only 2 out of 1,000 records are at risk due to uniqueness.

The use of the U_2 metric is sometimes justified by the argument that a smart adversary would focus on the sample unique records, and therefore we need to be concerned about these. However, even if we eliminate all sample uniques that are population uniques in the DF (i.e., $U_2 = 0$), an adversary can still have a very high probability of a successful match.

A more appropriate risk metric would then be:

$$U_3 = \frac{\sum_{j \in J} I\left(f_j = 1, F_j = 1\right)}{n} \tag{17.5}$$

In the 1,000-record example, this would give a risk of $U_2 = 0.002$, which corresponds to what one would expect intuitively. In this case we would use a decision rule similar to D_1, except that the threshold signifies the proportion of records that are at risk due to population uniqueness.

Another proposed metric still considers sample uniques only, but computes the probability of a correct match given that the identification database equivalence class may not be unique. Under one method of attack the adversary selects a record from the identification database and tries to match it with the disclosed data set [7]:

$$U_4 = \frac{\sum_{j \in J} I\left(f_j = 1\right)}{\sum_{j \in J} F_j I\left(f_j = 1\right)} \tag{17.6}$$

Alternatively, if the adversary selects a record from the disclosed data set and tries to match it with the identification database, we get:

$$U_5 = \frac{\sum_{j \in J} \left(I\left(f_j = 1\right) \Big/ F_j \right)}{\sum_{j \in J} I\left(f_j = 1\right)} \tag{17.7}$$

It is easy to show that both Equations (17.6) and (17.7) are special cases of the $_jR_c$ metric we discussed in the previous chapter when we focus only on sample uniques.

Summary

All of the uniqueness metrics only consider the unique records in the disclosed data set as having any re-identification risk, which will underestimate the overall re-identification risk for the disclosed data compared to the earlier metrics. This means that if they are high, then they can be informative, but if they are low, they would not be very informative by themselves.

In general, if risk is managed according to our risk metrics framework, then risk from uniqueness is also managed. Therefore there is no particular reason to focus on uniqueness by itself, since it is not a sufficient criterion to protect against identity disclosure.

On the other hand, estimating uniqueness under the journalist risk is a challenging statistical problem. This is particularly true when the sampling fractions are small or when the percentage of population uniques (in the identification database) is very high. In practice, this means that when our journalist risk metrics are operationalized, it may be necessary to consider uniqueness estimators in the decision rules as well.

References

1. Bethlehem J, Keller W, Pannekoek J. Disclosure control of microdata. *Journal of the American Statistical Association*, 1990; 85(409):38–45.
2. Sweeney L. Uniqueness of simple demographics in the US population. Carnegie Mellon University, Laboratory for International Data Privacy, 2000.
3. El Emam K, Brown A, Abdelmalik P. Evaluating predictors of geographic area population size cutoffs to manage re-identification risk. *Journal of the American Medical Informatics Association*, 2009; 16(2):256–266. PMID: 19074299.
4. Golle P. Revisiting the uniqueness of simple demographics in the US population. Workshop on Privacy in the Electronic Society, 2006.
5. El Emam K, Brown A, AbdelMalik P, Neisa A, Walker M, Bottomley J, Roffey T. A method for managing re-identification risk from small geographic areas in Canada. *BMC Medical Informatics and Decision Making*, 2010; 10(18).
6. Koot M, Noordende G, de Laat C. A study on the re-identifiability of Dutch citizens. Workshop on Privacy Enhancing Technologies (PET 2010), 2010.
7. Skinner G, Elliot M. A measure of disclosure risk for microdata. *Journal of the Royal Statistical Society (Series B)*, 2002; 64(Part 4):855–867.

Chapter 18

Modeling the Threat

This chapter describes how to model the threat from a re-identification attack. By modeling the threat we mean deciding on the final set of equations to use for measuring the risk of re-identification, and deciding on the list of quasi-identifiers in the data set.

The risk equations we presented earlier do not take into account the context of the disclosure. The context will modify the risk calculations significantly, and it provides a more realistic assessment of the overall risk.

Characterizing the Adversaries

We will start off by describing a set of general criteria that can be used to characterize an adversary. These criteria are good background information for some of the forthcoming analyses.

A useful way to categorize adversaries is in terms of how constrained they are. Five types of constraints to be considered are summarized below. Some of these were touched upon when we discussed the various definitions of identifiability in Chapter 12:

- **Financial constraints:** How much money will the adversary spend on a re-identification attack? Costs will be incurred to acquire databases (see the discussion in Chapter 16).

  Costs may also be incurred by the adversary when trying to verify that a particular re-identification has been successful. We know that the vast majority of publicly acknowledged re-identification attacks were verified [1].

- **Time constraints:** How much time will the adversary spend to acquire registries useful for a re-identification attack? For example, let's say that one of the registries that the adversary could use is the discharge abstract database from hospitals. Forty-eight states in the United States collect data on inpatients [2], and 26 states make their state inpatient databases (SIDs) available through the Agency for Healthcare Research and Quality (AHRQ) [3]. The SIDs for the remaining states would also be available directly from each individual state, but the process is more complicated and time-consuming. Would an adversary satisfy itself only with the AHRQ states, or would it put in the time to get the data from other states as well?

- **Willingness to misrepresent itself:** To what extent will the adversary be willing to misrepresent itself to get access to public or semipublic registries? For example, some states only make their voter registration lists available to political parties or candidates (e.g., California) [4]. Would an adversary be willing to misrepresent itself to get these lists? Also, some registries are available at a lower cost for academic use versus commercial use. Would an adversary misrepresent itself as an academic to reduce its registry acquisition costs?

- **Willingness to violate agreements:** To what extent would the adversary be willing to violate data sharing agreements or other contracts that it needs to sign to get access to registries? For example, acquiring the SIDs through the AHRQ requires that the recipient sign a data sharing agreement that prohibits re-identification attempts. Would the adversary still attempt a re-identification even after signing such an agreement?

- **Willingness to commit illegal acts:** To what extent would an adversary break the law to obtain access to registries that can be used for re-identification? For example, as noted earlier, privacy legislation and the Elections Act in Canada restrict the use of voter lists to running and supporting election activities [5]. There is at least one known case where a charity allegedly supporting a terrorist group has been able to obtain Canadian voter lists through deception for fund-raising purposes [6–8]. Although this was not a re-identification attack, it does demonstrate that adversaries can obtain voter registration lists from volunteers in election campaigns even if this is not allowed.

We can consider some examples where these criteria can be applied. If a DF will be disclosed publicly, say, as a public use file on the web, then we can examine a number of different adversaries.

First, there are the adversaries who would perform a demonstration attack on the data. These adversaries are interested in showing that an attack is possible. The motives for performing a demonstration attack vary, from embarrassing the data custodian, to illustrating a new attack method that they have developed, to gaining notoriety. A key characteristic of a demonstration attack is that it must be publicized to achieve its objective. All known demonstration re-identification attacks were performed by researchers or the media [9–20] (see the systematic review in [1]). This type of adversary is likely highly constrained with limited time and funds, an unwillingness to misrepresent itself, and an unwillingness to violate agreements and contracts.

In theory, one may assume that because of these constraints, a demonstration attack will not be performed on a data set that was part of a data breach, for instance, if a data recipient's network is hacked and a database is leaked on the Internet, or if an employee of the data recipient inadvertently posts the information online. However, it would not always be prudent to make such an assumption. Security researchers and professionals have sometimes used data sets that have been part of a data breach. A good example would be the use of stolen password lists that are posted on the Internet by security researchers and professionals. In the case of health data, it would seem unlikely that, say, a researcher would use a breached data set. There is a qualitative difference between unattributed password lists and individuals' health data.

Second are adversaries who would use the public data for commercial purposes. If the financial value of the data is high, then there would be ample reasons for these adversaries to put significant time and money into a re-identification attack. One can assume that such adversaries would not commit illegal acts.

For data sets that are public, however, there would also be expected to be adversaries out there who are willing to misrepresent themselves and commit illegal acts. Since the data are public, the data custodian cannot control what potential adversaries will do.

As another example, corporations that receive health data where they have had to sign a data sharing agreement prohibiting re-identification attempts as a condition for getting the data are not likely to attempt a re-identification attack; i.e., they would be unlikely to violate the agreement. Whether everyone within the corporation would follow the stipulations in the agreement will depend on the strength of the policies and their enforcement within the corporation. Just signing the agreement is a good start, but without internal processes to enforce the corporation's obligations, it would be difficult to fully trust that there would not be a re-identification attack by someone within the corporation.

Attempting a Re-Identification Attack

In the previous chapters we examined different metrics for assessing re-identification risk. However, these metrics do not take into account the attack scenario. We now consider plausible attack scenarios and adjust the metrics accordingly.

We need to capture the probability that the adversary will attempt to launch a re-identification attack. This determination is important because it allows us to more realistically model the overall re-identification probability.

The overall probability of re-identification can be expressed as [21]:

$$pr\left(re-identification, attempt\right) = pr\left(re-identification \middle| attempt\right) \times pr\left(attempt\right) \quad (18.1)$$

This means that the overall probability of re-identification will depend on whether an adversary will attempt re-identification to start off with. Quantifying *pr*(*attempt*) is difficult and is often not even attempted [21]. However, it may be possible to narrow down the possible range of values under different circumstances, as we discuss below.

To simplify notation, we will use the following from now on:

$$pr\left(re-identification\right) = pr\left(re-identification\middle|attempt\right) \times pr\left(attempt\right) \quad (18.2)$$

This should be understood to be the probability of an attempt and a re-identification.

In some risk assessments the authors assumed that *pr*(*attempt*) = 0 because there were no known re-identification attacks by an adversary on the specific type of DF [21]. We cannot make that very general assumption because a recent review of successful re-identification attacks on health data revealed that attacks on health data sets have occurred [1]; therefore we know that in some situations *pr*(*attempt*) > 0, and it is important to understand and model these. Other researchers in this area have noted that it is common, for the purposes of risk assessments, to assume that *pr*(*attempt*) = 1 [22]. Again, such a general assumption is not warranted because there will be situations where the value of *pr*(*attempt*) will be smaller than 1.

As is evident from Equation (18.2), the value of *pr*(*attempt*) is important for quantifying the overall risk. If it is low, then the overall re-identification probability could be reduced considerably, making an initially high risk acceptable.

Plausible Adversaries

We can now define two general classes of adversaries: (1) internal and (2) external. An internal adversary is one who is part of the staff at a known data recipient. An external one is outside the data recipient or unknown if the data are publicly available.

If a DF is used by or disclosed to a known data recipient, then both an internal and an external adversary are plausible. A known data recipient would be, for example, a researcher or a business partner. An internal adversary would be the researcher herself or a staff member of the researcher. If the data recipient is a business partner, then an internal adversary could be staff working for the business partner, say, employees or consultants.

An adversary is considered internal if there is no data breach at the data recipient. Should a data breach occur and the data become exposed external to the data recipient, then we need to worry about external adversaries. If the DF is disclosed publicly, say, as part of an open data initiative, then we would only worry about an external adversary.

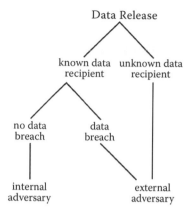

Figure 18.1   A decision tree to determine the type of adversary.

The determination of whether an adversary is internal or external is illustrated in the decision tree of Figure 18.1. This is a decision tree to determine which type of adversary is relevant and will drive the decision on which metrics to use.

An Internal Adversary

There are two general scenarios for a re-identification attack when the adversary is considered internal to the data recipient. The first scenario is when the data recipient deliberately attempts to re-identify the DF. If there is no contract or data sharing agreement between the data custodian and the data recipient prohibiting re-identification attacks, then one can assume that it is plausible that an internal adversary will attempt to re-identify the data. Not assuming that the data recipient will attempt a re-identification when it has no legal constraints on doing so would be naïve and difficult to defend. In such a case we can set $pr(attempt) = 1$ in Equation (18.2), and we can focus on the $pr(re\text{-}identification|attempt)$ term.

If there is a data sharing agreement in place, then the probability of a re-identification attempt will be reduced. How much this reduction would be will depend on how well the adversary is able to enforce the agreement and, in general, enforce good practices internally. This brings us back to the concept of "mitigating controls" that was discussed earlier. The stronger the mitigating controls that are in place, the lower the probability $pr(attempt)$. But also the "motives and capacity" dimension is important since if the internal adversary has no motive or technical or financial capacity to launch a re-identification attack, then the probability of an attempt would be low.

One way to model the relationship between "mitigating controls" and "motives and capacity" with the probability of a re-identification attack is to rely on subjective

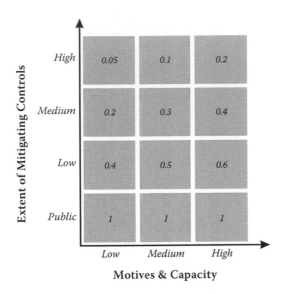

Figure 18.2 Matrix used to compute appropriate thresholds based on overall risk.

expert estimates. In the context of risk assessments, the use of subjective expert estimates is common [23]. To determine the value for $pr(attempt)$, we can use a matrix as shown in Figure 18.2. This matrix subjectively captures the likelihood that a re-identification attempt will be made. The values within the matrix were chosen to be consistent with precedents. As shown in Chapter 25, there are strong precedents for values of $pr(re\text{-}identification|attempt)$. These are re-identification probability values that have been used to disclose personal data under many different circumstances over the last couple of decades. Consistency with these precedents meant that the values in the matrix were chosen to ensure that $pr(re\text{-}identification)$ was below the various thresholds that are discussed in subsequent chapters.

Admittedly, the matrix in Figure 18.2 errs more on the conservative side. For example, if we characterize academic health researchers as having a "medium" value for mitigating controls and a "low" value for "motives and capacity," the matrix suggests that one in five will attempt a re-identification—this may be the researcher or her staff. There is evidence that health researchers do participate in re-identification attacks (see the comments in [1]), and therefore we know that $pr(attempt)$ should not be zero under these conditions. However, assuming that one in five health researchers will deliberately attempt an attack is also quite pessimistic. On the other hand, using a "cell size of five" rule, which is often applied in practice today (see the review in Chapter 25), also means that $pr(re\text{-}identification|attempt) \times pr(attempt) =$ 0.04, which is quite low.

The chapters in Section V of the book include the checklists for scoring these two dimensions and determining whether they are "low," "medium," or "high." That scoring mechanism has considerable face validity, as it has been in use in practice for the last five years.

If a data recipient is going to deliberately re-identify records in a DF, then she may attempt to re-identify as many records as possible. Alternatively, the data recipient may wish to perform a demonstration attack to embarrass the data custodian, in which case the re-identification of a single record would be sufficient. The risk metrics that the data custodian would then use are shown in Table 18.1. Sidebar 18.1 also provides an example where this approach is used to manage the re-identification risk for a population registry.

Table 18.1 Summary of the Re-Identification Risk Metrics when an Internal Adversary Deliberately Re-Identifies an Individual in a DF

Risk Type	Equation
Prosecutor	$$_pR_a = \frac{1}{n}\sum_{j\in J} f_j \times I\left(\left(\frac{1}{f_j} \times pr(attempt)\right) > \tau\right)$$ $$_pR_b = \frac{1}{\min_{j\in J}(f_j)} \times pr(attempt)$$ $$_pR_c = \frac{|J|}{n} \times pr(attempt)$$
Journalist	$$_jR_a = \frac{1}{n}\sum_{j\in J} f_j \times I\left(\left(\frac{1}{F_j} \times pr(attempt)\right) > \tau\right)$$ $$_jR_b = \frac{1}{\min_{j\in J}(F_j)} \times pr(attempt)$$ $$_jR_c = \max\left(\frac{|J|}{\sum_{j\in J} F_j}, \frac{1}{n}\sum_{j\in J}\frac{f_j}{F_j}\right) \times pr(attempt)$$
Marketer	$$_mR_1 = \frac{|J|}{N} \times pr(attempt)$$ $$_mR_2 = \frac{1}{n}\sum_{j\in J}\frac{f_j}{F_j} \times pr(attempt)$$

Sidebar 18.1: Re-Identification Risk for the BORN Registry with an Internal Adversary Who Deliberately Attempts a Re-Identification Attack

The BORN registry is a population registry of all births in the province of Ontario. That data set is disclosed to researchers mostly. All researchers are required to sign a data sharing agreement prohibiting re-identification. Therefore all data recipients are known. However, because of the wide variation of security and privacy practices at the researcher labs and institutions, the "mitigating controls" score is assumed to be medium. We also consider that the "motives and capacity" of Ontario researchers to re-identify a data set would be low. According to our risk matrix in Figure 18.2, we then use a value $pr(attempt) = 0.2$ when disclosing data from this population registry to researchers.

A plausible attack scenario is an adversary who is deliberately trying to re-identify an individual in the BORN DF. The target individual can be, say, a famous person who is known to have had a baby. Because all births are recorded in the registry, the appropriate risk metrics to use are prosecutor risk metrics rather than journalist risk metrics.

Taking a conservative approach, we can consider the maximum risk $_pR_b$. For data extracts that are not considered sensitive (i.e., the maternal health information does not contain any sensitive values), the data extracts are de-identified to ensure that for all j that $f_j \geq 5$. Therefore from Equation (18.2) we have $_pR_b = 0.2 \times 0.2 = 0.04$ as the overall risk of re-identification for the first attack scenario with an internal adversary.

For data extracts that are considered particularly sensitive, we set $f_j \geq 10$. With this value we have $_pR_b = 0.1 \times 0.2 = 0.02$ as the overall probability of a successful deliberate re-identification attack from an internal adversary.

If instead we consider the average risk, $_pR_c$, then we obtain a different result. Average risk is justified because the data custodian does not know which equivalence class will match the famous person's; then the risk across all equivalence classes can be considered.

Let us consider a DF with three quasi-identifiers: baby's date of birth, postal code, and mother's age. Where the baby's date of birth is generalized to month/year, the postal code to the first three characters, and the mother's age generalized to a five-year interval and top coded at 45 years and bottom coded at 19 years, the value calculated from an extract of the registry is $|J|/n = 0.2$. Therefore the overall risk is given by $_pR_c = 0.2 \times 0.2 = 0.04$. The risk values for prosecutor risk will by definition always be equal to or greater than marketer risk. Therefore managing prosecutor risk will also manage marketer risk.

The second scenario for the internal adversary is when someone employed by the data recipient spontaneously recognizes someone he or she knows in the DF. This individual would be someone who has access to the data, most likely a data analyst. During the analysis of the DF this individual recognizes a record belonging to someone in his or her circle of acquaintances. This can be modeled as

$$pr\left(re-identification\right) = pr\left(re-identification\,|\,acquaintance\right) \times pr\left(acquaintance\right) \quad (18.3)$$

where $pr(acquaintance)$ is the probability of the adversary having an acquaintance potentially in the data set. We assume that the adversary will also know the quasi-identifiers about this acquaintance. In this case we do not consider the probability of a re-identification attempt because the adversary is not attempting to launch an attack: This would be an inadvertent or accidental recognition of someone in the DF.

Let us consider an example where a data custodian is disclosing a cancer data set to a researcher. We then let

$$pr\left(acquaintance\right) = 1 - \left(1 - p\right)^m \quad (18.4)$$

where p is the prevalence of the type of cancer in the population, and m the number of people that the adversary knows (the number of acquaintances). Equation (18.4) is the probability that a random adversary knows a person who has that type of cancer. Figures 18.3 and 18.4 show the value for $pr(acquaintance)$ for oral and breast cancer based on prevalence data from the Surveillance Epidemiology and End Results (SEER) registry in the United States. Therefore, for someone who has 200 friends, her probability of having an acquaintance with oral cancer is approximately 0.07. However, for breast cancer, for someone with 200 friends that probability is close to 0.45. Because oral cancer is rarer than breast cancer, it is less likely that a re-identification through this type of attack will be successful because an adversary is less likely to know someone with oral cancer.

Equation (18.4) allows us to incorporate the notion of spontaneous re-identification of a record in the risk assessment. Because a spontaneous attack will affect a single data subject, only prosecutor and journalist risk metrics are relevant for evaluative purposes, and the appropriate risk equations are shown in Table 18.2.

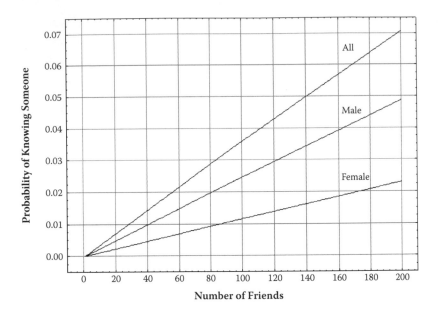

Figure 18.3 **The probability of having an acquaintance with oral cancer based on the number of friends one has.**

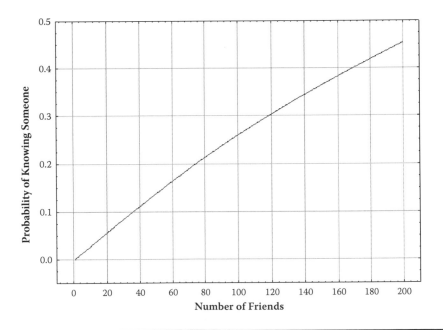

Figure 18.4 **The probability of having an acquaintance with breast cancer (assuming 50% of the friends are female) based on the number of friends one has.**

Modeling the Threat ■ 213

Table 18.2 Summary of the Re-Identification Risk Metrics when an Internal Adversary Spontaneously Re-Identifies an Individual in a DF

Risk Type	Equation
Prosecutor	$$_pR_a = \frac{1}{n}\sum_{j\in J} f_j \times I\left(\left(\frac{1}{f_j}\times\left(1-(1-p)^m\right)\right)>\tau\right)$$ $$_pR_b = \frac{1}{\min_{j\in J}(f_j)}\times\left(1-(1-p)^m\right)$$ $$_pR_c = \frac{|J|}{n}\times\left(1-(1-p)^m\right)$$
Journalist	$$_jR_a = \frac{1}{n}\sum_{j\in J} f_j \times I\left(\left(\frac{1}{F_j}\times\left(1-(1-p)^m\right)\right)>\tau\right)$$ $$_jR_b = \frac{1}{\min_{j\in J}(F_j)}\times\left(1-(1-p)^m\right)$$ $$_jR_c = \max\left(\frac{|J|}{\sum_{j\in J}F_j}, \frac{1}{n}\sum_{j\in J}\frac{f_j}{F_j}\right)\times\left(1-(1-p)^m\right)$$

A review of the literature on how many friends an individual would have is presented in Chapter 24. We assume that in order to know intimate health information about an acquaintance, that individual would need to be a friend. In general, choosing a value for m between an average of 150 and at the higher confidence interval a defensible value of 190 would fit within the most common estimates that have been produced in the literature. An application of this in the context of the BORN registry is provided in Sidebar 18.2.

Sidebar 18.2: BORN Registry Example of Spontaneous Recognition Risk

Out of all females in Ontario, the prevalence of births is approximately 0.019. If we use Dunbar's number of 150 and assume that half of a person's friends and acquaintances are female, we can set $m = 75$. The probability of an adversary knowing someone who has a baby in any single year is therefore 0.762.

For the case where we use maximum risk, we would need to set $f_j \geq 8$, and then we have $_pR_b = 0.125 \times 0.762 = 0.095$, which would be the risk from spontaneous recognition by a researcher who receives BORN data that are not considered highly sensitive. For data extracts that are considered highly sensitive, the risk calculation for setting $f_j \geq 15$ would be $_pR_b = 0.066 \times 0.762 = 0.05$.

When we consider average risk instead of maximum risk, and a data release where the baby's date of birth is generalized to quarter/year, the postal code to the first three characters, and the mother's age generalized to a ten-year interval and top coded at 45 years and bottom coded at 19 years, the value for $|J|/n = 0.06$, and therefore $_pR_c = 0.06 \times 0.762 = 0.0457$.

An External Adversary

If a data set is disclosed to a known data recipient, then an external adversary would be relevant if there is a data breach and the DF is inadvertently or deliberately exposed outside the data recipient. The appropriate general model would be

$$pr\left(re - identification\right) = pr\left(re - identification \big| breach\right) \times pr\left(breach\right) \quad (18.5)$$

Data for 2010 show that 19% of health care organizations suffered a data breach within the previous year [6]. More recent data for 2012 show that this number has gone up to 27% [7]. Therefore we have an average probability estimate for a breach occurring. The general equations for an external adversary when the data recipient is known are given in Table 18.3.

We can also consider a model such as

$$pr\left(re - identification\right) = pr\left(re - identification \big| breach, acquintance\right) \times$$
$$pr\left(acquaintance \big| breach\right) \times pr\left(breach\right) \quad (18.6)$$

This model accounts for the probability that an adversary would know someone who has the condition or procedure in the DF. However, the probability in Equation (18.6) will always be lower than the probability in Equation (18.5). Therefore we just need to manage the probability in Equation (18.5). An example of the application of risk assessment is provided in Sidebar 18.3.

Table 18.3   Summary of the Re-Identification Risk Metrics for an External Adversary Who Gets Access to the DF through a Breach

Risk Type	Equation
Prosecutor	$${}_pR_a = \frac{1}{n}\sum_{j\in J} f_j \times I\left(\left(\frac{1}{f_j}\times 0.27\right) > \tau\right)$$ $${}_pR_b = \frac{1}{\min_{j\in J}(f_j)}\times 0.27$$ $${}_pR_c = \frac{|J|}{n}\times 0.27$$
Journalist	$${}_jR_a = \frac{1}{n}\sum_{j\in J} f_j \times I\left(\left(\frac{1}{F_j}\times 0.27\right) > \tau\right)$$ $${}_jR_b = \frac{1}{\min_{j\in J}(F_j)}\times 0.27$$ $${}_jR_c = \max\left(\frac{|J|}{\sum_{j\in J}F_j}, \frac{1}{n}\sum_{j\in J}\frac{f_j}{F_j}\right)\times 0.27$$
Marketer	$${}_mR_1 = \frac{|J|}{N}\times 0.27$$ $${}_mR_2 = \frac{1}{n}\sum_{j\in J}\frac{f_j}{F_j}\times 0.27$$

Sidebar 18.3: Registry Breach and an External Adversary

Because BORN is a population registry, we again focus on the ${}_pR_b$ when considering maximum risk.

For a nonsensitive data set we can choose the threshold for the maximum risk to be $f_j \geq 8$ such that ${}_pR_b = 0.125 \times 0.27 = 0.033$, and for a sensitive data set at $f_j \geq 15$ we have ${}_pR_b = 0.0676 \times 0.27 = 0.018$.

When we consider average risk and a data release where the baby's date of birth is generalized to quarter/year, the postal code to the first three characters, and the mother's age generalized to a ten-year interval and top coded at 45 years and bottom coded at 19 years, the value for $_pR_c = 0.06 \times 0.27 = 0.0162$.

Because marketer risk will always be numerically lower than prosecutor risk, if we manage prosecutor risk we also manage marketer risk. We therefore do not consider marketer risk here.

In the case of a data set that has been made publicly available we do not consider breaches any more. In such a case the basic model is similar to Equation (18.1), except that we need to set *pr(attempt)* = 1. In such a case the risk equations are as shown in Table 18.4. For public data where there are no constraints on what can be done with the DF, one must assume that an attempted attack will occur. One ought to also consider that this could be a minimally constrained adversary with unlimited resources and funds who is willing to misrepresent itself and violate agreements and laws.

A summary of the four attacks and their associated equations is given in Table 18.5. In practice, because managing either prosecutor or journalist risk will automatically manage marketer risk, we will generally not directly deal with marketer risk. The marketer risk metrics are included here mostly for completeness.

What Are the Quasi-Identifiers?

In general, quasi-identifiers are variables that can be known by an acquaintance of a data subject or that can exist in a database and become known to an adversary. There are some authors who argue that, essentially, all fields in a database are quasi-identifiers because all fields in a database can be used to re-identify individuals [24]. This very broad argument is a significant oversimplification. For example, some fields are not even known by the patients themselves. Many patients will not know their own exact lab test values to one or two decimal places. That information cannot therefore be shared by the patient through his or her social network (physical or electronic). On the other hand, the lab result may exist in a database that belongs to the health care provider (such as the lab that did the test or the data subject's physician). Whether an adversary can get access to this database needs to be considered.

Other authors argue that only information in public databases should be considered quasi-identifiers [25]. However, this would not account for the knowledge that an adversary may have of acquaintances, as in attack T2. Some of that information would not be public. Also, one cannot discount the availability of commercial, nonpublic databases that can be used in an attack.

Table 18.4   Summary of the Re-Identification Risk Metrics for an External Adversary Who Gets Access to the DF through a Public Release of a Data Set

Risk Type	Equation
Prosecutor	$$_pR_a = \frac{1}{n}\sum_{j\in J} f_j \times I\left(\frac{1}{f_j} > \tau\right)$$ $$_pR_b = \frac{1}{\min_{j\in J}(f_j)}$$ $$_pR_c = \frac{|J|}{n}$$
Journalist	$$_jR_a = \frac{1}{n}\sum_{j\in J} f_j \times I\left(\frac{1}{F_j} > \tau\right)$$ $$_jR_b = \frac{1}{\min_{j\in J}(F_j)}$$ $$_jR_c = \max\left(\frac{|J|}{\sum_{j\in J} F_j}, \frac{1}{n}\sum_{j\in J}\frac{f_j}{F_j}\right)$$
Marketer	$$_mR_1 = \frac{|J|}{N}$$ $$_mR_2 = \frac{1}{n}\sum_{j\in J}\frac{f_j}{F_j}$$

Some examples of commonly used quasi-identifiers are given in Table 18.6 [26–28]. It should be noted that the final set of quasi-identifiers will have to be decided on a case-by-case basis. Examination of plausible sources of data can narrow down the list.

Sources of Data

An adversary may have background knowledge about the data subjects because she knows the data subjects personally, or because these individuals that the adversary is acquainted with have visible characteristics, such as facial wasting or physical

Table 18.5 Summary of the Plausible Attacks on a DF and Associated Risk That Needs to Be Managed

Attack Label	Adversary	Access to DF	Nature of Attack	Equation
T1	Internal	Legitimate	Deliberate	$pr(re-identification|attempt) \times pr(attempt)$ Probability of an attempt is defined through a checklist and a scoring matrix.
T2	Internal	Legitimate	Inadvertent	$pr(re-identification|acquaintance) \times pr(acquaintance)$ $= pr(re-identification|acquaintance) \times 1 - (1-p)^m$
T3	External	Breach	Deliberate	$pr(re-identification|breach) \times pr(breach)$ $= pr(re-identification|breach) \times 0.27$
T4	External	Legitimate	Deliberate	$pr(re-identification)$

Table 18.6 Examples of Common Quasi-Identifiers

Sex	Total income
Date of birth/age	Visible minority status
Geocodes (such as postal codes, census geography, information about proximity to known or unique landmarks, other location information)	Activity difficulties/reductions
	Profession
Home language	Event dates (admission, discharge, procedure, death, specimen collection, visit)
Ethnic origin	Codes (diagnosis, procedure, and adverse event)
Aboriginal identity	
Total years of schooling	Religious denomination
Marital status (legal)	Country of birth
Criminal history	Birth plurality

abnormalities. In such a case the adversary can determine the diagnosis, even at a high level, of the individuals.

The adversary may also be able to obtain private databases. These may be databases in the possession of the adversary, or databases that can be purchased from commercial data brokers. Note that an adversary may combine multiple sources together to construct a database useful for re-identification [26]. It is not necessary for the custodian to acquire all of these registries, but only to know what the variables are in these registries to be able to measure the probability of re-identification. Examples of public and semi-public registries that can be used for re-identification are:

- Voter registration lists, court records, obituaries published in newspapers or online, telephone directories, private property security registries, land registries, and registries of donations to political parties (which often include at least full address).
- Professional and sports associations often post information about their members and teams (e.g., lists of lawyers, doctors, engineers, and teachers with their basic demographics, and information about sports teams with their demographics, height, weight, and other physical and performance characteristics).
- Certain employers often post information about their staff online, for example, at educational and research establishments and at law firms. This is often a marketing exercise, but it does reveal personal information about the employees that can be useful for a re-identification attack.
- Individuals may reveal information about themselves on social networking sites, personal blogs, and Twitter feeds. In general, we would consider information that many people would post about themselves or that is commonly

posted. For example, few people post the Apgar score of their newborn babies on their Facebook wall, but they may tweet the baby's birth weight. If someone, exceptionally, does post an Apgar score, that does not make it a quasi-identifier.

■ Famous people (e.g., politicians and actors) will generally have more details about them (demographics and socioeconomic type of information) available in the public sphere.

For a registry to be useful as a potential source of quasi-identifiers, it must be plausible for the adversary to get access to it. By considering the constraints on the adversary, it is then possible to decide how plausible it is for the adversary to acquire each type of registry and for which province or state. For example, if the data to be disclosed are for patients in California, and it is assumed that the adversary is highly constrained, then the voter registration lists would not be available to the adversary for a re-identification attack (they are only available for parties, candidates, political committees, and scholarly or journalistic purposes). However, if the adversary is expected to misrepresent itself, then the adversary may pretend to be, say, a journalist and obtain the voter registration list for a re-identification attack.

We would generally not consider whether a characteristic is rare or not when deciding whether a particular variable is a quasi-identifier. This is an important point because it has been common practice to remove records with rare diagnoses during the de-identification process. For example, some diagnoses are rare. Their probability of re-identification will therefore be high. It is not necessary to pull these out explicitly and treat them in a different manner, as this rareness will be evident in the computed probability values.

Correlated and Inferred Variables

When selecting quasi-identifiers out of the set of variables in a data set, there are two issues that one must be aware of: correlated variables and inferences.

Correlated variables may occur within the same data set. For example, a birth registry may have the date of birth of the baby and the date of discharge. These two variables will be highly correlated. The date of birth of the baby is an obvious quasi-identifier. But it is important to select the date of discharge also as a quasi-identifier. The reason is that if the date of birth is generalized or is suppressed for a particular patient, a more specific value can be determined from the date of discharge, or can be imputed from the date of discharge. Another similar example occurs with the correlation between date of death and date of autopsy.

Correlations also occur across domains. For example, a health care professional can determine the drugs that a patient is likely to take from his or her diagnosis, and to some extent vice versa as well. Therefore generalization or suppression of pharmacy data may not be effective if diagnosis data are retained in the DF. In such a case both of those fields would need to be generalized or suppressed in a compatible way to confound predicting one from the other. It should be kept in mind that many pieces of information in a medical record will be correlated.

Another concern is inferences. If a field in the DF can be inferred from other information not in the DF, then that field should be considered a quasi-identifier. These can take multiple forms. An adversary can make inferences from the data set itself. Examples of inferences would be age and gender from a diagnosis or lab test code (for example, some lab tests are only performed on men or women often within a particular age range), age from year of graduation, and profession from payer (for professions that have a single insurer).

It may also be possible to make inferences about the data using general knowledge. For example, if a piece of general knowledge is that Japanese women are unlikely to have a heart attack, then that information can be used to narrow down the records that belong to a target data subject who is a Japanese woman. Under these circumstances, the diagnosis field would need to be considered a quasi-identifier to thwart such inferences.

References

1. El Emam K, Jonker E, Arbuckle L, Malin B. A systematic review of re-identification attacks on health data. *PLoS ONE*, 2011; 6(12):e28071.
2. Consumer-Purchaser Disclosure Project. *The state experience in health quality data collection.* 2004.
3. El Emam K, Mercer J, Moreau K, Grava-Gubins I, Buckeridge D, Jonker E. Physician privacy concerns when disclosing patient data for public health purposes during a pandemic influenza outbreak. *BMC Public Health*, 2010 (under second review).
4. Benitez K, Malin B. Evaluating re-identification risks with respect to the HIPAA privacy rule. *Journal of the American Medical Informatics Association*, 2010; 17(2):169–177.
5. El Emam K, Jabbouri S, Sams S, Drouet Y, Power M. Evaluating common de-identification heuristics for personal health information. *Journal of Medical Internet Research*, 2006; 8(4):e28. PMID: 17213047.
6. Bell S. Alleged LTTE front had voter lists. *National Post*, July 22, 2006.
7. Bell S. Privacy chief probes how group got voter lists. *National Post*, July 25, 2006.
8. Freeze C, Clark C. Voters lists "most disturbing" items seized in Tamil raids, documents say. *Globe and Mail*, May 7, 2008. http://www.theglobeandmail.com/servlet/story/RTGAM.20080507.wxtamilssb07/BNStory/National/home. Archived at http://www.webcitation.org/5Xe4UWJKP.
9. Bender S, Brand R, Bacher J. Re-identifying register data by survey data: An empirical study. *Statistical Journal of the United Nations*, 2001; ECE 18:373–381.
10. Narayanan A, Shmatikov V. Robust de-anonymization of large sparse datasets. Proceedings of the 2008 IEEE Symposium on Security and Privacy, 2008.
11. Frankowski D, Cosley D, Sen S, Terveen L, Riedl J. You are what you say: Privacy risks of public mentions. In *SIGIR '06*. Seattle: ACM, 2006.

12. Ochoa S, Rasmussen J, Robson C, Salib M. Reidentification of individuals in Chicago's homicide database: A technical and legal study. 2001. http://groups.csail.mit.edu/mac/classes/6.805/student-papers/spring01-papers/reidentification.doc. Archived at http://www.webcitation.org/5x9yE1e7L.

13. Supreme Court of the State of Illinois. *Southern Illinoisan v. the Illinois Department of Public Health*. 2006.

14. Gordin M and the Minister of Health and the Privacy Commissioner of Canada. Memorandum of fact and law of the privacy commissioner of Canada. Federal Court, 2007.

15. Elliot M. *The evaluation of risk from identification attempts*, 1–29. Manchester: University of Manchester, 2003.

16. El Emam K, Kosseim P. Privacy interests in prescription data, part II. *IEEE Security and Privacy*, 2009; 7(2):75–78.

17. Brownstein J, Cassa C, Mandl K. No place to hide—Reverse identification of patients from published maps. *New England Journal of Medicine*, 2006; 355(16):1741–1742.

18. Barbaro M, Zeller Jr. T90. A face is exposed for AOL searcher no. 4417749. *New York Times*, August 9, 2006.

19. Backstrom L, Dwork C, Kleinberg J. Wherefore art thou R3579X? Anonymized social networks, hidden patterns, and structural steganography. WWW 2007. Banff: ACM, 2007.

20. Narayanan A, Shmatikov V. De-anonymizing social networks. *Proceedings of the 30th IEEE Symposium on Security and Privacy* 2009; 173–187.

21. Marsh C, Skinner C, Arber S, Penhale B, Openshaw S, Hobcraft J, Lievesley D, Walford N. The case for samples of anonymized records from the 1991 census. *Journal of the Royal Statistical Society, Series A (Statistics in Society)*, 1991; 154(2):305–340.

22. Elliot M, Dale A. Scenarios of attack: The data intruder's perspective on statistical disclosure risk. *Netherlands Official Statistics*, 1999; 14(Spring):6–10.

23. Vose D. *Quantitative risk analysis: A guide to Monte Carlo simulation modeling*. New York: John Wiley & Sons, 1996.

24. Narayanan A, Shmatikov V. Myths and fallacies of "personally identifiable information." *Communications of the ACM*, 2010; 53(6):24–26. DOI: 10.1145/1743546.1743558.

25. Yakowitz J. *Tragedy of the commons*. Social Sciences Research Network, 2011. http://ssrn.com/abstract=1789749.

26. El Emam K, Jonker E, Sams S, Neri E, Neisa A, Gao T, Chowdhury S. *Pan-Canadian de-identification guidelines for personal health information*. 2007. http://www.ehealthinformation.ca/documents/OPCReportv11.pdf. Archived at http://www.webcitation.org/5Ow1Nko5C.

27. El Emam K, Brown A, Abdelmalik P. Evaluating predictors of geographic area population size cutoffs to manage re-identification risk. *Journal of the American Medical Informatics Association*, 2009; 16(2):256–266. PMID: 19074299.

28. ISO/TS 25237. *Health informatics: Pseudonymization*. Geneva: International Organization for Standardization, 2008.

Chapter 19

Choosing Metric Thresholds

Using the re-identification metrics and decision rules outlined previously requires that certain thresholds are set. In this chapter we will provide some guidance on setting thresholds for identity disclosure decision rules. Privacy statutes and regulations do not provide an explicit definition of what is an acceptable risk of re-identification. As noted earlier, many statutes use a reasonableness standard. For example, Ontario's PHIPA states that "identifying information means information that identifies an individual or for which it is reasonably foreseeable in the circumstances that it could be utilized, either alone or with other information, to identify an individual," and the U.S. HIPAA describes de-identified information where "there is no reasonable basis to believe that the information can be used to identify an individual." We can turn to precedents as a basis for deciding on acceptable risk levels for our three thresholds.

Choosing the α Threshold

The first threshold that needs to be set is α. There are a number of criteria that can be used for deciding on this value.

One can argue that if there is a re-identification of a single record, then that would be sufficient to cause extensive damage to the reputation of the data custodian and the trust of the public in that custodian. There are examples demonstrating severe consequences from the re-identification of a single individual:

- In the case of AOL, the company posted search queries on the web and *New York Times* reporters were able to re-identify one individual from these queries [1–3]. The bad publicity from this resulted in the CTO of the company resigning and the researcher who posted the data to lose his job.
- There was a highly publicized case of a researcher re-identifying the insurance claims transactions of the governor of Massachusetts [4]. The researcher linked insurance claims data made available by the state employees' insurer and the voter registration list for Cambridge. This resulted in restrictions on the disclosure of insurance claims data and influenced the de-identification guidelines in the HIPAA Privacy Rule.
- At Children's Hospital of Eastern Ontario there was an example of a commercial data broker requesting prescription records [5]. The data broker noted that 100 other hospitals had already provided the requested fields. A re-identification attack was able to re-identify a single patient. This resulted in restrictions on the types of fields that would be disclosed [6].
- A national broadcaster aired a report on the death of a 26-year-old female taking a particular drug [7]. She was re-identified from the adverse drug reaction database released by Health Canada. Subsequently Health Canada restricted access to certain fields in the adverse drug event database, and litigation between the two organizations continued for a number of years.

Alternatively, if a regulator will penalize a data custodian if there is a breach of a single record, then a re-identification of a single record would be considered harmful.

If the quasi-identifiers in the disclosed health data set can be linked with other data sets to determine an individual's identity, then this information would be useful to an adversary for committing financial fraud or (medical) identity theft. If the adversary wishes to commit, say, medical identity theft, then it only needs to successfully re-identify a single individual. There is evidence that a market for individually identifiable medical records exists [8, 9].

By the above logic, an appropriate value of α is zero. Then if any record is high risk, the decision would be that the whole data set is high risk.

One can also rely on precedents to set an α value higher than zero. Previous disclosures of cancer registry data have deemed thresholds of 5% and 20% of the population at risk as acceptable for public release and research use, respectively [10–12]. In that case we would set $\alpha = 0.05$ or $\alpha = 0.2$, depending on the nature of the data recipient. With that precedent, there is no reason not to have an intermediate value as well, such as $\alpha = 0.1$. However, having α values as high as 0.2 may be considered alarming by some members of the public.

We can also consider a method that ensures equivalence to the HIPAA Privacy Rule. The HIPAA Privacy Rule in the United States defines the Safe Harbor standard for creating data that have a low probability of re-identification. In analyzing the acceptable probability of re-identification during the consultations prior to issuing the regulation, a τ threshold of 0.5 was used. Studies have shown that in the United States, 0.04% of the records will have a probability of re-identification equal to or higher than 0.5 in population data sets [13, 14]. This also means that any random sample from the U.S. population would be expected to have 0.04% of the records with a re-identification probability greater than 0.5. Another study evaluated the proportion of records that can be re-identified in a sample and found that only 0.01% had a re-identification probability greater than 0.5 [15]. Both the 0.0004 and 0.0001 values are alternatives for α, which are the proportion of records that can acceptably have a high probability of re-identification.

Using a τ value equal to 0.5 would be considered quite high by most observers. However, it is possible to achieve a similar risk exposure as the Safe Harbor standard.

Risk exposure captures the amount of loss if a risk materializes multiplied by the probability of that loss occurring:

$$Risk\,exposure = Loss \times Probability \tag{19.1}$$

The risk exposure for Safe Harbor is the probability of a correct re-identification multiplied by the number of individuals that would experience that re-identification. If we have N individuals in a data set, then the risk exposure is $0.5 \times 0.0004 \times N$. Now, if we have a $\tau = 0.05$ and wish to use it to compute an α value that has the same maximum risk exposure as the HIPAA Safe Harbor standard, we would use

$$\alpha = \frac{0.5 \times 0.0004}{\tau} \tag{19.2}$$

which would give us a value of 0.004. In practice this equivalence to the Safe Harbor scheme will result in α values that are quite close to zero, and therefore its general practical utility may be questioned.

Choosing the τ and λ Thresholds

The τ threshold represents the acceptable maximum probability of an individual record being re-identified. The λ threshold represents the highest acceptable average probability of a record being re-identified. The maximum probability will be equal to or higher than average probability, and therefore τ represents a much more stringent standard. The data custodian has to select one of these two types of risk thresholds to use.

If we use general scientific precedents for when we trust empirical evidence, we can choose values of 0.05 or 0.1. These are values used to test hypotheses in scientific disciplines, and represent a common threshold for when evidence becomes convincing. Although the context of hypothesis testing is different from our context, the analogy is around how low the probability needs to be for us to trust the evidence.

If we consider attack T4, based on the review of precedents in Chapter 25, the largest threshold probability value used in Canada for a public use file is 0.05. Therefore setting, say, $\tau = 0.05$ at the low end is consistent with current practice. At the other end of the spectrum, if we consider attack T1 and a λ threshold of 0.05, a data recipient with high mitigating controls and a low motives and capacity would have a *pr(attempt)* value of 0.05 according to our recommendations. The highest probability value used, historically, for the release of data without taking context into account is 0.33, which in this case would result in an overall probability of re-identification below the λ threshold ($0.33 \times 0.05 = 0.016 < 0.05$).

Choosing the Threshold for Marketer Risk

Marketer risk pertains to the situation when the adversary will match the DF with another database. Let us denote that threshold value by ψ.

For a simple recommendation one can also rely on the previous cancer registry data thresholds of 5% and 20% noted above [10–12]. Similarly, we would set $\psi = 0.05$, $\psi = 0.1$, or $\psi = 0.2$.

Consider one scenario where an adversary is motivated to market a product to all of the individuals in the DF by sending them a flyer, an email, or by calling them. In that case the adversary uses a public registry, say, a voter registration list, to re-identify the individuals. The adversary does not need to know which records were re-identified incorrectly because the incremental cost of including an individual in the marketing campaign is low. As long as the expected number of correct re-identifications is sufficiently high, that would provide an adequate return to the adversary. A data custodian, knowing that a marketing potential exists, needs to adjust ψ down to create a disincentive for marketing. For example, one can argue that $\psi = 0.01$ may be a sufficiently low threshold to make it not worthwhile for the marketer.

A second scenario is when a data custodian, such as a provincial or national registry, is disclosing data to multiple parties. For example, the registry may disclose a data set A with ethnicity and socioeconomic indicators to a researcher and a data set B with mental health information to another researcher. Both data sets share the same core demographics on the patients. The registry would not release both ethnicity and socioeconomic variables, as well as mental health data to the same researcher because of the sensitivity of the data and the potential for group harm, but would do so to different researchers. However, the two researchers may collude and link A and B against the wishes of the registry. Before disclosing the data, the registry managers can evaluate the proportion of records that can be correctly linked/re-identified on the common demographics if the researchers colluded in linking data. The registry would want to set ψ such that there is a disincentive to link. Under those circumstances ψ = 0.6 may be sufficient to discourage such linking because then 40% of the matched records would be incorrectly matched, which would make any analysis on that linked data meaningless.

Some precedents exist that can be used to inform an absolute ψ threshold rather than a proportion or percentage of records at risk. We can, for example, rely on how the Department of Health and Human Services (HHS) in the United States classifies health data breaches, whereby they will not publicize breaches affecting less than 500 records [16]. This effectively sets two tiers of breaches, and one can argue that a re-identification affecting less than 500 records would be considered lower risk. With that argument one can set

$$\psi = \begin{cases} 500\!\!\big/\!n, & \text{if } n \geq 500 \\ 1, & \text{if } n < 500 \end{cases}$$

Proposed cyber-security legislation in the United States treated data breaches with more than 10,000 more strictly in terms of notification triggers than those with fewer, and similarly, the proposed Identity Theft Protection Act required notification when breaches involved more than 1,000 individuals [17]. These reflect different severity thresholds for an inadvertent disclosure of personal information.

If the adversary is financially motivated and wishes to sell patient identities, then the value of an identity is important. In the underground economy, the rate for the basic demographics of a Canadian has been estimated to be $50 [18]. Another study determined that full identities are worth $1 to $15 [19]. Therefore the re-identification of a single individual would not be financially lucrative, but the re-identification of a large database would be. Similarly, Symantec has published an online calculator to determine the worth of an individual record for an adversary interested in financial fraud, and it is generally quite low [20]. If not sold, this kind of identifiable health information can be monetized through extortion, as demonstrated recently with hackers requesting large ransoms [21, 22]. In one case, where the ransom amount is known, the value per patient's health information was $1.20 [22]. Given the low value of individual records, a disclosed database would only be worthwhile to such an adversary if a large number of records can be re-identified. If the ψ value is sufficiently small, then there would be less incentive for a financially motivated adversary to attempt re-identification.

Choosing among Thresholds

For each of the thresholds above there are a number of different values. Choosing among them would be a function of the invasion of privacy score. A checklist to assess this dimension and its scoring is provided in Chapter 26. The reasoning here is that a higher re-identification threshold would be acceptable if there was little invasion of privacy (e.g., the data were not sensitive or patient consent was obtained beforehand for the disclosure). A lower re-identification threshold would be used if the data had a high invasion of privacy potential (e.g., the data were more sensitive). This would be consistent with the expectations of the patients and other data subjects whose health information was being disclosed. In Sidebar 19.1 we summarize the thresholds that we use in practice.

Sidebar 19.1: Thresholds Used in Practice

The following are the thresholds that we have used in practice with the organizations we have worked with. Our extensive experience with these provides them with a considerable amount of face validity. They also are consistent with the data release precedents in Chapter 25 when coupled with our risk equations. Although note that there may be exceptions—for example, if a data custodian is compelled by a court order to release a DF with a particular threshold. In that case the data custodian would have to follow the court order.

α	Always set to zero
τ	0.05 — High invasion of privacy
	0.075 — Medium invasion of privacy
	0.1 — Low invasion of privacy
λ	0.05 — High invasion of privacy
	0.075 — Medium invasion of privacy
	0.1 — Low invasion of privacy
ψ	0.05 — High invasion of privacy
	0.1 — Medium invasion of privacy
	0.2 — Low invasion of privacy

Thresholds and Incorrect Re-Identification

Note that we did not consider any consequences from an incorrect re-identification when selecting a threshold. For example, if we have 1,000 records and the adversary matches all of them to a population registry, and let the expected number of records correctly re-identified be 50. But there will be 950 records that were incorrectly re-identified. The adversary would not know which 50 records were correctly re-identified.

If the adversary will be sending email spam to these 1,000 re-identified patients, then there is no real injury to the 950 patients. If the adversary was going to try to fraudulently use the health insurance policies of the 1,000 patients or open financial accounts in their names, there will be no injury to the 950 patients (because the re-identified identities will not match the actual identity information during the verification process, and therefore these attempts will fail). Under such conditions we would not consider the incorrect re-identifications as a problem.

On the other hand, if a reporter was going to expose a person in the media based on incorrect information, this could cause reputational harm to the patient. Or if employment, insurance, or financial decisions were going to be made based on the incorrectly re-identified data, there could be social or economic harm to the individuals.

Within the current framework we argue that if we make the probability (or expected proportion) of incorrect re-identification sufficiently high for the adversary, this would act as a deterrent to launching a re-identification attack. This argument is based on two assumptions: (1) An incorrect re-identification is detrimental to the adversary's objectives, and (2) the threshold that is used is published or known to the adversary to influence the adversary's behavior.

References

1. Hansell S. AOL removes search data on group of web users. *New York Times*, August 8, 2006.
2. Barbaro M, Zeller Jr. T. A face is exposed for AOL searcher no. 4417749. *New York Times*, August 9, 2006.
3. Zeller Jr. T. AOL moves to increase privacy on search queries. *New York Times*, August 22, 2006.
4. Sweeney L. Computational disclosure control: A primer on data privacy protection. PhD thesis, Massachusetts Institute of Technology, 2001.
5. El Emam K, Kosseim P. Privacy interests in prescription records. Part 2. Patient privacy. *IEEE Security and Privacy*, 2009; 7(2):75–78.
6. El Emam K, Dankar F, Vaillancourt R, Roffey T, Lysyk M. Evaluating patient re-identification risk from hospital prescription records. *Canadian Journal of Hospital Pharmacy*, 2009; 62(4):307–319.
7. Federal Court (Canada). *Mike Gordon v. the Minister of Health: Affidavit of Bill Wilson*. 2006.
8. Luck N, Burns J. Your secrets for sale. *Daily Express*, February 16, 1994.
9. Rogers L, Leppard D. For sale: Your secret medical record for 150. *Sunday Times*, November 26, 1995, sect. 2.
10. Howe H, Lake A, Shen T. Method to assess identifiability in electronic data files. *American Journal of Epidemiology*, 2007; 165(5):597–601.

11. Howe H, Lake A, Lehnherr M, Roney D. *Unique record identification on public use files as tested on the 1994–1998 CINA analytic file*. North American Association of Central Cancer Registries, 2002.

12. El Emam K. Heuristics for de-identifying health data. *IEEE Security and Privacy*, July/August 2008; 72–75.

13. National Committee on Vital and Health Statistics. *Report to the secretary of the US Department of Health and Human Services on enhanced protections for uses of health data: A stewardship framework for "secondary uses" of electronically collected and transmitted health data*. 2007.

14. Sweeney L. Data sharing under HIPAA: 12 years later. Workshop on the HIPAA Privacy Rule's De-Identification Standard, Department of Health and Human Services, 2010.

15. Lafky D. The Safe Harbor method of de-identification: An empirical test. Fourth National HIPAA Summit West, 2010.

16. Department of Health and Human Services, Office of Civil Rights. Breaches affecting 500 or more individuals. 2010.

17. Jones M. Data breaches: Recent developments in the public and private sectors. *I/S: A Journal of Law and Policy for the Information Society*, 2007–2008; 3(3):555–580.

18. Polsky S. Witness statement to the Standing Senate Committee on Legal and Constitutional Affairs. Parliament of Canada, 2007.

19. Symantec. Symantec global internet threat report—Trends for July–December 07. Symantec Enterprise Security, 2008.

20. Symantec. What is the underground economy? 2009. http://www.everyclickmatters.com/victim/assessment-tool.html.

21. Kravets D. Extortion plot threatens to divulge millions of patients' prescriptions. *Wired*, 2008.

22. Krebs B. Hackers break into Virginia health professions database, demand ransom. *Washington Post*, 2009.

PRACTICAL METHODS FOR DE-IDENTIFICATION

IV

Chapter 20

De-Identification Methods

Based on our experience, the de-identification methods that have the most acceptability among data recipients are generalization and suppression. In some instances sub-sampling is also an acceptable option.

Other methods, such as the addition of random noise, distort the individual-level data in ways that are sometimes not intuitive and may result in incorrect results if these distortions affect the multivariate correlational structure in the data. This can be mitigated if the specific type of analysis that will be performed is known in advance and the distortions can account for that. Nevertheless, they tend to have low acceptance among researchers and analysts [1]. Furthermore, random noise perturbation can be filtered out to recover the original data (see the discussion in Chapter 14 on this); therefore the effectiveness of noise addition can be questioned.

Alternative methods such as swapping and shuffling can also distort the data when applied in a manner that does not take into account the specific analyses that are anticipated. Because it is not always possible to anticipate all possible analyses, we have not found them to have high acceptability by the health data user community.

In this chapter we discuss generalization and suppression methods in more detail.

Generalization

Principles

Generalization reduces the precision in the data. As a simple example of increasing generalization, a patient's date of birth can be generalized to a month and year of birth, to a year of birth, or to a five-year interval. Allowable generalizations can be specified a priori in the form of a generalization hierarchy, as in the age example above.

Generalizations have been defined for SNP sequences [2] and clinical data sets [3]. Instead of hierarchies, generalizations can also be constructed empirically by combining or clustering sequences [4] and transactional data [5] into more general groups.

When a data set is generalized the re-identification probability can be measured afterwards. Records that are considered high risk are then flagged for suppression. When there are many variables the number of possible ways that these variables can be generalized can be quite large. Generalization algorithms are therefore used to find the best generalization.

Optimal Lattice Anonymization (OLA)

A commonly used de-identification criterion is k-anonymity, and many k-anonymity algorithms have been developed [6–15]. This criterion stipulates that each record in a data set is similar to at least another k − 1 record on the potentially identifying variables. For example, if k = 5 and the quasi-identifiers are age and gender, then a k-anonymized data set has at least five records for each value combination of age and gender. The k-anonymity criterion is equivalent to maximum risk. For example, for maximum prosecutor risk, $_pR_b$, if we want to ensure that $f_j \geq 5$ then we would set k = 5. This can similarly be extended to maximum journalist risk: $_jR_b$.

We will describe the OLA algorithm, which was designed as a k-anonymity algorithm for cross-sectional data [1], as an example of how optimal generalization would work. With only slight modifications, OLA can be used to manage all of the remaining risk metrics that have been presented thus far but we will only describe the default version of OLA here, which assumes that we are trying to manage maximum risk.

OLA has two steps: generalization and then suppression. During generalization certain records are flagged for suppression, and these go through a cell suppression algorithm in the second step.

Let us consider the simplified example where we have three quasi-identifiers: date of birth, gender, and date of visit. The domain generalization hierarchies for these quasi-identifiers are shown in Figures 20.1 through 20.3. These hierarchies describe how the precision of each quasi-identifier can be reduced during generalization.

All of the possible generalizations can be expressed in the form of a lattice as shown in Figure 20.4. In this lattice each possible generalization is represented by a

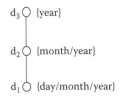

Figure 20.1   Domain generalization for date of birth.

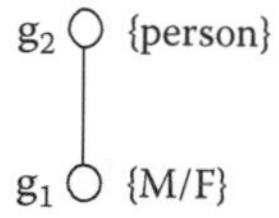

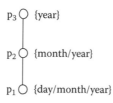

Figure 20.2   Domain generalization for gender.

p_3 {year}

p_2 {month/year}

p_1 {day/month/year}

Figure 20.3   Domain generalization for visit date.

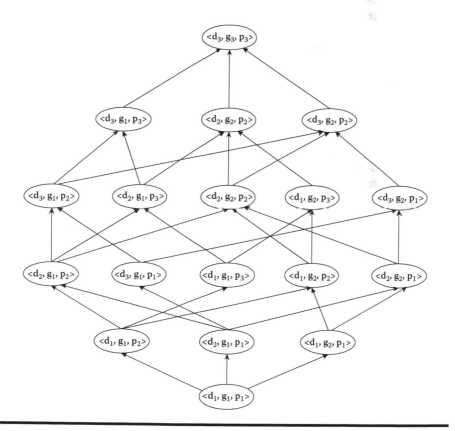

Figure 20.4   A lattice showing the possible generalizations of the three quasi-identifiers.

node starting from the original data set at the lowest node, $<d_1,g_1,p_1>$. As one moves up the lattice the quasi-identifiers are generalized. For example, node $<d_2,g_1,p_1>$ has the date of birth generalized to month and year. The objective of OLA is to find the best generalization (node) in that lattice.

In k-anonymization algorithms such as OLA, a maximum amount of suppression is specified: *MaxSup*. It means that if there is suppression in more than *MaxSup* records, that would not be an acceptable generalization and that node would not be considered a good solution and discarded. For example, if *MaxSup* is set to 5%, then the generalization algorithm will ignore all nodes with generalizations that will result in more than 5% of the records being flagged for suppression. This will also guarantee that no more than 5% of the records will have any suppression in them.

OLA will analyze each node in the lattice and within each node flag for suppression records that are in equivalence classes smaller than k. If the total number of patients flagged for suppression is less than *MaxSup*, then that node is a candidate for being the best solution. OLA implements an efficient method to evaluate all of the nodes in this lattice and compute how many records are flagged for suppression in each node.

After examining all of the nodes, OLA will choose the node with the smallest information loss among the candidate nodes. Information loss is used to measure the amount of distortion to the data. A simple measure of information loss is how high up the hierarchy the chosen generalization level is. However, this creates difficulties of interpretation, and other more theoretically grounded metrics that take into account the difference in the level of precision between the original data set and the generalized data have been suggested [1].

Therefore generalization is an optimization problem whereby the optimization algorithm tries to find the generalization for each of the quasi-identifiers that will ensure that (1) the probability of re-identification is at or below the threshold, (2) the percentage of records flagged for suppression is below *MaxSup*, and (3) information loss is minimized.

Tagging

The OLA search through the nodes is quite efficient because of a process of predictive tagging nodes. This means that it is possible to predict whether a node is a candidate solution or not without performing calculations on it.

A path between two nodes in Figure 20.4 indicates that one node is a generalization of another. For example, node $<d_2,g_1,p_1>$ is a generalization of node $<d_1,g_1,p_1>$. A path from the start node $<d_1,g_1,p_1>$ to the sink node $<d_3,g_2,p_3>$ is a *generalization strategy*.

If a node X is evaluated and it is determined that it is a candidate node, then all nodes above X on the generalization strategies that pass through X would also be candidate solutions. This is because a node that is a generalization of one that meets the *MaxSup* criterion will also meet the *MaxSup* criterion. This allows us to tag all nodes above X without evaluating them.

Similarly, if a node X does not meet the *MaxSup* criterion, then all nodes below X on the generalization strategies that pass through X would not. This allows us to tag all nodes below X without evaluating them.

Records to Suppress

A critical element in the application of OLA is computing the number (or percentage) of records that are flagged for suppression. The flagged records will depend on which derived metric is being used to measure re-identification risk.

Records are flagged for suppression based on their equivalence class risk; therefore we will talk about the equivalence classes flagged for suppression. Let J' denote the set of equivalence classes flagged for suppression.

For risk measured using R_b metrics, for example, the records flagged for suppression are all records in any equivalence class j where $\theta_j > \tau$. Therefore we have:

$$J'_b = \left\{ j \in J \mid \theta_j > \tau \right\} \tag{20.1}$$

This will guarantee that D_b is low.

For risk measured using R_a metrics, we first order the equivalence classes by θ_j such that the equivalence classes with the highest risk are at the top. At the outset the set J'_a is empty. We then start from the top and add the first equivalence class to J'_a. Let the number of records in the J'_a equivalence classes be denoted by n'_a such that

$$n'_a = \sum_{x \in J'_a} |x|$$

If the following inequality is true, then we stop:

$$\frac{1}{n'_a} \sum_{j \in J'_a} f_j \times I\left(\theta_j > \tau\right) \geq \left[\frac{1}{n} \sum_{j \in J} f_j \times I\left(\theta_j > \tau\right) \right] - \alpha \tag{20.2}$$

If the inequality is not satisfied, then we progress to the next equivalence class down and add it to J'_a, and so on until Equation (20.2) is satisfied. This approach suppresses the highest-risk equivalence classes first. In practice these will often be the smallest equivalence classes in the data set, but not always.

For the marketer risk metrics, we need to consider two situations. Let's consider the $_mR_1$ metric. We first create an empty set J'_1, and order the equivalence classes in the data set by their size such that the smallest equivalence classes are on top. Let the number of records in the J'_1 equivalence classes be denoted by n'_1 such that

$$n'_1 = \sum_{x \in J'_1} |x|$$

We then start from the top and add the first equivalence class to J'_1. If the following inequality is true, then we stop:

$$|J'_1| - \psi n'_1 \geq |J| - \psi n \tag{20.3}$$

If the inequality is not satisfied, then we progress to the next equivalence class down and add it to J'_1, and so on until Equation (20.3) is satisfied. With this approach we first suppress the smallest equivalence classes.

For $_mR_2$ we first order the equivalence classes by their $(f_j \times 1/F_j)$ score such that the equivalence classes with the highest scores are at the top. Let the number of records in the J'_2 equivalence classes be denoted by n'_2 such that

$$n'_2 = \sum_{x \in J'_2} |x|$$

At the outset the set J'_2 is empty. We then start from the top and add the first equivalence class to J'_2. If the following inequality is true, then we stop:

$$\frac{1}{n'_2} \sum_{j \in J'_2} f_j \times \frac{1}{F_j} \geq \left(\frac{1}{n} \sum_{j \in J} f_j \times \frac{1}{F_j} \right) - \psi \tag{20.4}$$

If the inequality is not satisfied, then we progress to the next equivalence class down and add it to J'_2, and so on until Equation (20.4) is satisfied. With this approach we first suppress the equivalence classes that have the highest expected number of records that would be re-identified.

Suppression Methods

Overview

Usually suppression is applied to the specific records flagged for suppression. Suppression means the removal of values from the data. There are three general approaches to suppression: (1) casewise deletion, (2) quasi-identifier removal, and (3) local cell suppression.

Casewise deletion removes the whole patient or visit record from the data set. This results in the most distortion to the data because the sensitive variables are also removed, even though those do not contribute to an increase in the risk of identity disclosure.

Quasi-identifier removal only removes the values on the quasi-identifiers in the data set. This has the advantage that all of the sensitive information is retained.

Local cell suppression is an improvement over quasi-identifier removal in that fewer values are suppressed. Local cell suppression applies an optimization algorithm to find the least number of values on the quasi-identifiers to suppress [16]. All of the sensitive variables are retained, and in practice considerably fewer of the quasi-identifier values are suppressed compared to casewise and quasi-identifier deletion.

Fast Local Cell Suppression

Local suppression is an optimization problem because the algorithm needs to find the fewest cells to suppress to ensure that the maximum risk level can be maintained. However, because of the large search space, current algorithms use heuristics in their search and do not produce globally optimal solutions. Consequently, different algorithms will produce different amounts of cell suppression on the same data set.

One suppression algorithm had a $3k(1 + \log 2k)$ approximation to k-anonymity with a $O(n^{2k})$ running time [17], where n is the number of records flagged for suppression. Another had a $6k(1 + \log m)$ approximation and $O(mn^2 + n^3)$ running time [17], where m is the number of variables. An improved algorithm with a $3(k - 3)$ algorithm has been proposed [16] with polynomial running time. Because of its good approximation, the latter algorithm has been used in the past on health data sets [1, 3].

However, all of the above suppression algorithms require the computation of a pairwise distance among all pairs of records in a data set. This means $n(n - 1)/2$ distances need to be computed because they require the construction of a complete graph with n vertices (the rows flagged for suppression) and the edges are weighted by a distance metric (the number of cells that differ between the two nodes). Such algorithms can realistically only be used on relatively small data sets, when the number of records flagged for suppression is small, or when the analyst can wait for a long time for an answer (i.e., instantaneous answers are not expected). Algorithms that require the computation of all pairwise distances between records are impossible to practically use on large data sets (for example, when $n = 100,000$, which is not a particularly large data set). Therefore there is a clear need for new suppression algorithms that can handle large data sets efficiently.

Available Tools

A series of recent reports provide a summary of free and supported commercial tools for the de-identification of structured clinical and administrative data sets [18, 19]. Also, a review of text de-identification tools has recently been published [20], although many of these text de-identification tools are experimental or still only used in research settings, and may not be readily available.

Case Study: De-Identification of the BORN Birth Registry

General Parameters

In this example we will go through the steps for a complete de-identification of a data set. We will work with a data extract from the BORN Birth Registry. We assume that a researcher has requested four quasi-identifiers: baby's date of birth, mother's date of birth, maternal postal code, and baby's sex. The researcher has also requested some fields that are considered sensitive. When we performed the "Invasion of Privacy" assessment on the requested data, the score came back as HIGH because of the data sensitivity and because the data were not being disclosed with consent. Because this is a population registry, we are only interested in prosecutor risk (managing prosecutor risk automatically manages marketer risk). We will use average risk to decide on how to de-identify this data set. The relevant metric for us then is $_pR_c$. Therefore, according to our thresholds, we have $\lambda = 0.05$. The last parameter we used as *MaxSup* = 5%, which ensured that no more than 5% of the records will have some suppression applied to them.

The DF will be provided to a known data recipient. This means that we need to manage attacks T1, T2, and T3. We will examine each in order below. We will use the notation $_pR_c$ (*T1*), $_pR_c$ (*T2*), and $_pR_c$ (*T3*) to signify the risk values for each of the three attacks.

Also, 1.08% of the records in the original data set had some missingness in them. The missingness in the original data was as summarized in Table 20.1.

Table 20.1 The Original Missingness in the BORN Data Extract Used in Our Example Case Study

Quasi-identifier	Original Missingness
Baby DoB	0%
Mother DoB	0%
Postal code	1.023%
Baby sex	0.061%

Attack T1

For attack T1, we need to evaluate the probability that an attempted attack will occur. When the mitigating controls and motives and capacity analyses were performed on the requesting researcher, the scores were medium and low. This means that $pr(attempt) = 0.2$. When we measured the risk from the original data set we found that $_pR_c$ (T1) = 0.198, which is higher than our threshold.

When we ran the OLA algorithm on this data set we obtained the results in Table 20.2. As can be seen, there was no suppression in this result. The $_pR_c$ (T1) = 0.04, which is lower than our threshold.

In general, it is always good to present data users with multiple options that illustrate the tradeoffs, and let them make the tradeoffs themselves. Therefore we generated a number of other solutions that meet the threshold under attack T1. In one solution we tried to keep more detail in the postal code. This solution is shown in Table 20.3. Again we see that there was no suppression necessary, but we lost more precision on the date of birth variables. The risk here is given by $_pR_c$ (T1) = 0.04.

We considered a final option under this attack where we keep more information for the mother's date of birth. This result is illustrated in Table 20.4, which has $_pR_c$ (T1) = 0.03.

The above three options illustrate the tradeoffs that one may need to make. The three alternative data sets had different levels of generalization, but they were all below our threshold.

Table 20.2   Option 1 Results under Attack T1

Quasi-identifier	Generalization	Original Missingness + Suppression
Baby DoB	None	0%
Mother DoB	5-year interval	0%
Postal code	First character	1.023%
Baby sex	None	0.061%

Table 20.3   Option 2 Results under Attack T1

Quasi-identifier	Generalization	Original Missingness + Suppression
Baby DoB	Month/year	0%
Mother DoB	10-year interval	0%
Postal code	First three characters	1.023%
Baby sex	None	0.061%

Table 20.4 Option 3 Results under Attack T1

Quasi-identifier	Generalization	Original Missingness + Suppression
Baby DoB	Quarter/year	0%
Mother DoB	5-year interval	0%
Postal code	First three characters	1.023%
Baby sex	None	0.061%

Attack T2

For attack T2, we already saw in a previous chapter that the probability of knowing a new mother in any single year is 0.762; therefore $_pR_c$ (*T2*) = 0.75 for the original data set, which is quite a high probability of inadvertent re-identification. Just because of such a high value of risk, one would expect more distortion to the data. The first option is given in Table 20.5, and this gives $_pR_c$ (*T2*) = 0.03.

In another option we try to retain more postal code information. This gives us the result in Table 20.6 with $_pR_c$ (*T2*) = 0.046. This data set had a bit more suppression applied to it in order to ensure that the overall risk is kept below the threshold.

Table 20.5 Option 1 Results under Attack T2

Quasi-identifier	Generalization	Original Missingness + Suppression
Baby DoB	Week/year	0%
Mother DoB	5-year interval	0%
Postal code	First character	1.023%
Baby sex	None	0.061%

Table 20.6 Option 2 Results under Attack T2

Quasi-identifier	Generalization	Original Missingness + Suppression
Baby DoB	Year	3.063%
Mother DoB	5-year interval	3.063%
Postal code	First three characters	4.08%
Baby sex	None	3.066%

Table 20.7   Option 1 Results under Attack T3

Quasi-identifier	Generalization	Original Missingness + Suppression
Baby DoB	None	0%
Mother DoB	5-year interval	0%
Postal code	First character	1.023%
Baby sex	None	0.061%

Table 20.8   Option 2 Results under Attack T3

Quasi-identifier	Generalization	Original Missingness + Suppression
Baby DoB	Quarter/year	0%
Mother DoB	5-year interval	0%
Postal code	First three characters	1.023%
Baby sex	None	0.061%

Attack T3

Under the third attack, T3, the overall probability of re-identification is $_pR_c$ (*T3*) = 0.267, which is still quite a bit higher than the threshold. A first attempt to produce a de-identified data set produced Table 20.7, where $_pR_c$ (*T3*) = 0.043. Note that these are the same generalizations as one of the T1 attack results. For the same data set, the re-identification probability can still be different under different attacks.

A data set that retained more geographic information was evaluated as well, and this is shown in Table 20.8, where $_pR_c$ (*T3*) = 0.0405.

Summary of Risk Assessment and De-Identification

Based on these results, we need to select a subset of the options that would work under the three attacks. In this case we saw that the alternative results under attack T3 were a subset of the results under attack T1. The most distortion was performed to the data set under attack T2. We would therefore present the two options from the T2 attack to the researcher and allow her to choose which particular data set is most appropriate for the analysis that she wishes to perform. The results from the T2 attack will also satisfy the threshold under the T1 and T3 attacks.

References

1. El Emam K, Dankar F, Issa R, Jonker E, Amyot D, Cogo E, Corriveau J-P, Walker M, Chowdhury S, Vaillancourt R, Roffey T, Bottomley J. A globally optimal k-anonymity method for the de-identification of health data. *Journal of the American Medical Informatics Association*, 2009; 16:670–682.
2. Lin Z, Hewett M, Altman R. Using binning to maintain confidentiality of medical data. Proceedings of the American Medical Informatics Association Annual Symposium, 2002.
3. El Emam K, Dankar F, Vaillancourt R, Roffey T, Lysyk M. Evaluating patient re-identification risk from hospital prescription records. *Canadian Journal of Hospital Pharmacy*, 2009; 62(4):307–319.
4. Malin B. Protecting genomic sequence anonymity with generalization lattices. *Methods of Information in Medicine*, 2005; 44:687–92.
5. Loukides G, Gkoulalas-Divanis A, Malin B. Anonymization of electronic medical records for validating genome-wide association studies. *Proceedings of the National Academy of Sciences*, 2010; 107:7898–7903.
6. Samarati P, Sweeney L. Protecting privacy when disclosing information: k-Anonymity and its enforcement through generalisation and suppression. Menlo Park, CA: SRI International, 1998.
7. Samarati P. Protecting respondents' identities in microdata release. *IEEE Transactions on Knowledge and Data Engineering*, 2001; 13(6):1010–1027.
8. Sweeney L. Achieving k-anonymity privacy protection using generalization and suppression. *International Journal of Uncertainty, Fuzziness and Knowledge-Based Systems*, 2002; 10(5):571–588.
9. Ciriani V, De Capitani di Vimercati SSF, Samarati P. k-Anonymity. In *Secure data management in decentralized systems*. New York: Springer, 2007.
10. Bayardo R, Agrawal R. Data privacy through optimal k-anonymization. Proceedings of the 21st International Conference on Data Engineering, 2005.
11. Iyengar V. Transforming data to satisfy privacy constraints. Proceedings of the ACM SIGKDD International Conference on Data Mining and Knowledge Discovery, 2002.
12. Du Y, Xia T, Tao Y, Zhang D, Zhu F. On multidimensional k-anonymity with local recoding generalization. IEEE 23rd International Conference on Data Engineering, 2007.
13. Xu J, Wang W, Pei J, Wang X, Shi B, Fu A. Utility-based anonymization using local recoding. ACM SIGKDD International Conference on Knowledge Discovery and Data Mining, 2006.
14. Wong R, Li J, Fu A, Wang K. (alpa,k)-Anonymity: An enhanced k-anonymity model for privacy-preserving data publishing. ACM SIGKDD International Conference on Knowledge Discovery and Data Mining, 2006.
15. Aggarwal G, Feder T, Kenthapadi K, Motwani R, Panigrahy R, Thomas D, Zhu A. Approximation algorithms for k-anonymity. *Journal of Privacy Technology*, November 2005.
16. Aggarwal G, Feder T, Kenthapadi K, Motwani R, Panigrahy R, Thomas D, Zhu A. Anonymizing tables. In *Proceedings of the 10th International Conference on Database Theory (ICDT05)*. New York: Springer, 2005.
17. Meyerson A, Williams R. On the complexity of optimal k-anonymity. Proceedings of the 23rd Conference on the Principles of Database Systems, 2004.

18. Fraser R, Willison D. Tools for de-identification of personal health information. Canada Health Infoway, 2009. http://www2.infoway-inforoute.ca/Documents/Tools_for_De-identification_EN_FINAL.pdf. Archived at http://www.webcitation.org/5xA2KBoMm.
19. Health System Use Technical Advisory Committee—Data De-Identification Working Group. *"Best practice" guidelines for managing the disclosure of de-identified health information*. 2011. http://www.ehealthinformation.ca/documents/Data%20De-identification%20Best%20Practice%20Guidelines.pdf. Archived at http://www.webcitation.org/5x9w6635d.
20. Meystre S, Friedlin F, South B, Shen S, Samore M. Automatic de-identification of textual documents in the electronic health record: A review of recent research. *BMC Medical Research Methodology*, 2010; 10(1):70.

Chapter 21

Practical Tips

In this chapter we present a set of practical techniques that have been found helpful when measuring re-identification probabilities and de-identifying data sets in the real world. These will allow you to maximize the utility of the data that are disclosed and to address some of the practical questions that may come up.

Disclosed Files Should Be Samples

If an adversary is trying to re-identify a single individual, the re-identification risk when the adversary knows that the individual is in the DF will always be higher than if the adversary does not know that. By ensuring that the DF is a sample, then the adversary would not have that knowledge. Sampling protects against individuals self-revealing that they are in the DF.

If individuals in the DF know that their data are in the DF, then the data custodian cannot realistically assume that none of them will self-reveal that fact. The data custodian can ask the individuals to keep that fact a secret; otherwise, their risk of re-identification will rise. In such a case, if an individual self-reveals that fact, then one can argue that he or she has been forewarned. This, however, may not be an appropriate approach if individuals are volunteering their data or have been compelled to provide their data. Therefore sampling reduces the re-identification risk without putting an additional burden on the individuals.

The exact size of the sample should be sufficient to ensure that there is uncertainty about who is in the DF. Sample size will of course also be driven by the need for the DF to retain utility for any subsequent data analysis.

Disclosing Multiple Samples

Disclosing multiple samples means that more than one sample data set will be created from the same population data set. For example, the data custodian may have disclosed the first sample last year and decided to disclose a second sample this year. The data custodian is disclosing multiple different data sets because the probability of re-identification of a single data set that combines the information from all disclosed samples is too high.

The assumption is that a data recipient will attempt to match the samples to gain new or additional information about the individual. Therefore the data custodian needs to ensure that the correct match rate is sufficiently low.

There are two scenarios where a data custodian will disclose multiple samples. To simplify the explanations we will assume that there are two data sets being disclosed, A and B.

The first situation is when data sets A and B have different sets of variables, but the two data sets pertain to the same individuals. This is a rather simple scenario because there are no overlapping variables among the two recipients.

The way to handle this particular scenario is to shuffle the records in each sample. This way, if a recipient tries to match the two records, it cannot use the positional information for that purpose.

The data recipient may try a random match. If the two data sets pertain to exactly the same individuals and they are both of size N, then if a recipient tries to match the records randomly, the proportion of records that would be correctly matched will be $1/N$, on average.

If sample A had N records on N people and sample B had n records on n people, where $n < N$ and B's records are a subset of A's records, then the proportion of B's records that would be correctly matched is still $1/N$, on average, and the proportion of A's records that would be matched correctly is n/N^2, on average. Therefore the more records in the data sets that are disclosed, the more the proportion of correct matches decreases. Furthermore, it should be noted that under this scenario the adversary would not know which records were correctly matched, only that a certain proportion of them were correctly matched.

If the proportion of records that will be matched successfully after shuffling is small, and if the recipients will not know which records were matched successfully, then this acts as a strong disincentive to match the two samples. Therefore always shuffle your data before disclosure.

Under the second scenario the two samples have some overlapping variables; for example, they may both have the individuals' date of birth and postal code.

If the two disclosed samples each have N records, and they have the same individuals in them, then the proportion of records that can be correctly matched, if the recipient tries, to the data sets is $|J|/N$, which is the $_mR_1$ metric.

If one of the samples is a subset of the other, with the smaller sample having n records, with $n < N$, then the proportion of the records in the smaller data set that will be correctly matched is given by the $_mR_2$ metrics.

Note that the recipient will not know which records were successfully matched. For example, if the proportion produced by either of these two metrics is, say, 0.4, then it is not known which 40% of the records are correctly matched.

Creating Cohorts

Cohorts are subsets of a full data set that have specific characteristics. In some situations the data custodian may want to disclose a cohort as a DF rather than the full data set. For example, if the full data set consists of births, then a cohort may be births of premature babies or births by young mothers. The manner in which the probability of re-identification is measured for a cohort will be a function of how the cohort is defined.

We will consider three scenarios for creating the cohort. These differ by whether the variables that are used to define the cohort consist of quasi-identifiers or not. For example, let us consider a birth registry with two quasi-identifiers: age of mother and gender of the baby. The three scenarios based on this example would be:

- The cohort is defined as all births to teenage mothers, in which case that cohort is defined using a quasi-identifier.
- The cohort is defined as all births of premature babies, in which case that cohort is not defined using a quasi-identifier.
- The cohort is defined as all premature births to teenage mothers, in which case that cohort is defined using both a non-quasi-identifier and a quasi-identifier.

These distinctions are important because an adversary has background information about the quasi-identifiers. Therefore if a cohort is defined using quasi-identifiers, then an adversary would know who is in the cohort. For example, if the cohort consists of teenage mothers, and the adversary has background knowledge about Alice, who is an 18-year-old mother, then the adversary would know that Alice is in the cohort.

For each one of these scenarios, we consider how to measure the probability of re-identification. In the descriptions below we refer to the full population data set as the original data that the data custodian has. The DF that is created is a cohort from that full data set.

Cohort Defined on Quasi-Identifiers Only

Under this condition the adversary would know who is in the DF, and therefore the metrics that are suitable under the prosecutor risk assumptions would need to be used: $_pR_a$, $_pR_b$, and $_pR_c$. In this case the sampling fraction or the size of the cohort would not matter in the computation of the metric values.

Cohort Defined on a Non-Quasi-Identifier

Under this condition the adversary would not know whether or not any particular individual is in the cohort because the cohort was not constructed based on any of the adversary's background knowledge. Therefore the DF could be treated as a sample from the full data set, and the prosecutor risk metrics $_pR_a$, $_pR_b$, and $_pR_c$ would not apply. The remaining risk metrics would apply; however, the computation of the sampling fraction has to be done carefully.

We will let π_1 denote the sampling fraction of the full data set from some population. If the full data set is itself a population, then we can say $\pi_1 = 1$. If the cohort represents a sampling fraction of π_2 from the full data set, then the correct sampling fraction for the cohort is $\pi_1 \times \pi_2$.

If $\pi_1 = 1$, then for the computation of $_jR_a$, $_jR_b$, and $_jR_c$ and the F_j values (representing the equivalence class sizes in the population) can be computed directly from the full data set. Otherwise, estimators would need to be used.

Cohort Defined on Non-Quasi-Identifiers and Quasi-Identifiers

This situation is the most complex, and requires two steps. In the first step it is necessary to create a subset of the full data using only the quasi-identifiers. For example, this would be our data set consisting of teenage mothers only. Let us say that the number of records in this data set is n_1. Because this is based on quasi-identifiers, we assume that the adversary will know if the target individual(s) is in this subset.

In the second step, from that subset we would create the cohort of records for premature babies. Let the number of records in this cohort be n_2.

The metrics that are relevant here are exactly the same ones as for the case when the cohort is defined on a non-quasi-identifier, except that the appropriate sampling fraction to assume for any estimates is n_2/n_1.

Impact of Data Quality

All of the techniques discussed this far assume that the data are of high quality. This will not necessarily be the case. Data quality problems arrive due to transcription errors, optical character recognition (OCR) errors, missing data, and inaccuracies in creating linked data sets. They manifest themselves as misspellings, data entered in the wrong fields, a different way of expressing the same thing, and inaccurate numeric values. The effectiveness of re-identification attacks will be reduced when there are data quality problems. Furthermore, measures of the probability of re-identification will be higher than what will occur in practice because the measures do not account for matching errors due to low-quality data.

In reality many data sets will have quality problems. These will include the original data sets as well as any identification database that is used for matching. The consequence will be that the re-identification risk assessments that are performed using the methods described here will tend to be conservative. Measurement techniques that take into account errors are an area of active research, and new metrics are expected to become available in the next few years to adjust for such errors.

At the same time, many data collection systems are being automated. This means that instead of data having to be transcribed manually as it is being transferred from one system to the other (or printed and scanned into another system), this data transfer is being automated and hence reducing the chances of additional errors being introduced. Furthermore, automated edit checks are now expected as a standard feature of data collection systems. These kinds of improvements are, over time, reducing the amount of data quality problems as well.

Publicizing Re-Identification Risk Measurement

We noted earlier that a general equation characterizing the overall probability of a re-identification attack is

$$pr\left(re-identification\right) = pr\left(re-identification\,\middle|\,attempt\right) \times pr\left(attempt\right) \quad (21.1)$$

This equation is meaningful in the context where an adversary may deliberately attempt to re-identify a data set.

It is generally assumed that if the probability of re-identification is small, then this would act as a deterrent for an adversary to attempt re-identification to start off with. Similarly then, if the probability of re-identification is high, then that would make re-identification attempts more likely. Therefore there is a negative correlation between these two values.

The implication of this is that it is better for the data custodian to publicize a low probability of re-identification value (i.e., the *pr(re-identification|attempt)* value). To the extent that this value is small, it will act as a deterrent to an attempted re-identification attack.

Adversary Power

A cross-sectional data set may have many quasi-identifiers. A data subject in a longitudinal data set can have multiple visits or claims. It is not reasonable, or plausible for that matter, for an adversary to have background information on all of these quasi-identifiers or visits. For example, if a cross-sectional data set has 30 quasi-identifiers, say, a survey, it is not reasonable to assume that an adversary will know 30 things about an individual in the data set—that is just too much background information. The situation gets less plausible for longitudinal data where a data subject may have ten or more visits or hundreds of claims. We therefore assume that an adversary would only have information on a subset of these quasi-identifiers or visits, respectively. This is known as the power of the adversary.

The power of the adversary reflects the number of quasi-identifiers or visits that the adversary would have background information about. We denoted the power of the adversary as p.

In a cross-sectional data set, the value of p would be the number of quasi-identifiers that the adversary has background knowledge of, where p is a number smaller than the number of quasi-identifiers in the data set. In the case of longitudinal data, the value of p indicates the number of visits about which the adversary would have background information that can be used for an attack.

Previous research that considered the power of the adversary always assumed that the power is fixed for all data subjects [1–5]. However, intuitively it makes sense that the adversary would have different amounts of background knowledge, or power, for different data subjects. For example, everything else being equal, it is easier to have background information about a patient with a large number of visits than about a patient with few visits. Therefore we would expect power to increase monotonically with the number of visits that a patient has.

Also, it is likely that certain pieces of background information are more easily knowable than others by an adversary, making it necessary to treat the quasi-identifiers separately when it comes to computing the power of an adversary. For example, it would be easier to know a diagnosis value for patients with chronic conditions whose diagnoses keep repeating across visits. In such a case, if the adversary knew the information in one visit, then it would be easier to predict the information in other visits, increasing the amount of background knowledge that the adversary can have. In this case the diversity of values on a quasi-identifier across a patient's visits becomes an important consideration. Therefore we expect the power of an adversary to decrease monotonically with the diversity of values on the quasi-identifiers.

By taking into account the power of the adversary it is possible to allow the use and disclosure of more detailed information in a defensible way. To operationalize this concept, however, one must decide on a value of p. Historically, we have used $p = 5$, and then performed a sensitivity analysis on the resulting risk measurements to determine the impact if that value was increased.

Levels of Adversary Background Knowledge

An adversary is not likely to know or have background knowledge that is quite detailed about individual data subjects. This is particularly true under attack scenarios where the adversary is not using an existing clinical database to launch an attack.

For example, most patients do not know their own ICD-9 diagnosis codes, or have sufficient knowledge of their condition to determine what that ICD-9 code is. Similarly, an adversary is unlikely to know the detailed ICD-9 codes. However, the adversary may know a higher-level version of that diagnosis code.

This allows us to perform the analysis assuming the adversary only knows the high-level diagnosis code, in this example, but allows the disclosure of the full ICD-9 code. When launching an attack on the data, the adversary would have to generalize the ICD-9 codes in the DF to the higher level that he or she knows in order to perform the matching. This kind of approach has been used in the past for the de-identification of health data [6].

De-Identification in the Context of a Data Warehouse

The implementation of data warehouses by health data custodians is increasing. This allows the integration in a single place of data from multiple sources in the organization. When the data warehouse has been created for secondary purposes, such as research, there is no need to have identifiable information in it. However, creating a fully de-identified data warehouse will result in a significant loss of data utility. The main reason for this is that there will be a very large number of variables, potentially thousands. There will also be many quasi-identifiers, potentially hundreds. Furthermore, all of the data recipients will not be known precisely up front. The de-identification of such a large and complex data set for a set of unknown data recipients means that one has to be conservative and de-identify the data making worst-case assumptions.

A more practical strategy is to mask the data in the data warehouse so that they do not have any direct identifiers. The data will still have a high risk of re-identification, and therefore strong policies and procedures should be in place to manage them, and the organization must have the authority to create a data warehouse of identifiable health information. When there is a request for data from the data warehouse, then the extracts must be de-identified one by one using the methods described earlier. This approach will maximize the quality of the data that are included in the DF, and also means that the effort to create a de-identified data set will not be excessive.

This approach is not always possible because sometimes the organization does not have the authority to create a data warehouse that has health information with a high risk of re-identification. In such a case it may be necessary to segment the data and de-identify each segment separately. This also means that data extracts must be within data segments rather than across data segments. For example, the data may be segmented by disease. The data recipients would then only be able to pull extracts within each segment.

De-identification technology is improving all of the time. Therefore over time it may be possible to have effective de-identification applied to a complete data warehouse across multiple domains.

References

1. Terrovitis M, Mamoulis N, Kalnis P. Privacy-preserving anonymization of set-valued data. *Proceedings of the VLDB Endowment*, 2008; 1:115–125.
2. Xu Y, Fung B, Wang K, et al. Publishing sensitive transactions for itemset utility. In *Eighth IEEE International Conference on Data Mining (ICDM '08)*, 1109–1114. Los Alamitos, CA: IEEE Computer Society, 2008.
3. Xu Y, Wang K, Fu AW-C, et al. Anonymizing transaction databases for publication. In *Proceedings of the 14th ACM SIGKDD International Conference on Knowledge Discovery and Data Mining*, 767–775. New York: ACM, 2008.
4. Liu J, Wang K. Anonymizing transaction data by integrating suppression and generalization. In *Advances in knowledge discovery and data mining*, ed. M Zaki, J Yu, B Ravindran, 171–180. Berlin: Springer, 2010.
5. He Y, Naughton JF. Anonymization of set-valued data via top-down, local generalization. *Proceedings of the VLDB Endowment*, 2009; 2:934–945.
6. El Emam K, Paton D, Dankar F, et al. De-identifying a public use microdata file from the Canadian National Discharge Abstract Database. *BMC Medical Informatics and Decision Making*, 2011; 11.

END MATTER

Chapter 22

An Analysis of Historical Breach Notification Trends

The objective of this chapter is to determine the trends in medical data breach notification in the United States during the period of 2007–2010. Counts of breaches inform law enforcement, regulators, and legislators of the extent of the problem.

After September 2009 mandatory national breach notification laws came into effect in the United States, and information about breaches was published regularly by the DHHS. It reported 207 breaches by health information custodians involving 500 or more records, and more than 25,000 data breaches involving less than 500 records [1].

Prior to September 2009, state breach notification statutes were in place; however, there was no central location where these breaches were published. But multiple public breach lists gathered media reports and information from attorneys general and law enforcement, and provided an updated catalog of medical data breaches as they occurred. The breach lists are our primary source of pooled national information about medical data breaches prior to 2010. Recent studies have analyzed the distributions and trends in these data to draw conclusions about security risks to personal information [2–6].

But many of these lists were also incomplete in that they do not capture all breaches that are disclosed—many disclosed breaches appear in only one list, and many disclosed breaches are not included in any breach list, as we show below. Even in cases where notification is mandatory and covers the whole country, breach lists are still incomplete. For example, at the time of writing there were 14 breaches that met the notification criteria and appeared in our data set but did not appear in the DHHS list [7]. Other analysts have found similar inconsistencies [8].

Variations among lists in their breach counts are driven by two factors: those related to measurement and those related to the number of actual breaches disclosed. Measurement artifacts mean that the lists undercount and will have different counts. These are due to (1) the effort the list owners expend to collect information about breaches (the more effort expended, the higher the count), (2) the media's willingness to report on breaches (it has been argued that there is increasing media fatigue with breach stories [9–11], and within any single year we found at least 80% of breaches in our data set were reported in the media; therefore media fatigue could have an important impact on lists), (3) the ease of gathering information from regulators, law enforcement, and attorneys general about breaches, (4) some lists do not capture certain types of breaches (e.g., the public DHHS list does not include breaches involving less than 500 records), and (5) the extent to which custodians notify in all jurisdictions (e.g., notifying multiple state and federal authorities).

It is only possible to meaningfully examine historical trends in medical data breaches if the measurement artifacts are accounted for. For example, if the number of breaches captured by a list is decreasing over time, does that indicate media fatigue (measurement artifact), list curators spending less time collecting data (measurement artifact), list curators having difficulty getting the information from regulators, law enforcement, or attorneys general (measurement artifact), or a reduction in breaches that actually occur (substantive trend)?

In this chapter we solve the list incompleteness problem by providing an estimate of the total number of disclosed medical data breaches in the United States over the three-year period 2007–2009. Our estimate compensates for the measurement artifacts above by accounting for them—effectively addressing the measurement problem. The resulting estimates can be used to assess and interpret changes in historical reported breach counts due to variations in notification factors. We then examine the three-year data to draw conclusions about historical medical data breach trends.

Methods

Definitions

We are concerned with *disclosed breaches*, which are breaches that do occur and where the appropriate individuals and organizations have been notified as required by the relevant law. Not all breaches that occur will be disclosed. We used public breach lists as our main data source. A breach that is included in a list is considered *captured* by that list. Only disclosed breaches can be captured. The difference between all breaches and disclosed breaches is illustrated in Figure 22.1.

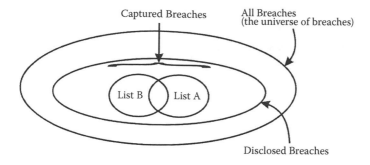

Figure 22.1   The differences among the types of breaches.

Breach Lists

Because breach lists are incomplete, we use the data from three breach lists to estimate the total number of disclosed breaches. The three breach lists do not necessarily have to be independent. Data were gathered from the three lists between February 2010 and April 2010.

Original Data Sources

The three lists are the Dataloss database (www.datalossdb.org), the POGO websites (www.pogowasright.org, www.databreaches.net, and www.phiprivacy.net) (henceforth the POGO list), and the Identity Theft Resource Center breach reports posted at http://www.idtheftcenter.org (henceforth the ITRC list). The exact data sources for the three lists are summarized in Table 22.1.

Table 22.1   Data Sources for the Three Lists

	Lists		
Sources	*POGO*	*Dataloss*	*ITRC*
Media reports	✓	✓	✓
Websites (other listings, blogs, company websites, etc.)	✓	✓	✓
Notification lists (states' attorneys general offices and federal agencies)	✓	✓	✓
FOIA requests/open records requests	✓	✓	
Individual contributors	✓	✓	✓

For POGO, the data are collected and verified by one individual. The breach reports are compiled from published mainstream media reports, notifications to states' attorneys general posted on the states' websites, notifications obtained under the Freedom of Information Act (FOIA) or open records requests, information submitted by readers of the websites (which is verified), other web resources that report or track incidents, and information released by the organizations that have experienced the breaches.

The Dataloss database is managed by four curators and requires that breaches come from publically available sources, such as online news feeds, blogs and other websites, media reports, and government agencies. The curators also regularly submit FOIA requests to state governments in order to obtain primary source information on reported breaches. FOIA requests can also reveal breaches that were not reported by the publically available sources.

ITRC lists breaches reported by various media sources as well as publically available notification lists from state government agencies. ITRC only lists publically available information, and does not use FOIA requests as a source. Each breach incident must have been published by a credible public source or sources, or the item will not be included in the listings.

All three lists originate in the United States. POGO and the Dataloss database also report on international incidents, but the ITRC does not include any reports of breaches occurring outside of the United States. The ITRC also limits its reporting to breaches of information that could be used for the purposes of identity theft.

Sponsors of Lists

POGO was created by a health care worker concerned with patient privacy. This person does not accept any sponsorship for maintaining these lists.

The Dataloss list is maintained by the Open Security Foundation. Supporters of the foundation range from individual donors to larger organizations that provide both financial and material support. Their corporate sponsors are data security-related companies.

ITRC is sponsored by government departments, corporate sponsors, foundation grants, and donations. At the time of writing, its government sponsors included the Department of Justice in the United States. Its corporate sponsors include both security- and identity theft-related companies.

Data Quality

For the purpose of our analysis, the lists do not need to be comprehensive in that they report all disclosed breaches. It is only necessary that the listed breaches are real breaches.

We contacted the list curators and examined the process descriptions on the list websites to determine the amount of quality assurance performed on the information that they contain.

In terms of verification by the list curators of public sources of breaches that make it onto their lists, media reports are included in the lists if they cite the source of the information on which they are reporting (e.g., a corporate spokesperson, someone in law enforcement, a press release from the entity). Where a breach listing had a link to an information source, we also checked the information source to confirm the details of the breach.

Notification letters are obtained from states' attorneys general offices that receive written notification of breaches from the breached entities, and also from federal agencies that publicly list breach reports that they have received from organizations. Other trusted sources would include press releases from a U.S. Attorney's office, information posted on the breached organization's website, and information obtained by way of FOIA requests sent to state governments.

Breaches from untrusted sources (e.g., tips or blogs) are also verified manually. For example, POGO contacts the entities to ask them to confirm or deny the allegation. If confirmed, POGO interviews them by phone or email and then includes a statement on the breach report as to what the corporate spokesperson said. In some cases, POGO may include a statement they email to the curator. In cases of phone interviews, these are reported in the breach incident description. The entities are alway free to send the curator any requested corrections if they think POGO misunderstood or misreported something. According to the POGO curator, that's happened twice at the most in the past 4 years.

Estimating the Number of Disclosed Breaches

Estimates were made using a capture-recapture (CR) model. A CR model can estimate the total population of disclosed breaches, including those missed by the breach lists. CR models have been used in the biological sciences to estimate the size of animal populations [12, 13], and in epidemiology to estimate birth and death rates [14, 15], as well as the size of diseased populations [16]. The basic principle is that animals are caught on multiple occasions and marked/identified. Using the information on the number of animals caught/not caught on the multiple occasions, a complete capture history of animal capture is known. Methods have been developed to estimate the total population size from such capture histories. CR models are a general estimation technique; they have also been used in other disciplines where the underlying assumptions can be met, such as estimating the number of defects in software from multiple independent inspections and code reviews [17, 18].

Table 22.2   Example of an Ascertainment Matrix

		List A		
		Included	Not Included	
List B	Included	n_{11}	n_{12}	N_{1+}
	Not Included	n_{21}	n_{22}	N_{2+}
		N_{+1}	N_{+2}	

There are two general types of CR models. The first are open models that account for changes in animal populations over the estimation period, such as migration and birth/death. The second are closed models that assume that the populations are fixed during the estimation period. We use only closed models since it is reasonable to assume that within a single year the total number of breaches that occur is a fixed number that needs to be estimated (for example, breaches that were reported at one point do not disappear or die).

The analogy to our problem would be that each list is considered a capture occasion and each breach is an animal that is caught. Assuming we have two lists that capture breaches independently, intuitively, if there are many breaches that overlap these two lists, then we would expect that the total number of breaches would be close to the number of unique breaches in the two lists. Also, if the overlap is small, then we would expect that the total number of breaches would be much higher than the number of unique breaches.

As an example, let us assume that the data from the two lists can be represented by a 2 × 2 ascertainment matrix, as shown in Table 22.2. The rows represent the number of breaches captured in list B, and the columns the number of breaches captured by list A. The value of n_{22} is unknown, as it represents the number of breaches that are not captured by any list, and therefore needs to be estimated.

The correlation between the two lists is given by [19]

$$r = \frac{n_{11}n_{22} - n_{12}n_{21}}{\sqrt{\left(n_{11}+n_{12}\right)\left(n_{21}+n_{22}\right)\left(n_{11}+n_{21}\right)\left(n_{12}+n_{22}\right)}} \qquad (22.1)$$

If the two lists are independent, then $r = 0$. Under such an assumption we have $n_{11}n_{22} = n_{12}n_{21}$, and can therefore estimate

$$\hat{n}_{22} = \frac{n_{12}n_{21}}{n_{11}}$$

and the total population size is given by

$$\hat{N} = n_{11} + n_{12} + n_{21} + \frac{n_{12}n_{21}}{n_{11}} = \frac{N_{+1}N_{1+}}{n_{11}}$$

This estimator is known as the Lincoln-Peterson estimator and is an instance of the general maximum likelihood estimate of population size with two methods of ascertainment [12]. An estimator has been developed in the case where the correlation between the two lists is not zero [15]. However, this still assumes that all breaches have an equal probability of being captured, which is not a reasonable assumption. The accuracy of the estimator will be a function of the dependencies and the variation in capture probabilities that it can model. Therefore it is important to understand possible dependencies in the data set and ensure that the estimation model can account for these.

Models have been developed that are suitable for more than two lists and that take into account three different types of dependencies and sources of variation that occur in the real world [20–23]. We explain these dependencies below in the context of our problem:

1. *The lists have different probabilities of capturing a breach.* This assumption implies that the breach list owners will exert a different amount of effort to capture information about breaches that occur, and therefore the probability of a breach being reported will vary by list. The analogy to animal populations is that capture probabilities of animals might vary. For example, small mammals tend to stay in their dry homes during rainy weather. Therefore the probability of capturing a small mammal is higher for days with fine weather than for days with rainy weather. Estimation models that make this assumption assume variation in capture probabilities over *occasions* [12].

   Models that only take into account variation across occasions assume that every list i has the probability p_i of capturing every breach. Thus all different breaches have the same capture probability, but the lists have different capture capabilities. Hence with this source of variation accounted for, a model allows for lists with differing "general capability to capture breaches." Note that this general capability affects all breaches. The Lincoln-Peterson estimator noted above makes this assumption.

2. *Breaches do not have equal probabilities of being captured by a list.* For example, one would expect that breaches affecting more records and individuals are more likely to be captured than those involving only a handful of records. This may be because they are likely to be reported in more media outlets, for example. The animal analogy is that different animals vary in their capture probability. For example, older animals are less mobile than younger ones and stay more often in their homes. Therefore the probability of capturing an old animal is smaller than that of capturing a young animal. Estimation models that make this assumption assume *heterogeneity* in capture probabilities for individual animals [12].

Models that only take heterogeneity into account assume that every breach j has the probability of p_j being captured by a list, which is the same for every list. Thus different breaches can vary in their capture probability, but all lists have the same capture capability.

3. *The lists are not independent.* This may be because some lists gather information from other lists, so if a breach is captured in one list, then a second list is likely to notice that breach and the breach will be captured in that second list. This means that if a breach is captured in list A, then there is a non-negligible chance that it will also be captured in list B. The animal analogy is that if an animal is caught on one occasion, that will have an impact on its probability of being caught on a future occasion (e.g., animals become trap shy or trap happy because of the availability of food in traps, and therefore the probability to get caught for the first time is less than the probability for subsequent captures). Estimation models that make this assumption consider behavioral changes across capture occasions [12]. However, in animal populations there is an order to trapping, whereas in our case there is no meaningful order [24]. Furthermore, if the capture probabilities among breaches are heterogeneous (effect 2 above), this may also induce dependencies among the lists [25].

The different assumptions above can be combined. For example, a model may assume that every breach j has the probability p_j of being captured, and that every list has the probability p_i of capturing breaches. The probability p_{ij} that list i captures breach j is computed as $p_{ij} = p_i \times p_j$. This allows for different capture probabilities for the different breaches and lists. Note that if one of the sources of variation above does not exist in the data, then the estimate that accounts for the source of variation or dependency would still give valid results. For instance, if there is no variation among list capture probabilities in the data, then the joint probability becomes $p_{ij} = P \times p_j$, where P is the common probability of capturing a breach across all lists. On the other hand, if a source of variation exists in the data and is not captured by the model, then the results may not be valid. Therefore if sufficient data are available, it is better to use a model that captures all three sources of variation.

A number of commonly used ecological estimators have been developed that take multiple dependencies into account (using maximum likelihood and jackknife methods, for example) [12, 13]. However, they generally require more than three lists (or capture occasions) to give reliable estimates.

Initially, we attempted to use an estimator suitable for three lists that also took into account covariates (for example, the number of records implicated in a breach would be a covariate since we hypothesized that larger breaches are more likely to be disclosed) [26–28]. The conclusions drawn were quite similar to the results we present using a simpler model that does not account for the covariates. Therefore, we do not present the covariate model results.

We therefore use an estimator based on sample coverage that is suitable for three lists and that takes into account the three effects mentioned above, without using covariates [24, 29]. We estimate the disclosed breach population size and a bootstrap 95% confidence interval for each of the three years.

Data Collection

All breaches in the United States from the three lists over the period January 2007 to December 2009 inclusive were collected. They were initially filtered by two people to extract only the types of breaches of interest to us (see below), and to de-duplicate breaches that were mentioned more than once. Any discrepancies were addressed during a face-to-face meeting.

There were two types of medical data breaches of interest: (1) those that occur at a health information custodian (e.g., a hospital or an organization that handles medical data, such as a medical insurance claims processor firm), and (2) those where the data themselves consist of medical records. The two types are not the same. For example, a breach of financial records from a hospital would be of the former type, and the loss of prisoner medical records from a sheriff's office would be an example of the latter type. We will refer to these as *custodian breaches* and *record breaches*, respectively.

We considered only reported custodian breaches. This seems more appropriate given that most breach notification laws during the period of analysis did not cover medical records specifically, and therefore there was not compelling incentive to report only medical record breaches in most of the country.

Interrater Agreement

To determine the reliability of the coding of breaches an inter-rater agreement analysis was performed. To determine how many breaches need to be rated by a second rater, we performed a power analysis for using the kappa statistic [30]. To determine the expected kappa value for the power analysis, we can rely on generally accepted benchmarks for kappa values. General guidelines for moderate to good agreement vary from 0.4 to 0.75 [31–34]. To err on the conservative side, we will assume that our value of kappa will be at least 0.5. At that level of agreement and 80% power to reject a null hypothesis comparing kappa to agreement by chance, the second rater needed to code 32 breaches [35, 36].

Two coders performed two sets of ratings as custodian breach or not, and record breach or not. Both values of kappa were above 0.9.

Results

There were 579 unique breaches disclosed in the three lists. Only 189 breaches were reported in all three lists (33%). Table 22.3 shows the actual number of breaches

Table 22.3   Number of Breaches Captured in Each List and the Union of Breaches in the Three Lists

	Less than 500 Individuals			500 or More Individuals		
	Dataloss	POGO	ITRC	Dataloss	POGO	ITRC
2007	18	69	36	69	111	82
2008	48	118	64	97	136	111
2009	40	108	59	56	82	70

Table 22.4   Overlap among the Data Sources Overall for the Three Years

	Dataloss	POGO	ITRC
Dataloss		209	229
POGO			291

Table 22.5   Actual and Estimates of the Number of Disclosed Medical Data Breaches over the 2007–2009 Period

	Less than 500 Individuals			500 or More Individuals		
	Captured	Population Estimate (95% CI)	Undercount	Captured	Population Estimate (95% CI)	Undercount
2007	39	147 (145–153)	73%	82	85 (83–93)	3.5%
2008	75	112 (85–212)	33%	93	95 (93–101)	2%
2009	80	110 (87–211)	27%	52	53 (52–59)	2%

captured by each of the three lists. The overlap in breaches among the three lists is shown in Table 22.4. The CR estimates are shown in Table 22.5 for the two types of breaches. This table also shows the actual and the percentage of undercount between the estimated total disclosed breaches and the actual count of captured breaches from the three lists.

Discussion

Summary of Main Results

None of the three lists had all of the captured breaches; therefore each list under-counts. However, the POGO list comes closest to having the most breaches that are captured. This is not surprising since that list focuses on health information.

There are also large differences among the lists. For example, Dataloss captured 81 custodian breaches for 2007, whereas POGO captured 141. The individual lists exhibit inconsistent trends. Some show a decrease between 2008 and 2009, whereas others suggest a plateau is reached (e.g., POGO for record breaches). Therefore across the lists there is considerable variation in counts and trends.

Our estimated numbers of disclosed breaches are higher than the numbers captured in the breach lists. The trends over time indicate a peak in 2008 with a subsequent decline in estimated disclosed breaches in 2009 for both breaches involving 500 or more records and those involving less than 500 records. Then there is a dramatic jump again in 2010 from our estimate of 110 small breaches to more than 25,000, and from our estimate of 53 large breaches to 207.

Post Hoc Analysis

In 2010 DHHS had been notified of 207 breaches involving 500 or more records, and more than 25,000 involving less than 500 records. This suggests that breaches involving less than 500 records are much more likely to occur than larger breaches.

We constructed a cumulative odds logistic regression model [37] whereby the number of lists that a breach appears in was the ordinal outcome, and a binary variable indicating whether a breach involved more than 500 (coded as 1) or not (coded as 0).

The results of this model are shown in Table 22.6. The chi-square value for the model as a whole was significant, indicating that the model is better than the model with no predictors. The proportionality test is not significant, which means that our data meet the assumption of proportional odds, and therefore this type of ordinal regression model is suitable. For large custodian breaches the odds are 8.4 that

Table 22.6 Results of the Ordinal Logistic Regression Model

	Custodian Breaches
Model chi-square	120 ($p < 0.001$)
Proportionality of odds across response categories chi-square	0.32 ($p = 0.57$)
Coefficient (odds ratio, 95% CI)	8.4 (5.6–12.6)

one or more list will capture that breach. Such a strong effect size provides strong evidence that the lists are much more likely to capture large breaches (greater than 500 records) than small breaches.

References

1. Office for Civil Rights. *Annual report to Congress on breaches of unsecured protected health information for calendar years 2009 and 2010.* U.S. Department of Health and Human Services, 2011.
2. Hsasn R, Yurcik W. Beyond media hype: Empirical analysis of disclosed privacy breaches 2005–2006 and a dataset/database foundation for future work. Workshop on the Economics of Securing the Information Infrastructure, 2006.
3. Hasan R, Yurcik W. A statistical analysis of disclosed storage security breaches. 2nd International Workshop on Storage Security and Survivability (StorageSS '06), 2006.
4. Curtin M, Ayres L. *Using science to combat data loss: Analyzing breaches by type and industry.* Interhack Corporation, 2009.
5. Widup S. *The leaking vault: Five years of data breaches.* Digital Forensics Association, 2010.
6. Hourihan C. *An analysis of breaches affecting 500 or more individuals in healthcare.* HITRUST Alliance, 2010.
7. Department of Health and Human Services—Office of Civil Rights. *Breaches affecting 500 or more individuals.* 2010. http://www.hhs.gov/ocr/privacy/hipaa/administrative/breachnotificationrule/postedbreaches.html.
8. Schwartz M. ITRC: Why so many data breaches don't see the light of day. Dark Reading, 2010. http://www.darkreading.com/security/attacks/showArticle.jhtml?articleID=225702908. Archived at http://www.webcitation.org/5sdi4aNei.
9. Schneier B. Breach notification laws. Schneier on Security, 2009. http://www.schneier.com/blog/archives/2009/01/state_data_brea.html.
10. Open Security Foundation. Where did the breach go? 2010. http://datalossdb.org/where_did_it_go.
11. MacSweeney G. When risk managers cry wolf. Wall Street and Technology, 2006. http://www.wallstreetandtech.com/blog/archives/2006/11/when_risk_manag.html. Archived at http://www.webcitation.org/5tvLAV11b.
12. Otis D, Burnham K, White G, Anderson D. Statistical inference from capture data on closed animal populations. *Wildlife Monographs*, 1978; 62:1–135.
13. White G, Anderson D, Burnham K, Otis D. Capture-recapture and removal methods for sampling closed populations. Los Alamos National Laboratory, 1982.
14. Chandra Sekar C, Edwards Deming W. On a method of estimating birth and death rates and the extent of registration. *Journal of the American Statistical Association*, 1949; 44(245–248):101–115.
15. Greenfield C. On the estimation of a missing cell in a 2×2 contingency table. *Journal of the Royal Statistical Society, Series A*, 1975; 138:51–61.
16. Hook E, Regal R. Capture-recapture methods in epidemiology: Methods and limitations. *Epidemiologic Reviews*, 1995; 17(2):243–264.
17. El Emam K, Laitenberger O. Evaluating capture-recapture models with two inspectors. *IEEE Transactions on Software Engineering*, 2001; 27(9):851–864.

18. Briand LC, El Emam K, Freimut BG, Laitenberger O. A comprehensive evaluation of capture-recapture models for estimating software defect content. *IEEE Transactions on Software Engineering*, 2000; 36(6):518–540.
19. Sheskin D. *Handbook of parametric and nonparametric statistical procedures*. Boca Raton, FL: CRC Press, 1997.
20. Seber G. *The estimation of animal abundance and related parameters*. 2nd ed. Charles Griffin & Company, 1982.
21. Seber G. A review of estimating animal abundance. *Biometrics*, 1986; 42:267–292.
22. Seber G. A review of estimating animal abundance II. *Statistical Review*, 1992; 60:129–166.
23. Schwarz C, Seber G. A review of estimating animal abundance III. *Statistical Science*, 1999; 14:427–456.
24. Chao A, Tsay P, Lin S-H, Shau W-Y, Chao D-Y. The application of capture-recapture models to epidemiological data. *Statistics in Medicine*, 2001; 250:3123–3157.
25. Hook E, Regal R. Effect of variation in probability of ascertainment by sources ("variable catchability") upon "capture-recapture" estimates of prevalence. *American Journal of Epidemiology*, 1993; 137(10):1148–1166.
26. Huggins R. On the statistical analysis of capture experiments. *Biometrika*, 1989; 76(1):133–140.
27. Yip P, Huggins R, Lin DY. Inference for capture-recapture experiments in continuous time with variable capture rates. *Biometrika Trust*, 1995; 83(2):477–483.
28. Huggins R. Some practical aspects of a conditional likelihood approach to capture experiments. *Biometrics*, 1991; 47:725–732.
29. Chao A, Tsay P. A sample coverage approach to multiple-system estimation with application to census undercount. *Journal of the American Statistical Association*, 1998; 93(283–293).
30. Cohen J. A coefficient of agreement for nominal scales. *Educational and Psychological Measurement*, 1960; XX(1):37–46.
31. Hartmann D. Considerations in the choice of interobserver reliability estimates. *Journal of Applied Behavior Analysis*, 1977; 10(1):103–116.
32. Landis J, Koch G. The measurement of observer agreement for categorical data. *Biometrics*, 1977; 33:159–174.
33. Altman D. *Practical statistics for medical research*. London, UK: Chapman & Hall, 1991.
34. Fleiss J. *Statistical methods for rates and proportions*. New York: Wiley, 1981.
35. Sim J, Wright C. The kappa statistic in reliability studies: Use, interpretation, and sample size requirements. *Physical Therapy*, 2005; 85(3):257–268.
36. Flack V, Afifi A, Lachenbruch P. Sample size determinations for the two rater kappa statistic. *Psychometrika*, 1988; 53(3):321–325.
37. O'Connell A. *Logistic regression models for ordinal response variables*. Sage, 2006.

Chapter 23

Methods of Attack for Maximum Journalist Risk

In this chapter we describe three methods of attack that represent journalist risk. Under all three methods the simple re-identification risk metric for journalist risk is the same.

Method of Attack 1

Under this method of attack the adversary will start from the disclosed data set and select a record to re-identify. The adversary does not care which record, although he will choose strategically. The most likely records to be re-identified are those in the smallest equivalence classes in the disclosed data set. Therefore the adversary would randomly select one of those records.

Assume that an adversary draws a record randomly from the smallest equivalence classes in the disclosed data set and tries to match it with its corresponding record in the identification database, and assume without loss of generality that $f_1, \ldots, f_m$ are the smallest equivalence classes in the disclosed data set (i.e., they all contain the same number of records, and it is the smallest compared to the other equivalence classes); then the probability of correctly identifying the record is denoted by θ_{max} and is calculated as follows:

θ_{max} = P(correctly identifying a record drawn at random from the smallest equivalence classes in the sample)

= P(choosing a record from f_1 and correctly identifying it ∨ choosing a
record from f_2 and correctly identifying it ∨ ... ∨ choosing a record
from f_m and correctly identifying it)

$$= \sum_{i=1}^{m} P(\text{choosing a record from } f_i \text{ and correctly identifying it})$$

$$= \sum_{i=1}^{m} P(\text{choosing a record from } f_i) \; P(\text{correctly identifying the record given i was chosen from } f_i)$$

$$= \sum_{i=1}^{m} \frac{f_i}{mf_i} \frac{1}{F_i}$$

$$= \frac{1}{m} \sum_{i=1}^{m} \frac{1}{F_i}$$

$$= \frac{\sum_{i=1}^{m} \frac{1}{F_i}}{m}$$

$$= \frac{1}{m} \cdot \frac{m}{F_1} = \frac{1}{F_1} = \frac{1}{\min_{j \in J}(F_j)}$$

Method of Attack 2

Under this method of attack the adversary selects a record from the identification
database and tries to match it with the records in the disclosed data set. The most
likely record to be re-identified is one in the smallest equivalence class, and therefore the adversary would select a record from the smallest equivalence classes in the
identification database.

Assume the adversary draws at random a record from the smallest identification
database equivalence classes and tries to match it with the records in the sample.
And assume without loss of generality that $F_1, ..., F_m$ are the smallest equivalence
classes in the identification database (i.e., they all contain the same number of
records, and it is the smallest compared to the other equivalence classes). Then the
probability of correctly identifying the record is calculated as follows:

P(correctly linking a record drawn at random from the smallest equivalence classes in the subset of the population defined above)

$=$ P(choosing a record from F_1 and correctly identifying it $\vee$ choosing a record from F_2 and correctly identifying it $\vee$ ... $\vee$ choosing a record from F_m and correctly identifying it)

$$= \sum_{i=1}^{m} P(\text{choosing a record from } F_i \text{ and correctly identifying it})$$

$$= \sum_{i=1}^{m} P(\text{choosing a record from } F_i) \, P(\text{correctly identifying the record given it was chosen from } F_i)$$

$$= \sum_{i=1}^{m} P(\text{choosing a record from } F_i) \, P(\text{the record chosen is included in the sample given it was chosen from } F_i) \, P(\text{the record is correctly matched given it is included in the sample and given that it was chosen from } F_i)$$

$$= \sum_{i=1}^{m} \left(\frac{F_i}{mF_i} \frac{f_i}{F_i} \frac{1}{f_i} \right)$$

$$= \frac{1}{m} \sum_{i=1}^{m} \left(\frac{1}{F_i} \right)$$

$$= \frac{1}{m} \frac{m}{F_1} = \frac{1}{F_1} = \frac{1}{\min_{j \in J} \left(F_j \right)}$$

Method of Attack 3

Under this method of attack the adversary has a specific target person in mind, and therefore does not rely on an identification database. However, the adversary does not know whether that target individual is in the disclosed data set or not. Therefore the probability is given by:

P(the target record is included in the sample) P(the record is correctly matched given it is included in the sample)

We assume that the target record matches the equivalence class j; then:

$$= \frac{f_j}{F_j} \frac{1}{f_j} = \frac{1}{F_j}$$

However, the data custodian does not know which equivalence class the target individual will come from, and therefore it would be necessary to make a worst-case assumption in that it comes from the smallest equivalence class; hence we have

$$
1 \Big/ \min_{j \in J} \big(F_j \big)
$$

Chapter 24

How Many Friends Do We Have?

An important consideration in operationalizing risk measurements that take into account the number of friends one has is to get a good estimate of m, which is the number of friends that an individual would, on average, have. We consider the literature here, which informs our choice of m.

In 1993, Dunbar extrapolated the theory that group size in non-human primates is dependent upon neocortex size to the human context. The concept is that the "current neocortex size sets a limit on the number of relationships that it [an animal] can maintain through time, and hence limits the maximum size of its group" [1]. Dunbar applied this to humans, suggesting that the number of relationships we can keep track of in a social network is dependent upon our current neocortex size. Using an equation developed to predict primate mean group size, the best-fit reduced major axis regression equation between neocortex ratio and mean group size, he finds a predicted group size of 147.8 (95% CI = 100.2–231.1). Dunbar himself admits that in using this equation he is "extrapolating well beyond the range of neocortex ratios on which it is based" [1], and therefore the large confidence interval was not unexpected. However, using other equations based on neocortex size, he found similar results ranging from 107.6 to 248.6.

Looking at anthropological evidence of hunter-gatherer societies, Dunbar provides some support for this number. He found that historically hunter-gatherer groups contained a hierarchy of groups from small bands of 30–50, to intermediate clan groupings of 100–200, and larger tribal units of up to 2,000. The intermediate grouping seems to function along the lines of what would be found in nonhuman primates: It is based on regular interaction with and direct personal knowledge of group members, and forms a "coalitionary support" network that can be called upon to defend against attack by other groups [1]. He found that the average size of the intermediate groupings in these societies was 148.4 [1]. He also found similar group sizing among contemporary Hutterite communities, which view 150 as the maximum group size prior to groups being divided off into separate communities; as well as academic communities, with groupings of sub-disciplines averaging around 200; and professional armies with a basic unit of around 150 [1].

Since the introduction of this theory, also called the social brain hypothesis, there have been several studies examining social network size in humans. Dunbar himself has conducted studies to help support the number 150 for human social network size. In 2003, Dunbar and Hill conducted a survey examining the exchange of Christmas cards among British citizens [2]. They chose Christmas because they believed it "represents the one time of year when individuals make an effort to contact all those individuals within their social network whose relationships they value" [2]. The results of their survey were a mean network size of 153.5 (±84.5) when everyone in the household to whom the cards were sent was included, and 124.9 (±68) when limited to individuals who were actively contacted [2].

Another survey, examining the closeness of ties within social networks in Belgium, found a mean network size of 71.84 (SD = 33.07) [3]. The inclusion of people in one's network was limited to all relatives and unrelated people with whom there was a personal relationship and for whom these conditions applied: "(i) they have contact details; (ii) they have had some sort of contact within the last 12 months; (iii) they feel they would wish the relationship to continue" [3]. The second limitation of contact within the past 12 months may explain the lower mean in this study, as one may have people in their social network with whom one has not been in touch in the past year but to whom one still feels close ties.

Two studies of social networking sites undertook by Dunbar and colleagues show that there is no correlation between the use of social networking sites and the size of one's offline social network [4, 5]. In fact, having a large number of friends on Facebook is not the norm. According to Dunbar, Facebook's statistics put the average number of friends around 130 [5]. Another study of Facebook found that the average active Facebook user had 190 friends in his or her network, and the median friend count was 99 [6]. An active user was defined as someone who had "logged into the site in the last 28 days from our time of measurement in May 2011 and had at least one Facebook friend" [6]. The authors point out that this definition differs from Facebook's definition of an active user, which would explain the difference in numbers. However, both numbers hover around Dunbar's original estimate of ~150.

Gonçalves, Perra, and Vespignani studied Twitter conversations to validate Dunbar's number [7]. They analyzed "genuine social interaction" by looking at active communication between users. "We introduce the weight w_{ij} of each edge, defined as the number of times user i replies to user j as a direct measurement of the interaction strength between two users and stable relations will be those with a large weight" [7]. They found that the average weight of each outward connection increased until a maximum, which falls between 100 and 200 friends, was reached. This is in line with Dunbar's estimation, especially if the confidence interval (100.2–231.1) is taken into consideration.

One study by McCarty et al. took a different approach for estimating network size in humans [8]. They used both a "scale-up method" and a "summation method" to estimate the size of personal social networks. The scale-up method "is based on the assumption that the number of people a person knows in a particular subpopulation is a function of, among other things, the number of people known overall" [8]. This method assumes that the probability that a member of a person's network is part of a subpopulation, for example, people who are left-handed, will be equivalent to the probability of a person from the general population being in that subpopulation. So if one-fourth of the people in the population are left-handed, then one-fourth of a given person's network should be left-handed as well. A person would be included in one's network if "you know the person and they know you by sight or by name; you can contact them in person, by telephone or by mail; and you have had contact with the person in the past two years" [8]. To test this method, they performed a survey in which people were asked to estimate the number of people that they know in 29 different subpopulations. From these answers, the size of the person's social network was calculated. They found that the average personal network size of survey respondents was 286. The summation method asks respondents to count the number of people who are of certain relations to the individual (family, friends, co-workers, etc.). These relation types are then used to estimate overall network size. In a separate survey, they found that the two methods were well correlated, producing similar results. They found a mean network size of 290.7 (SD = 258.8) for the summation method and 290.8 (SD = 264.4) for the scale-up method [8]. In a follow-up survey, the authors found a network size of 291.2 (SD = 259.3) for the scale-up method and 281.2 (SD = 255.4) for the summation method [8].

McCarty's estimation appears to be well above Dunbar's original estimate. It seems the difference may originate in who is being included in the definition of a network. Dunbar appears to stress not only a reciprocal nature of the relationships within one's social network, but also a value given to the relationships by the individual. In the Christmas card study, he mentions that people send cards to those "whose relationships they value" [2]. Similarly, in the Belgian study, they use a criteria of wanting to continue the relationship with a person as a condition of being included in one's social network [3]. This seems to indicate stronger ties between the people in Dunbar's network than in the personal network proposed by McCarty. In McCarty's study, they included relation types such as "people at work but don't work with directly" and "people who provide a service" [8]. These appear to be people with whom one would not be likely to have very strong ties. McCarty et al. acknowledge this issue in their paper, stating that prior studies looking at network size produced varying results "due in part to the definition of who should be included in a respondent's network" [8].

References

1. Dunbar RIM. Coevolution of neocortical size, group size and language in humans. *Behavioral and Brain Sciences*, 1993; 16(4):681–693.
2. Hill RA, Dunbar RIM. Social network size in humans. *Human Nature*, 2003; 14(1):53–72.
3. Roberts SGB, Dunbar RIM, Pollet TV, Kuppens T. Exploring variation in active network size: Constraints and ego characteristics. *Social Networks*, 2009; 31(2):138–146.
4. Dunbar RIM. Social cognition on the Internet: Testing constraints on social network size. *Philosophical Transactions of the Royal Society B: Biological Sciences*, 2012; 367(1599):2192–2201.
5. Pollet TV, Roberts SGB, Dunbar RIM. Use of social network sites and instant messaging does not lead to increased offline social network size, or to emotionally closer relationships with offline network members. *Cyberpsychology, Behavior and Social Networking*, 2011; 14(4):253–258.
6. Johan U, Brian K, Lars B, Cameron M. *The anatomy of the Facebook social graph*. Ithaca, NY: Cornell University Library, arXiv:111.4503. Available from: http://arxiv.org/abs/111.4503. 2011.
7. Gonçalves B, Perra N, Vespignani A. Modeling users' activity on Twitter networks: Validation of Dunbar's number. *PLoS One*, 2011; 6(8):e22656–e22656.
8. McCarty C, Killworth P, Bernard HR, Johnsen E, Shelley GA. Comparing two methods for estimating network size. *Human Organization*, 2001; 60(1):28–39.

Chapter 25

Cell Size Precedents

Historically, data custodians have used the "cell size of five" rule as a threshold for deciding whether to de-identify data [1–12]. This rule has been applied originally to count data in tables. However, count data can be easily converted to individual-level data; therefore these two representations are in effect the same thing. A minimum "cell size of five" rule would translate into a maximum probability of re-identifying a single record of 0.2. Some custodians use a cell size of 3 [13–17], which is equivalent to a probability of re-identifying a single record of 0.33. For the public release of data, a cell size of 11 has been used in the United States [18–22], and a cell size of 20 for public Canadian and U.S. patent data [23, 24].

In commentary about the de-identification standard in the HIPAA Privacy Rule, the DHHS notes in the *Federal Register* [11, 12] "the two main sources of disclosure risk for de-identified records about data subjects are the existence of records with very unique characteristics (e.g., unusual occupation or very high salary or age) and the existence of external sources of records with matching data elements that can be used to link with the de-identified information and identify data subjects (e.g., voter registration records or driver's license records) ... an expert disclosure analysis would also consider the probability that a data subject who is the target of an attempt at re-identification is represented on both files, the probability that the matching variables are recorded identically on the two types of records, the probability that the target data subject is unique in the population for the matching variables, and the degree of confidence that a match would correctly identify a unique person." Unique records are those that make up a cell count of 1. It is clear that the DHHS considered unique records to have a high risk of re-identification, and records that are not unique to have an acceptably low risk of re-identification. This translates to a minimal cell size of 2, although cell sizes less than 3 are explicitly not recommended in the disclosure control literature [25].

<3 (>0.33)	3 (0.33)	5 (0.2)	11 (0.09)	20 (0.05)
identifiable data	highly trusted data disclosure			highly untrusted data disclosure

Figure 25.1 The different levels of risk that have been used in practice in terms of minimal cell size across Canada and the United States.

It is clear that the most popular threshold in practice is 5. However, for highly sensitive information, the thresholds used have not been consistent. For example, a minimal count of 3 has been recommended for HIV/AIDS data [15], and a cell size of 5 for abortion data [6]. Public data releases have used different cell sizes in different jurisdictions. Part of the variability has to do with tolerance for risk, the sensitivity of the data, whether a data sharing agreement will be in place, and the nature of the data recipient.

A minimum cell size criterion amounts to a maximum risk value. For example, for a minimal cell size of 5 we are saying that no record should have a probability of re-identification that is higher than 0.2. Therefore, the maximum risk is 0.2. In some cases this is too stringent of a standard or may not be an appropriate reflection of the type of attack. In such a case one can use average risk, which averages the probability across all records. The average risk will always be lower than or equal to maximum risk. This means that if one were to use the average risk then one can use less stringent values than the ones presented here. For example, if a cell size of 5 is an appropriate threshold for maximum risk, then a cell size of 5 or even smaller than 5 would be appropriate for average risk. This makes the review of cell size thresholds suitable for both types of risk metrics.

It is possible to construct a decision framework based on these precedents with five "bins" representing five possible thresholds, as shown in Figure 25.1. At one extreme would be data sets that would be considered identifiable, where the cell size is smaller than 3. Next to that are data that are de-identified with a minimal cell size of 3. Given that this is the least de-identified data set, one would disclose such data sets to trusted entities only where the risks are minimal (for example, there is a data sharing agreement in place and the data recipient has good practices in place). At the other end of the spectrum is the minimal cell size of 20. That high level of de-identification would be used in situations where the data is publicly released with no restrictions or tracking of what is being done with the data and who has accessed the data.

If the extreme situations cannot be justified in a particular disclosure, then an alternate process is needed to choose one of the intermediate values. In Figure 25.1 this is a choice between a value of 5 and 10.

The above framework does not preclude the use of other values (for example, a data custodian may choose to use a threshold value of 25 observations per cell). However, this framework does ground the choices based on precedents on actual data sets.

References

1. Cancer Care Ontario data use and disclosure policy. Cancer Care Ontario, 2005.
2. Security and confidentiality policies and procedures. Health Quality Council, 2004.
3. Privacy code. Health Quality Council, 2004.
4. Privacy code. Manitoba Center for Health Policy, 2002.
5. Subcommittee on Disclosure Limitation Methodology, Federal Committee on Statistical Methodology. *Working paper 22: Report on statistical disclosure control.* Office of Management and Budget, 1994.
6. Statistics Canada. Therapeutic abortion survey. 2007. http://www.statcan.ca/cgi-bin/imdb/p2SV.pl?Function=getSurvey&SDDS=3209&lang=en&db=IMDB&dbg=f&adm=8&dis=2#b9. Archived at http://www.webcitation.org/5VkcHLeQw.
7. Office of the Information and Privacy Commissioner of British Columbia. Order 261-1998. 1998.
8. Office of the Information and Privacy Commissioner of Ontario. Order P-6441994, 1994. http://www.ipc.on.ca/images/Findings/Attached_PDF/P-644.pdf. Archived at http://www.webcitation.org/5inrVJyQp.
9. Alexander L, Jabine T. Access to social security microdata files for research and statistical purposes. *Social Security Bulletin*, 1978; 41(8):3–17.
10. Ministry of Health and Long Term Care (Ontario). Corporate Policy 3-1-21. 1984.
11. Department of Health and Human Services. Standards for privacy of individually identifiable health information. 2000. http://aspe.hhs.gov/admnsimp/final/PvcFR06.txt
12. Department of Health and Human Services. Standards for privacy of individually identifiable health information. Federal Register. 2000. http://aspe.hhs.gov/admnsimp/final/PvcFR05.txt
13. de Waal A, Willenborg L. A view on statistical disclosure control for microdata. *Survey Methodology*, 1996; 22(1):95–103.
14. Duncan G, Jabine T, de Wolf S. Private lives and public policies: Confidentiality and accessibility of government statistics. Washington, DC: National Academies Press, 1993.
15. National Center for Education Statistics. NCES statistical standards. U.S. Department of Education, 2003.
16. Office of the Privacy Commissioner of Quebec. *Chenard v. Ministere de l'agriculture, des pecheries et de l'alimentation (141).* 1997.
17. Centers for Disease Control and Prevention. Integrated guidelines for developing epidemiologic profiles: HIV prevention and Ryan White CARE Act community planning.
18. Centers for Medicare and Medicaid Services. BSA inpatient claims PUF. 2011.
19. 2008 Basic Stand Alone Medicare Claims Public Use Files. http://www.cms.gov/Research-Statistics-Data-and-Systems/Statistics-Trends-and-Reports/BSAPUFS/Downloads/2008_BSA_PUF_Disclaimer.pdf
20. Erdem E, Prada SI. Creation of public use files: lessons learned from the comparative effectiveness research public use files data pilot project. 2011.http://mpra.ub.uni-muenchen.de/35478/ (accessed 9 Nov2012).
21. Baier P, Hinkins S, Scheuren F. The Electronic Health Records Incentive Program Eligible Professionals Public Use File. 2012.http://www.cms.gov/Regulations-and-Guidance/Legislation/EHRIncentivePrograms/downloads/EP-PUF-Statistical-Cert-Final.pdf

22. INSTRUCTIONS FOR COMPLETING THE LIMITED DATA SET ATA USE AGREEMENT (DUA) (CMS-R-0235L). http://www.cms.gov/Medicare/CMS-Forms/CMS-Forms/Downloads/CMS-R-0235L.pdf

23. El Emam K, Paton D, Dankar F, et al. De-identifying a Public Use Microdata File from the Canadian National Discharge Abstract Database. BMC Medical Informatics and Decision Making 2011;11.http://w14.biomedcentral.com/1472-6947/11/53

24. El Emam K, Arbuckle L, Koru G, Eze B, Gaudette L, Neri E, et al. De-identification methods for open health data: The case of the Heritage Health Prize claims dataset. *Journal of Medical Internet Resea*rch, 2012; 14(1):e33-e.

25. Willenborg L, de Waal T. *Elements of statistical disclosure control.* New York: Springer-Verlag, 2001.

Chapter 26

Assessing the Invasion of Privacy Construct

The objective of this chapter is to define a way to measure the invasion-of-privacy construct. Invasion of privacy is a subjective criterion that can be used by the data custodian (DC) to influence his or her choice of the re-identification metric thresholds. If the invasion of privacy is deemed to be high, then that should weigh the decision more toward a lower threshold. On the other hand, if the invasion of privacy is deemed to be quite low, then a higher threshold would be acceptable.

There are degrees of invasion of privacy, and the items in this section determine that degree. By measuring the extent of the potential invasion of privacy, it will be possible for the DC to decide how much de-identification needs to be done. For example, if data on a stigmatized disease are disclosed to a data requestor, then that would score higher on invasion of privacy than disclosing data on common allergies. In both cases there would be an invasion of privacy, but in terms of degree, the latter would be greater, and therefore the data require more de-identification.

In our definition of invasion of privacy we make two important assumptions:

- An invasion of privacy can only occur if the data that are disclosed/used are identifiable. Therefore all of the items below are based on the assumption that all of the data are identifiable by the data requestor. The custodian may have disclosed identifiable data, the disclosed data were de-identified, and the data requestor was able to re-identify them somehow, or the data requestor is using identifiable information provided by the custodian. When we talk about data in the context of this construct, then, we are referring to personal information or personal health information.

■ The disclosure/use will not entail going back to the data subjects and seeking their consent.

With the above assumptions, an invasion of privacy can occur under three conditions:

■ If the custodian inappropriately discloses the data to the data requestor or there is an inappropriate use of the data
■ If the data requestor inappropriately processes the data (e.g., in terms of the analysis performed on it)
■ There is a data breach at the data requestor site (whether it is deliberate or accidental)

The items below are intended to assess the different dimensions of invasion of privacy if any of the three conditions above are satisfied.

The data custodian is expected to be able to respond to/assess all of the items below. In some cases the DC may have to exercise his or her best judgment in order to respond.

It is assumed that it would be possible to make general assessments about all of the data subjects covered by the data, even if this is an approximation. For example, some data subjects may care if they have been consulted if their data is disclosed/used for secondary purposes, while others may not. However, if a nontrivial proportion of the data subjects would have cared, then the particular item would be rated closer to the affirmative.

Definitions

Data	This is identifiable or potentially identifiable information. The data can be identifiable if it explicitly contains identity information, such as names and phone numbers. The data are potentially identifiable if it is relatively easy for the data requestor to assign identity to the data, for example, if the identity information was replaced by pseudonyms and the data requestor is able to reverse engineer the pseudonyms because he or she has the pseudonym-to-identity mappings or can get them. Alternatively, the data requestor may have the power to compel the release of identity information. For example, if the data have an IP address and the data requestor is a law enforcement agency, then the agency may be able to compel the ISP to reveal the name and address associated with the IP address at the specified date and time.
Purpose	This is the purpose for which the data requestor has requested the data.

Dimensions

The invasion of privacy construct has three dimensions:

- The sensitivity of the data: The greater the sensitivity of the data, the greater the invasion of privacy.
- The potential injury to data subjects from an inappropriate disclosure/use/breach/processing: The greater the potential for injury, the greater the invasion of privacy.
- The appropriateness of consent for disclosing/using the data: The less appropriate the consent, the greater the invasion of privacy.

These are detailed further below.

Sensitivity of the Data

A1	**The personal information in the data is highly detailed.**
	More detail could mean many variables and/or the granularity/precision of the variables in the data is quite high. For example, instead of a general diagnosis it would contain a very specific diagnosis. For instance, a high-level diagnosis would be "disorders of the thyroid gland," whereas a more detailed diagnosis would be "nontoxic nodular goiter," and "absence of teeth" can be generalized to "diseases of oral cavity, salivary glands, and jaws."
	Precondition: None.
	Response categories: Yes/no (yes = more invasion of privacy; no = less invasion of privacy).
A2	**The information in the data is of a highly sensitive and personal nature.**
	This could mean, for example, information about sexual attitudes, practices, and orientation; use of alcohol, drugs, or other addictive substances; illegal activities; suicide; sexual abuse; sexual harassment; mental health; certain types of genetic information; and HIV status.
	Information about a stigmatized disease/condition or that can adversely affect a data subject's business dealings, insurance, or employment would also be considered sensitive.
	The following areas were highlighted as topics of concern in a letter from the National Committee on Vital and Health Statistics (NCVHS) to the Department of Health and Human Services (DHHS) dated November 10, 2010: "Re: Recommendations Regarding Sensitive Health Information." Especially sensitive data can include, but are not limited to: *(continued)*

- Psychotherapy notes
- Mental health information (including psychiatric diagnoses, descriptions of traumatic events, description or analysis of reports by the patients of emotional, perceptual, behavioral, or cognitive states)
- Substance abuse treatment records
- Information about HIV or other sexually transmitted diseases
- Information about sexuality (including sexual activity, sexual orientation, gender dysphoria or sexual reassignment, sexual dysfunction)
- Information surrounding reproductive health (including abortion, miscarriage, past pregnancy, infertility, use of reproduction technologies, the fact of having adopted children)
- Records of children

In addition, there are three specific circumstances where it is advisable to deem the entire patient record to be considered sensitive:

1. In cases of domestic violence or stalking, where an abuser or stalker might be able to use information in the record to locate the victim.
2. Records of public figures or celebrities may invite speculation, harassment, or undesired attention.
3. Records of adolescents may require special treatment in states where parent/guardian and adolescent access to records differs. An example would be a desire of adolescents to keep issues related to sexuality or reproductive health to themselves.

Precondition: None.

Response categories: Yes/no (yes = more invasion of privacy; no = less invasion of privacy).

Potential Injury to Data Subjects

B1   Many people would be affected if there was a data breach or the data were processed inappropriately by the data requestor.

This item pertains to the number of data subjects covered by the data. More data subjects would be injured if there was, say, a breach of data on 10,000 data subjects than a breach of data on 10 data subjects. In both cases it is an undesired outcome, but the former is more severe.

The new U.S. HITECH Act stipulates that any breach involving 500 or more individuals must be reported to the Department of Health and Human Services. This can be used as a guide for what is considered a large number of people.

If an inappropriate disclosure would affect a defined community (e.g., a minority group living in a particular area), then the number of people affected would be larger than the data subjects covered by the data.

Precondition: None.

Response categories: Yes/no (yes = more invasion of privacy; no = less invasion of privacy).

B2	If there was a data breach or the data were processed inappropriately by the data requestor that may cause direct and quantifiable damages and measurable injury to the data subject.

Damages and injury would include physical injury, such as due to stalking or harassment; emotional or psychological harm; social harm such as stigmatization, humiliation, damage to reputation or relationships; financial harm such as (medical) identity theft and financial fraud; and if the data can be used in making a decision that is detrimental to the data subjects, for example, a business, employment, or insurance decision. The damages and injury can occur to the data subjects themselves, their family unit, or to a defined group/community (e.g., neighborhood, minority groups, band leaders, Aboriginal people, people with disabilities).

Precondition: None.

Response categories: Yes/no (yes = more invasion of privacy; no = less invasion of privacy).

B3	If the data requestor is located in a different jurisdiction, there is a possibility, for practical purposes, that the data sharing agreement will be difficult to enforce.

It is assumed that there is some form of data sharing agreement between the custodian and the data requestor. For example, if the data requestor is an employee of the custodian, then there would be obligations in employment contracts. If the data requestor is a different company, then there would be a contract between the custodian and that company. If the data requestor is a researcher in a different institution, then a data sharing agreement would be signed by the data requestor.

This particular item becomes relevant under the circumstances where the data requestor is in a different jurisdiction than the custodian; for example, in the United States the PATRIOT Act compels custodians to disclose data in secret. In that case a law in a different jurisdiction effectively overrides the provisions in the data sharing agreement. (*continued*)

In some jurisdictions enforcing contracts in courts is difficult or exceedingly slow that for practical purposes the data sharing agreement cannot be enforced in that jurisdiction.

Precondition: None.

Response categories: Yes/no (yes = more invasion of privacy; no = less invasion of privacy).

Appropriateness of Consent

C1 **There is a provision in the relevant legislation permitting the disclosure/use of the data without the consent of the data subjects.**

In some cases there will be legislative authority to disclose the data without consent. For example, when the data are being disclosed to a medical officer of health at a public health authority. But if the data requestor was a commercial data broker, then there is no exception allowing the disclosure without consent. Compelling disclosures, such as in the case of a court order to release data, would also be considered as providing authority to disclose the data without consent.

In Ontario, custodians can disclose data to prescribed entities without the patient's consent. In the case of research, a research ethics board (REB) is permitted in most jurisdictions to disclose the data without consent. If the REB elects not to do so, the response to this question would still be yes.

Uses of data by sub-contractors and business associates (called agents in Ontario) without consent are permitted in many jurisdictions. Therefore, all subsequent items in this section pertain to disclosures only.

Precondition: None.

Response categories: Yes/no (yes = less invasion of privacy; no = no change in invasion of privacy).

C2 **The data were unsolicited or given freely or voluntarily by the data subjects with little expectation of it being maintained in total confidence.**

This would pertain, for example, to data subjects posting their data on a public website as part of a discussion group. It is not always obvious that when data subjects post their data on the web there is an expectation of privacy, but in some cases they may not understand the privacy settings or policies of the website, or the organization running the website may change its policy after the data were collected in unexpected ways. Therefore the response to this question must take into account the specific context and history of the location where the data subjects posted their information.

Precondition: If item C1 is endorsed, then this item would not apply.

Response categories: Yes/no (yes = less invasion of privacy; no = no change in invasion of privacy).

C3	**The data subjects have provided express consent that their data can be disclosed for this secondary purpose when it was originally collected or at some point since then.**

This item refers to obtaining explicit consent from the data subjects (opt-in or opt-out). The consent may have been for the data requestor's specific project (for example, in the case of data subjects consenting for the data that were collected during the provision of care to also be used for a specific research analysis), or may have been broad to encompass a class of projects that include the data requestor's purpose for processing the data (for example, the data subjects consented for their data to be used for research on cardiovascular diseases, without knowing in advance what the possible research questions may be).

Precondition: If items C1 and C2 are endorsed, then this item would not apply.

Response categories: Yes/no (yes = less invasion of privacy; no = more invasion of privacy).

C4	**The Data Custodian has consulted well-defined groups or communities regarding the disclosure of the data and had a positive response.**

This item would be endorsed yes if these well-defined groups or communities did not raise objections to the particular disclosure/use. If they did consult and the outcome was negative, then the item is scored no. Well-defined groups or communities include neighborhood members, minority groups, band leaders, Aboriginal people, people with disabilities, consumer associations, community representatives, privacy oversight bodies, and patient advisory councils.

The assumption with this item is that a nontrivial proportion of data subjects care what their group/community thinks about the disclosure and that they be consulted. The underlying assumption here is that the community would have some consensus view that can be represented.

Precondition: If items C1, C2, and C3 are endorsed, then this item would not apply.

Response categories: Yes/no (yes = less invasion of privacy; no = more invasion of privacy).

C5	A strategy for informing/notifying the public about potential disclosures for the data requestor's secondary purpose was in place when the data were collected or since then.

The custodian may have given notice of potential disclosures for secondary purposes, for example, through well-located posters at its site. The notice does not need to explicitly mention the particular data requestor's purpose, but should describe potential purposes that include the data requestor's purpose.

This is an example of obtaining implicit consent when there are no legislative exceptions and express consent was not obtained.

Precondition: If items C1, C2, C3, and C4 are endorsed, then this item would not apply.

Response categories: Yes/no (yes = less invasion of privacy; no = more invasion of privacy).

C6	Obtaining consent from the data subjects at this point is inappropriate or impractical.

For example, making contact to obtain consent may reveal the data subject's condition to others against his or her wishes, the size of the population is too large to obtain consent from everyone, many data subjects have relocated or died, there is a lack of existing or continuing relationship with the data subjects, the consent procedure itself may introduce bias, there is a risk of inflicting psychological, social, or other harm by contacting data subjects and/or their families in delicate circumstances, it would be difficult to contact data subjects through advertisements and other public notices, and undue hardship that would be caused by the additional financial, material, human, organizational, or other resources required to obtain consent. (*continued*)

This assessment may be contextual. For example, obtaining consent may be difficult for a researcher with limited funds, but if a large organization is requesting the data and it is expected to generate a large amount of revenue from processing the data, then the custodian may be able to convince the data requestor that it is worth its while to invest in obtaining consent.

Precondition: If items C1, C2, C3, C4, and C5 are endorsed, then this item would not apply.

Response categories: Yes/no (yes = less invasion of privacy; no = more invasion of privacy).

Chapter 27

Assessing the Mitigating Controls Construct

Introduction

The "mitigating controls" assessment instrument (henceforth the MCI) is used to evaluate the security and privacy practices of a data requestor (the requestor) from a custodian (the custodian). This information is critical for evaluating the overall risk to the custodian of disclosing the data to the requestor, and drives the amount of de-identification that needs to be applied to the data before they may be disclosed. The purpose of this chapter is to describe the workings of the MCI.

Origins of the MCI

The MCI was constructed based on a review of the recommended and mandated practices of more than a dozen health information custodians across the United States and Canada. Therefore it is based on a descriptive summary of what are considered good security and privacy practices. Because of its origins, its scope is health information in the U.S. and Canadian contexts. However, since health data are some of the most sensitive information about data subjects, whatever methods were deemed adequate to safeguard health information should be suitable for most other data types.

As will be seen below, we have also mapped these practices to existing professional, international, and U.S. and Canadian government regulations, standards, and policies, including ISO/IEC 27002, where appropriate. There are other practices in those standards that are not covered within the MCI. The reason is that we are only concerned with the health subset of these standards. It is also the case that for security-only standards there will be MCI controls that do not have corresponding practices in security standards—for similar reasons.

Subject of Assessment: Data Requestor versus Data Recipient

When an individual or organization asks for data from the custodian they are a *data requestor*. The MCI is used to assess the practices of the data requestor. But there are situations where two other types of organizations/individuals may be assessed:

- Potential data requestors—Using the MCI before making a data request.
- Data recipients—The MCI is used to check their compliance to the conditions in the data sharing agreement.

Therefore the same entity can play any one of these three roles at different points in time. In general, the MCI is worded for a requestor being assessed. However, it should be noted that, depending on the context, it may be one of the other two roles that is the subject of the assessment, and the MCI is still applicable.

Applicability of the MCI

There are two general kinds of data disclosure situations: (1) where the data requestor is requesting the data for its own uses and will limit the disclosure of the data to other entities unless aggregated or otherwise de-identified as specified in a data sharing agreement (DSA) with the custodian, and (2) where the requestor may make the data publicly available (e.g., on the Internet). MCI applies only to the first situation. In the second scenario, the custodian has no control over what happens to the data and what practices the data recipients will have in place. The MCI would not be meaningful in such a case.

Structure of the MCI

The MCI is divided into three sections:

- Controlling access, disclosure, retention, and disposition of personal data
- Safeguarding personal data
- Ensuring accountability and transparency in the management of personal data

Each section has a series of questions. If a question has multiple response categories, then they are intended to be mutually exclusive. This means that only one response category should be applicable to the requestor. If it seems that more than one response category is applicable, then the closest one must be chosen.

Scoring

After completion of the MCI, the end user gets an assessment that is low, medium, or high—referring to the capability of the requestor to meet data protection commitments. This assessment is rolled up from the scores for the individual questions. All questions must be answered to obtain a final assessment from the MCI. If any response is missing, then a global MCI assessment cannot be produced.

The questions are scored such that initial response categories test for low capabilities and subsequent response categories test for higher capabilities. There may be more than one question that is scored low and/or high. These are all detailed in the scoring algorithm below and next to each question.

The questions are framed in such a way that a true statement at a lower level (low or medium) would make irrelevant true statements at a higher level (medium or high). Therefore if the respondent endorses a low response category, it becomes impossible to get a high score for that question. This reflects the fact that baseline, or reference, capabilities are a prerequisite for more effective practices.

Which Practices to Rate

The MCI is intended to score the practices that will be in place when the data are disclosed to the requestor. It is not intended to assess current practices if these practices are going to change before the requestor receives the data. Let us consider four examples:

■ The simplest case is when a requestor is completing the MCI with reference to the practices that it has in place today. In that case the MCI acts as a standard assessment tool.

■ A start-up company is using the MCI and does not yet have all its security and privacy practices in place yet. The MCI should be answered with respect to the practices that will be in place in the future when the company receives the data. The responses to the MCI become an obligation by the company to demonstrate implementation of these practices before it receives the data from the custodian.

■ A requestor is negotiating with the custodian about the disclosure of some data. The requestor agrees to implement some additional practices to reduce its risk and hence have less de-identification applied to the data that it will get. In that case the MCI is answered with respect to practices that will be implemented in the future. The custodian must demonstrate implementation of the new practices endorsed in the MCI as a condition for getting the data.

■ In some cases a custodian is completing the MCI on behalf of potential requestors. For instance, consider a registry that discloses health information to researchers. The custodian does not wish to have every researcher requesting data to complete the MCI. The custodian then completes the MCI on behalf of all of the researchers that typically request data and uses that as the basis for its risk decision. Such an approach needs to average across all of the researchers. In such a case the endorsed practices still become obligations on the researchers, and will be reflected in their data sharing agreements. The researchers with weak practices will then have to make some improvements to meet those criteria.

If a situation occurs that is substantially different from the examples given above, then the requestor and custodian need to make a decision on how to score the MCI and document that.

Third-Party versus Self-Assessment

The MCI can be completed by a third party on a requestor's behalf to determine what its score should be. This third party would likely be a privacy consultant or a professional auditor, and the score would be reported back to the custodian to decide what level of de-identification needs to be applied to the data.

A third party may also perform an assessment using the MCI as part of the compliance check by the custodian. For example, as part of disclosing a data set to a researcher, the researcher had agreed to maintain a certain score on the MCI by implementing a specific set of practices. One year later the custodian may commission an audit of that researcher to determine compliance.*

The MCI may be used in a self-assessment mode. In this case the requestors may evaluate themselves and report to the custodian their score, which the custodian then uses to decide on the extent of de-identification to apply. Usually when this kind of self-assessment is performed, the custodian also has an audit function (say, by third-party auditors) that audits the self-assessors randomly (or using some other defensible criterion) to ensure the integrity of the self-assessment process.

Finally, the MCI can be used in self-assessment mode by the requestor just so that it would know what its score would be without reporting to the custodian. This may be done in anticipation of making a request to the custodian. For example, a custodian may stipulate that only those with a high score on the MCI can apply for the data. In that case potential requestors may self-assess to determine where they stand.

---

* The custodian in such a case may need to verify that the MCI is current in the event that new versions may be released.

Scoring the MCI

The MCI consists of questions, and many questions have multiple sections (e.g., one section on policies and one section on incidents). The MCI is scored at different levels:

Response categories. Scores on response categories affect the sections. Each response category can be scored as a low, medium, or high. In general these can be taken to mean a low, medium/normal, or high capability to meet the requirements of the category. The exact scoring is provided next to each response category below. Some response categories will force the section score to a certain level irrespective of the other section. A forceLow scoring rule means that this whole question must be scored low, irrespective of what the other section scores are. Such a scoring rule is used when a response category is critical for other things to work properly—a building block requirement. A forceMedium score means that the section score can be either a medium or a low, but cannot be a high because the endorsed practice would preclude a high, irrespective of the other section scores. Response categories that have a "none" next to them have no impact on scoring. These will be "not applicable" types of responses. If a question is a check box, then it is scored only if endorsed; otherwise, it would have no impact on the scoring.

Questions. All response categories within a section are mutually exclusive, meaning that only one response can be selected per section. Each section will take the score of the endorsed response category. The whole question will use a rule based on the section scores:

- Low1High1: If one section response is scored low, then the whole question is scored low; otherwise, if one section response is scored high, then the whole question is scored high. Otherwise, the question is scored medium.
- Low1High2: If one section response is scored low, then the whole question is scored low; otherwise, if two section responses are scored high, then the whole question is scored high. Otherwise, the question is scored medium.

Interpreting the MCI Questions

For each of the MCI questions there are additional explanations of the rationale and how to interpret them. In this section we address some general issues that come up repeatedly across multiple questions.

Notes and Annotations

There will be situations where the notes and annotations need to be attached to the responses that are selected. Some common examples are:

■ Response categories may not capture the exact situation at the requestor's site. In such a case the respondent may choose the closest response category. A note explaining this discrepancy and why that particular response category was chosen should be included with the response.
■ Some response categories have "escapes" for exceptional circumstances. In these cases the respondent may use these with a note explaining. These are further elaborated upon below, and will have "[with annotations]" at the end of the question to make clear that such a response requires an explanation.

The respondent is encouraged to use notes and annotations to explain the responses in case questions are raised at a later point about why a particular response was chosen.

General Justifications for Time Intervals

Some of the response categories mention certain expected time intervals for things to happen. These expected time intervals are justified based on legislation, bylaws, or precedent. Below we provide some of the background related to those intervals.

Legislative Requirements

Doctors must retain clinical records for 10 years from the date of last activity according to the Ontario Public Hospitals Act, R.R.O. 1990, Reg. 965, s.20(3). This sets out the general rule of 10 years from the last activity in the file of adult data subjects, or 10 years after the 18th birthday of children. This is echoed in the College of Physicians and Surgeons of Ontario—Policy Statement 5-05: Medical Records. See no. 6 on p. 11 and Appendix A.

Once data are copied from a clinical setting to a research setting, it is assumed to no longer be a part of the clinical record of that data subject. This makes the general retention rules for doctors and hospitals (10 years in Ontario) moot, but does provide a reference point.

Three pieces of legislation do apply: Ontario's Personal Health Information Protection Act (PHIPA), Ontario's Limitations Act, and the Federal Food and Drug Regulations:

PHIPA: While data disclosed to a researcher are no longer a clinical record, PHIPA does provide guidance in Section 44, "Disclosure for Research." Section 44(5) requires the researcher to enter into an agreement with the custodian. This agreement may impose conditions and restrictions with respect to use, security, disclosure, return, or disposal of the information. PHIPA is silent on the length of retention; however, a reading of Principle 5.3 ("Limiting Use, Disclosure, and Retention") in the federal PIPEDA makes clear that retention should be the shortest period of time that fulfills the purposes for which the data were disclosed. Such purposes include not only the length of time of the research project, plus the necessary retention to allow appropriate scholarly review.

Limitations Act: The Ontario Limitation Act, 2002, places a basic limitation for actions of two years (s.4). As a matter of prudence, therefore, the default retention period for records used by researchers should be two years after the last use or reference to the data.

Food and Drug Regulations: Division 5, C.05.012(4) states that records for clinical trials must be retained for 25 years.

Practical Requirements

The purpose of the MCI is to determine if the requestor can reasonably be expected to fulfill its requirements for use, disclosure, and retention of the data that it will receive. As a practical matter, having a policy in and of itself is necessary but insufficient for positive assurance of capability. For that reason data requestors will be asked to demonstrate through logs, reports, audits, assessments, or inspections that they have implemented their policies. The practical question is: What amount of time is sufficient to demonstrate this capability? By applying the Limitations Act minimum of two years, it is reasonable to assume that the organization can demonstrate both retention (for two years) and disposal (the year following the expiry of the limitation) in a three-year time frame. This is the minimal practicable time for which both questions can be answered. A period longer than this minimal time would be overly prejudicial to new organizations and researchers. Note that these timelines are only required for the highest level of assurance, and organizations that may be unable to demonstrate this because they are newer organizations may still obtain high scores by the quality of their other assurances.

It is the case that an organization may be able to demonstrate instances of the application of an expiry of retention deadline and the appropriate disposal of records within a shorter time frame than three years. However, this might be the result of a newly developed and applied policy and does not necessarily provide evidence of an organizational culture of compliance. For this reason as well (demonstration of a consistent culture of compliance), two years was selected as a reasonable time period to provide reasonable due diligence assurance that the potential requestor has consistently self-applied its policies.

Remediation

Some questions inquire about whether the requestor is enforcing a policy, and there is a response category that the policy is partially enforced with remediation (for the instances when the policy is not enforced). It is easier to explain the interpretation of these types of questions and responses with an example. Consider the following two response categories:

1. There is a new role-based or "need-to-know" policy being developed, but it is not yet implemented
2. a. The data requestor has a role-based data access policy, but it is not always enforced or audited, and remediation is under way.
   OR
   b. The data requestor has a role-based data access policy but it is not always enforced or audited, and the requestor has chosen to accept the risk.

Under response category 1 the requestor has not implemented the policy. Whether there is a plan to implement it or not does not matter. If the policy is not implemented, then the first response category in this example needs to be selected.

The second response category is for situations where the policy is partially implemented. In this case the requestor may have identified the reasons why there is only partial implementation and prepared a plan for addressing the gaps between policy requirements and the organization's practice (remediation), and the execution of this plan is under way. In this case response 2.a would be valid. If the requestor has a remediation plan but has not actually started implementing it, but does have the intention to implement it soon, then response 2.a would be acceptable with a note attached to the response indicating this fact.

Plans for remediation may involve the transfer of risk due to partial implementation, say, through an insurance policy. Therefore remediation does not necessarily mean changing the practices of the organization to make sure that the policy is followed all of the time, although, in such cases, it would be advisable to add a note or annotation explaining that the plan is to transfer the risk. The requestor should not be surprised to find that its choice to transfer rather than reduce risk may be unacceptable.

The requestor may choose not to implement a remediation plan. For example, the cases where the policy was not followed were truly exceptional and their causes outside the control of the requestor, and therefore the expense of remediation for such a rare event may not be appropriate. In that case response 2.b would be appropriate. However, response 2.b always requires an explanation associated with it to explain why this response was chosen.

In some situations endorsing response 2.b would not be acceptable, for example, if the policy is a compliance requirement and compliance is necessary for the requestor's business. In such a case only option 2.a would be acceptable. This highlights the need for any annotations or notes attached to a response 2.b to justify that the partial compliance to the policy does not compromise the satisfaction of any compliance requirements.

Controlling Access, Disclosure, Retention, and Disposition of Personal Data

The Requestor Allows Only Authorized Staff to Access and Use Data on a "Need-To-Know" Basis (i.e., When Required to Perform Their Duties) (Low1High2)

While the "need-to-know" principle is relatively self-explanatory, it is important to note that the "need" referred to is defined in the context of the data and by any consent directives or legislative requirements that are associated with that data. Need does not refer to the requestor's desire for the information for its own purposes. It might more properly be called "justification for access."

Note: Incidents should be the first point of query.

Response Categories

   i. General
     1. Access to information resources is based on the rule that "access is generally disallowed, unless expressly allowed" (medium).
  ii. Access Policies
     1. The data requestor either has no procedures or policies/processes for role-based access to data, or it is ad hoc (low).
     2. There is a new role-based or need-to-know policy being developed, but it is not yet implemented (low).
     3. The data requestor has implemented a role-based data access policy, but it is not always enforced, and remediation is under way to ensure regular enforcement (medium).
       OR
       The data requestor has a role-based data access policy, but it is not always enforced, and the requestor has chosen to accept the risk [with annotations] (medium).
     4. The data requestor has implemented an appropriate role-based data access policy with policy enforcement and periodic access audits (high).
 iii. Retention [if ii.4 is endorsed]
     1. Records of the periodic audits are kept, or will be kept, for a minimum of two years (high).
 iv. Incidents
     1. There are recorded incidents where need-to-know was not enforced and disclosure may have taken place without subsequent remediation; usually taken to mean actions to both address any harms resulting from the incident and actions taken to prevent a repetition or a related incident (low).

2. The requestor has identified cases where role-based access rules were not applied (unauthorized use occurred). However, unauthorized disclosure did not occur, and could not occur without prior authorization (medium).
3. There are no recorded incidents where an existing role-based data access policy was not enforced (high).

References to Standards

- **Access control policy** [Section 11.1.1] in ISO/IEC 27002:2005. International Organization for Standardization and International Electrotechnical Commission (2005). Section 11.1 requires organizational control over information assets. Measures of control should be documented in an access control policy, including role-based access control.
- **Protection of organizational records** [Section 15.1.3] in ISO/IEC 27002:2005. International Organization for Standardization and International Electrotechnical Commission (2005). Section 15.1.3 requires that retention schedules should be established identifying types of records and periods of time the records should be maintained.
- **User account management** [Section DS5.4, p. 118] in *COBIT 4.1: Framework, Control Objectives, Management Guidelines, Maturity Models.* IT Governance Institute (2007). Deliver and Support 5.4 (DS5.4) addresses user provisioning, including user access privileges. Such access privileges should be approved, documented, and regularly reviewed.
- **Security for privacy criteria** (Principle 8) in *Generally Accepted Privacy Principles* (GAPP) [practitioner version, pp. 48–56]. American Institute of Certified Public Accountants, Inc. and Canadian Institute of Chartered Accountants (2009). This fragment of the GAPP provides detailed guidelines on how an entity should protect personal information against unauthorized access (both physical and logical), specifically, reference 8.2.2 (logical access controls) as well as references to access control in Sections 1 and 10 of GAPP.
- **Privacy incident and breach management** [Section 1.2.7] in *Generally Accepted Privacy Principles* [practitioner version]. American Institute of Certified Public Accountants, Inc. and Canadian Institute of Chartered Accountants (2009). Section 1.2.7 provides detailed instructions on privacy incident and breach management programs.

Government of Canada Sources

- **Safeguards for use and disclosure** [Sections 6.2.17, 6.2.18, 6.2.19] in Directive on Privacy Practices. Treasury Board of Canada Secretariat (2010). Federal government agencies need to identify work positions with legitimate purposes to access personal information, and to limit this access to individuals occupying those positions. Measures to address inappropriate access should also be implemented.

■ **Retention and disposition of personal information** [Section 6.2.23] in *Directive on Privacy Practices.* Treasury Board of Canada Secretariat (2010). Section 6.2.23 requires the application of retention schedules for records containing personal information.

■ **Limiting access** in *Guidance Document: Taking Privacy into Account before Making Contracting Decisions.* Treasury Board of Canada Secretariat (2010). The document requires that the principle of least privilege be used, limiting access to the minimum information required to perform legitimate duties.

■ **How to respond to a privacy breach** in *Guidelines for Privacy Breaches.* Treasury Board of Canada Secretariat. This section of the guidelines provides detailed instructions on how to respond to incidents of unauthorized access.

Government of U.S. Sources

■ **HIPAA Security Rule*** **45 CFR §164.308(a)(3)(i).**
  Standard: workforce security. A covered entity must implement policies and procedures to ensure that any and all staff, employees, and workforce members have appropriate, and only appropriate, access to electronic personal heath information (ePHI), and to prevent the staff, employees, and workforce members who do not have access to ePHI from obtaining access to ePHI. For implementation specifications for this standard see §164.308(a)(3)(ii).

■ **HIPAA Security Rule 45 CFR §164.308(a)(4)(i).**
  Standard: information access management. An organization must implement policies and procedures that authorize staff, employees, and workforce to access ePHI, and to provide protection for the use and disclosure of the ePHI. For implementation specifications for this standard see §164.308(a)(4)(ii).

  One of the safeguards under this section is ensuring that the staff, employees, and workforce members' duties be separated so that only the minimally necessary ePHI based on the specific job description is made available upon request (NIST HIPAA Security Rule Toolkit).

---

* The following note applies to all HIPAA references in this document: According to 45 CFR §164.308(d)(3), a covered entity must implement a required standard or implementation specification. However, some specifications are addressable, in which case a covered entity must either (1) implement the specification if reasonable and appropriate, or (2) if implementing the specification is not reasonable and appropriate, document the reasons why it is not reasonable and appropriate and implement an equivalent alternative measure if appropriate and reasonable.

- **HIPAA Security Rule 45 CFR §164.312(a)(1).**
  Standard: access control. The covered entity must make sure only authorized users have access to ePHI.

  One of the safeguards under this standard is the concept of "least privilege" when assigning access, allowing only authorized access for users, and process acting on behalf of users, which are necessary to accomplish the user's assigned tasks (NIST HIPAA Security Rule Toolkit).

A Data Sharing Agreement between Collaborators and Subcontractors Has Been (or Will Be) Implemented (Low1High2)

Data sharing agreements establish the parameters of data sharing and particularly with whom the data may be shared. They additionally provide information on the restrictions and conditions that apply to the data and should set out the consequences for failing to meet the conditions set out therein.

Response Categories

    i. Data Sharing Agreements (DSAs)
1. The data requestor does not use, or has not, used DSAs (low).
2. A DSA template exists (or one is being developed), but it has yet to be implemented (low).
3. The data requestor has a DSA template, but it is not always used or audited, and remediation is under way (medium).
   OR
   The data requestor has a DSA template, but it is not always used or audited, and the requestor has chosen to accept the risk [with annotations] (medium).
4. The data requestor has a DSA template that is always used, with periodic audits to check that the requestor is complying with its provisions (high).

   ii. Retention [if i.4 is endorsed]
1. Signed agreements are retained until a minimum of two years after the expiration of the DSA (high).

  iii. Collaborators and Subcontractors
1. Some collaborators or subcontractors are currently working without a data sharing agreement in place (low).
2. Data sharing agreements were signed by subcontractors but not all collaborators (medium).
3. All collaborators and subcontractors have signed data sharing agreements (high).

References to Standards

- **Addressing security in third-party agreements** [Section 6.2.3] in ISO/IEC 27002:2005. International Organization for Standardization and International Electrotechnical Commission (2005). Section 6.2 requires that information security should not be diminished by the introduction of a third party. Risks should be assessed and mitigated in such cases.
- **Manage third-party services** [Section DS2, p. 105] in *COBIT 4.1: Framework, Control Objectives, Management Guidelines, Maturity Models.* IT Governance Institute (2007). An organization should formalize relationship management, risk management, and performance monitoring processes with each supplier to ensure suppliers' ability to effectively deliver services in a secure manner.
- **Disclosure to third parties criteria** [Section 7.2.2] in *Generally Accepted Privacy Principles* [practitioner version] (2009). American Institute of Certified Public Accountants, Inc. and Canadian Institute of Chartered Accountants. Section 7.2.2 requires privacy agreements and monitoring procedures to be in place between data sharing organizations to ensure the protection of personal information according to pertinent laws and regulations.
- **Safeguarding personal data** [Section 7.2.1] in *CIHR Best Practices for Protecting Privacy in Health Research* (2005). Data sharing agreements between the researcher/institution and all involved should be signed prior to providing any access to data.
- **Data sharing agreements** [Section 8.3] in *CIHR Best Practices for Protecting Privacy in Health Research* (2005). Section 8.3 provides detailed information about elements concerning privacy that should be considered in data sharing agreements.

Government of Canada Sources

- **Safeguards for use and disclosure** [Section 6.2.20] in Directive on Privacy Practices. Treasury Board of Canada Secretariat (2010). Section 6.2.20 provides a list of requirements to be met when personal information is disclosed to another public or private sector institution.
- **Definition of an information sharing agreement** [Section 1.2] in *Guidance on Preparing Information Sharing Agreements Involving Personal Information.* Treasury Board of Canada Secretariat (2010). The document recommends that government agencies should prepare information sharing agreements when sharing personal information with other parties.

Government of U.S. Sources

■ **HIPAA Security Rule CFR 45 §164.308(b)(1).**
Standard: business associates contracts and other arrangements. A covered entity must have legal agreements called business associate agreements with contractors and vendors who do work for the organization using or creating ePHI.

Some of the safeguards under this standard are (1) ensuring that an organization's business associate agreements (as written and executed) contain sufficient language to ensure that required information types are protected, including the 2009, 2010, and 2011 HITECH Act updates and inclusions, and (2) ensuring that the organization's agreements and other arrangements meet all security requirements under the HIPAA Security Rule as per HITECH Act (NIST HIPAA Security Rule Toolkit).

Explanations

■ The acronym *DSA* is used for data sharing agreement.
■ The term *collaborators* is used mostly in cases where the requestor is a researcher, and there may be other researchers in the same or a different institution who are collaborators. Under current practice it is not common to have formal agreements with collaborators. However, when personal information is disclosed, such formal agreements would be necessary. Relationships with subcontractors tend to be more formal, and it is unlikely to have a subcontracting relationship without an agreement in place.
■ The terms *subcontractor* and *contractor* are used interchangeably. The reason is that within the context of this assessment they would be treated the same way.
■ The concern is with collaborators and subcontractors who may have access to the disclosed data. If they do not, then they would not be of concern in this assessment.
■ The requirement that "signed agreements are retained until a minimum of two years after the expiration of the agreement" is based on the two-year limit for civil actions.
■ Audits in the context of DSAs are intended to check for compliance with the DSA.

A Nondisclosure or Confidentiality Agreement (Pledge of Confidentiality) Is in Place (or Will Be) for All Staff, Including External Collaborators and Subcontractors (Low1High2)

Whereas a DSA provides assurances between entities, a nondisclosure agreement (NDA) or a confidentiality agreement (CA) provides assurances about the individual(s) who sign it. Every person at the requestor's organization that may have access to the requested data should have signed an appropriate NDA or CA with the requestor. If not, then the custodian must supply its own NDA or CA for individuals with access to requestor data to sign.

Response Categories

i. NDA and Confidentiality Policy
1. The data requestor does not have a policy with respect to nondisclosure agreements (NDAs) or confidentiality agreements (CAs) (low).
2. NDAs and/or CAs are signed, but only when requested by the data requestor's legal counsel (low).
3. The data requestor has an NDA and/or CA policy, but it is not always enforced or audited, and remediation is under way (medium).
   OR
   The data requestor has an NDA and/or CA policy, but it is not always enforced or audited, and the requestor has chosen to accept the risk [with annotations] (medium).
4. The data requestor has an NDA and/or CA policy that is enforced and audited (high).

ii. NDA/CA Signing
1. There are staff, collaborators, or subcontractors currently working that have not signed an NDA or CA (low).
2. All staff, external collaborators, and subcontractors sign an NDA or CA at the start of employment or contract, but not necessarily ever again (medium).
3. NDAs and/or CAs are re-signed on a regular basis (e.g., annually) to ensure complete coverage and awareness (high).

References to Standards

- **Confidentiality agreements** [Section 6.1.5] in ISO/IEC 27002:2005. International Organization for Standardization and International Electrotechnical Commission (2005). Section 6.1.5 states that confidentiality or nondisclosure agreements should be in place and regularly reviewed. They should reflect organizational needs for information protection.
- **Terms and conditions of employment** [Section 8.1.3a] in ISO/IEC 27002:2005. International Organization for Standardization and International Electrotechnical Commission (2005). All employees, contractors, and third-party users who are given access to sensitive information should sign a confidentiality or nondisclosure agreement prior to being given access to information processing facilities.
- **Data sharing agreements** [Section 8.3, para. 2] in *CIHR Best Practices for Protecting Privacy in Health Research* (2005). Data sharing agreements should

include a statement that the researcher will not use data for any other purpose without prior authorization of the data provider.

- **Contracted staff policies and procedures** [Section PO 4.14]. COBIT 4.1.
- **Staffing of roles** [Section PO 7.3]. COBIT 4.1.
- **Qualification of internal personnel** [Section 1.2.9]. GAPP.

Government of Canada Sources

- **Safeguards for use and disclosure** [Section 6.2.20] in Directive on Privacy Practices. Treasury Board of Canada Secretariat (2010). Section 6.2.20 states that an agreement or arrangement with adequate safeguards must be established between the government institutions and other corporate entities (public or private).

Government of U.S. Sources

- **HIPAA Security Rule 45 CFR §164(a)(3)(ii)(A).**
  Standard: workforce security; implementation specification: authorization and/or supervision. A covered entity must develop and implement procedures for authorization and/or supervision for staff, employees, and workforce members who work with ePHI or in locations where it may be accessed.

  Some of the safeguards under this specification are (1) ensuring that individuals requiring access to the organization's information and information systems sign appropriate access agreements prior to being granted access, and (2) periodically reviewing/updating the access agreements (NIST HIPAA Security Rule Toolkit).

Explanations

- The term *collaborators* is used mostly in cases where the requestor is a researcher, and there may be other researchers in the same or a different institution who are collaborators. Under current practice it is not common to have formal agreements with collaborators. However, when personal information is disclosed, such formal agreements would be necessary.
- The terms *subcontractor* and *contractor* are used interchangeably. The reason is that within the context of this assessment they would be treated the same way.
- The concern is with staff, collaborators, and subcontractors who may have access to the disclosed data. If they do not, then they would not be of concern in this assessment.
- The underlying assumption here is that any agreement with a collaborator and/or subcontractor who has access to the data would pass on the security and privacy provisions in the agreement between the requestor and the

custodian. This means that the custodian would consider the NDA or CA to meet its standards and not set a lower standard for handling the data. This may be something the custodian wishes to check or require.

■ If a collaborator and/or subcontractor is a signatory to the DSA between the requestor and the custodian, then a separate NDA or CA may not be needed. In such a case the responses to this question would be similar to the responses to the question on DSAs (question 2).

■ Audits in the context of enforcing NDAs and CAs entail confirming that staff, collaborators, or subcontractors are actually following the provisions in those agreements.

■ The requirement for an annual re-signing of agreements helps develop a culture of privacy within the organization by showing that management cares about these issues. It also serves to remind collaborators and subcontractors of their obligations. It is not unusual for collaborators and subcontractors to forget the details of their obligations as time passes by, and this annual act serves as a reminder. Alternative means to achieve the same thing, such as training, may be acceptable and may be documented in the notes attached to the responses. The requestor may also make the case that annual re-signing is too often and that this needs to be done less frequently. Again, this can be documented in the annotations accompanying the response.

The Data Requestor Only Publishes or Discloses Aggregated Data That Do Not Allow the Identification of Data Subjects (Low1High2)

Not all researchers are aware of the rich research on re-identification of data and may have an incorrect appreciation of the work necessary to ensure anonymity in released data. This section ensures that precautions are in place irrespective of the requestor's understanding of the risks of re-identification.

Response Categories

i. Disclosure Policy
1. The data requestor does not have a data disclosure policy or processes (including publication rules) (low).
2. The data requestor is developing a data disclosure policy or process, but it is not yet implemented (low).
3. The data requestor has a data disclosure policy or process, but it is not always applied and remediation is under way (medium).
OR
The data requestor has a data disclosure policy or process, but it is not always applied, and the requestor has chosen to accept the risk [with annotations] (medium).

4. The data requestor has a data disclosure policy with policy enforcement and periodic publication audits (high).

ii. Published Data

1. The data requestor has published potentially identifiable data (e.g., no small cell rules were applied), without explicit consent, and has not remediated the situation (low).

2. The data requestor has deliberately published, to date, only aggregated data and applied small cell rules (i.e., informal process is correct, but is not substantiated by policy or documentation) (medium).

3. The data requestor has a formal process for creating aggregate data and keeps a record of publications as an audit trail of compliance with data disclosure policy (high).

References to Standards

■ **Personal information** in *Generally Accepted Privacy Principles* [practitioner version, p. 5] (2009). American Institute of Certified Public Accountants, Inc. and Canadian Institute of Chartered Accountants. Nonpersonal information ordinarily is not subject to privacy protection because it cannot be linked to an individual. However, some organizations may still have obligations over nonpersonal information due to other regulations and agreements (for example, clinical research and market research).

■ **Information exchange policies and procedures** [Section 10.8.1]. ISO/IEC 27002:2005. International Organization for Standardization and International Electrotechnical Commission (2005).

■ **Exchange of sensitive data** [Section DS 5.11]. COBIT 4.1.

■ **Disposal, destruction, and redaction of personal information** [Section 5.2.3] in *Generally Accepted Privacy Principles* [practitioner version] (2009). American Institute of Certified Public Accountants, Inc. and Canadian Institute of Chartered Accountants. Section 5.2.3 states that personal information no longer subject to retention should be anonymized or destroyed in a manner that prevents loss, misuse, or unauthorized access.

■ **Controlling access and disclosure of personal data** [Section 8.1] in *CIHR Best Practices for Protecting Privacy in Health Research* (2005). Nonidentifiable data about individuals and aggregated data are made available to the general scientific community and for public use after appropriate scrutiny to minimize or avoid risks of inadvertent disclosure of individuals' identities.

■ **Provincial legislation (Ontario). Collection, use, and disclosure of personal health information** [Part IV, S 44(6)c] in Personal Health Information Protection Act, S.O. 2004, c3 (Ontario). The act specifically requires that personal health information used for research purposes cannot be published in a form that could reasonably enable a person to establish the identity of the individual.

Government of U.S. Sources

■ None in Security Rule.

Explanations

■ The underlying assumption of this question is that aggregated data have a low probability of re-identification and would therefore not be considered personal information.
■ Publication may mean externally or internally within the requestor's organization. The intent is that information is made available to a broad audience who were not authorized to have access to the raw data (and potentially has a high risk of re-identification).
■ In the questions, "small cell rules" is used only as a simple example of the kinds of things that one would do to reduce the probability of re-identification for aggregate data, but this does not mean that applying such rules is the only action needed when creating aggregate data.

Long-Term Retention of Personal Data Is Subject to Periodic Audits and Oversight by Independent Bodies (Low1High2)

Implicit in the requirement for audits and oversight is that data retention should be governed by retention policies supported by retention schedules and disposal procedures. The use of independent bodies, such as an internal audit department or an external consultant, will provide assurance to an entity that it is meeting its own policy goals. The requirement above sets the high standard, while the existence of policies and procedures is required for the medium standard.

Response Categories

i. Data Retention Policy
  1. The data requestor does not have a data retention policy for records (low).
  2. The data requestor is developing data retention policies, but has not implemented them (low).
  3. The data requestor has a data retention policy, but it is only partially observed, and remediation is under way (medium).
     OR
     The data requestor has a data retention policy, but it is only partially observed, and the requestor has chosen to accept the risk [with annotations] (medium).
  4. The data requestor has a data retention policy that is applied, measured, and audited (high).

ii. Enforcement
   1. The data requestor has personal data that have been kept longer than is required, or can't determine if that is the case (low).
   2. The data requestor does not retain personal data on a long-term basis, but cannot document the practice based on policy or other reasonable metrics (medium).
   3. The data requestor is able to provide proof of enforcement of data retention policies for the last three years (high).

References to Standards

- **Retention of personal data** [Section 9.1.2] in *CIHR Best Practices for Protecting Privacy in Health Research* (2005). Any long-term retention of personal data established for general health research purposes should be subject to periodic audits and effective oversight by independent third parties, including research ethics boards (REBs).
- **Disposal, destruction, and redaction of personal information** [Section 5.2.3] in *Generally Accepted Privacy Principles* [practitioner version] (2009). American Institute of Certified Public Accountants, Inc. and Canadian Institute of Chartered Accountants. Section 5.2.3 states that personal information no longer subject to retention should be anonymized or destroyed in a manner that prevents loss, misuse, or unauthorized access.
- **Independent review of information security** [Section 6.1.8] in ISO/IEC 27002:2005. International Organization for Standardization and International Electrotechnical Commission (2005). Section 6.1.8 states that information security should be independently reviewed at planned intervals.
- **Storage and retention arrangements** [Section DS11.2, p. 142] in *COBIT 4.1: Framework, Control Objectives, Management Guidelines, Maturity Models*. IT Governance Institute (2007). Section DS11.2 states that an organization should implement procedures for data retention to meet business objectives, the organization's security policy, and regulatory requirements.

Government of Canada Sources

- **Retention and disposition of personal information** [Section 6.2.23] in Directive on Privacy Practices. Treasury Board of Canada Secretariat (2010). Heads of government institutions or their delegates are responsible for applying the retention and disposal standards associated with the personal information and reporting the length of the retention period in the relevant personal information bank.
- **Requirements** [Section 6.1.3] in Directive on Recordkeeping. Treasury Board of Canada Secretariat (2009). The departmental IM senior official designated by the deputy head is responsible for establishing, implementing, and

maintaining retention periods for information resources of business value, as appropriate.

- **Personal information** in *Retention Guidelines for Common Administrative Records of the Government of Canada.* Library and Archive Canada (2007). In establishing retention periods for records containing personal information, federal institutions must ensure that the Privacy Act and Privacy Act Regulations are applied.

Government of U.S. Sources

- **HIPAA Security Rule 45 CFR §164.316(b)(2).**
  Standard: documentation. According to NIST HIPAA Security Rule Toolkit, an organization should have a data retention policy and procedure(s) that consider all HIPAA retention requirements.

Explanations

- The term *records* in this question means electronic or physical records.
- Examples of data retention metrics would be the average number of weeks by which data were kept beyond that allowed by policy, and how many copies of the data the organization has (including backup copies).
- The three-year data retention requirement allows for the possibility of demonstrating consistent application of data retention rules.
- The HIPAA rule meets the policy, but not the actual enforcement standard— in other words, it does not provide for oversight.

Data Will Be Disposed of After a Specified Retention Period (Low1High2)

Retention periods can only be demonstrated by the timely disposal of data at the end of the defined period. Timely disposal of electronic data can be difficult to prove, since copies of data may easily be made without a record of the copy having been made. Disposal can mean physical destruction, electronic wiping, a return of media containing data to the supplier, or in some cases the transfer of information to governmental archives.

Response Categories

   i. Data Destruction Procedures
1. The data requestor does not have data destruction procedures for records (low).
2. The data requestor is developing data destruction procedures, but has not implemented them (low).

3. The data requestor has data destruction procedures, but it is only partially observed, and remediation is under way (medium).
OR
The data requestor has data destruction procedures, but it is only partially observed, and the requestor has chosen to accept the risk [with annotations] (medium).
4. The data requestor has data destruction procedures that are regularly applied, measured, and audited (high).

ii. Data Destruction
1. The data requestor has personal data that should have been destroyed, or can't determine if that is the case (low).
2. The data requestor regularly destroys personal data, but cannot document the practice based on policy or other reasonable metrics (medium).
3. The data requestor is able to provide proof of enforcement of personal data destruction policies for the last three years (high).

References to Standards

■ **Disposal of media** [Section 10.7.2] in ISO/IEC 27002:2005. International Organization for Standardization and International Electrotechnical Commission (2005). Section 10.7.2 states that disposal of records in various media should be logged and controlled. Procedures should be defined for securely handling, transporting, and storing backup media and system documentation.

■ **Disposal of electronic records** [Section 6.9.2] in CAN/CGSB-72.34-2005: *Electronic Records as Documentary Evidence.* National Standard of Canada (2005). Section 6.9.2 states that the disposal of electronic records requires documented proof such as an audit log, a certificate, or evidence of disposal. It should identify the records disposed, the nature of records, the date the records were created or received, the person who authorized the disposal, and the time and date of disposal.

■ **Storage and retention arrangements** [Section DS 11.2]. COBIT 4.1.

■ **Implementing disposition** [Section 9.9] in ISO 15489-1: *Information and Documentation—Records Management Part 1.* International Organization for Standardization (2001). Section 9.9 states that records destruction should be carried out in a manner that preserves confidentiality of information contained in them. All copies and backups, including security copies of records authorized for destruction, should be destroyed.

■ **Disposal, destruction, and redaction of personal information** [Section 5.2.3] in *Generally Accepted Privacy Principles* [practitioner version] (2009). American Institute of Certified Public Accountants, Inc. and Canadian Institute of Chartered Accountants. Section 5.2.3 states that personal information no longer subject to retention should be anonymized or destroyed in a manner that prevents loss, misuse, or unauthorized access.

Government of Canada Sources

- **Retention and disposition of personal information** [Section 6.2.23] in Directive on Privacy Practices. Treasury Board of Canada Secretariat (2010). Heads of government institutions or their delegates are responsible for applying the retention and disposal standards associated with the personal information in the relevant personal information bank.
- **Requirements** [Section 6.1.3] in Directive on Recordkeeping. Treasury Board of Canada Secretariat (2009). The departmental IM senior official designated by the deputy head is responsible for developing and implementing a documented disposition process for all information resources, and performing regular disposition activities for all information resources.
- **Destruction of assets** [Section 10.2] in *Operational Security Standard on Physical Security*. Treasury Board of Canada Secretariat (2008). Protected and classified information with no historical or archival value for which the retention period has expired must be promptly destroyed, including surplus copies, drafts copies, and waste. HIPAA Security Rule 164.310(d)(2)(i).

Government of U.S. Sources

- **HIPAA Security Rule 45 CFR §164.310(d)(2)(i).**
  Standard: device and media controls; implementation specification: disposal. An organization must have a documented process for the final disposal of ePHI and the hardware and other electronic media on which ePHI is stored.
- **HIPAA Security Rule 45 CFR §164.310(d)(2)(ii).**
  Standard: device and media controls; implementation specification: media reuse. According to NIST HIPAA Security Rule Toolkit, an organization should have one individual or department responsible for coordinating data disposal and reuse of hardware and software across the enterprise.

Explanations

- The term *records* in this question means electronic or physical records.
- The three-year data retention requirement allows for the possibility of demonstrating consistent application of data destruction rules.

Information Is Not Processed, Stored, or Maintained Outside of Canada, and Parties Outside of Canada Do Not Have Access to the Data (Low1High2)

This question is moot if the requestor is himself or herself outside of Canada and the data supplier has ensured that there is no regulatory or other impediment to the disclosure of data to an entity outside of Canada. Some jurisdictions in Canada do prohibit the sharing of health data in this manner. If a data supplier outside of Canada is using the MCI tool, the wording should be modified to be appropriate for the data's country of origin.

Response Categories

i. General
1. The data requestor is outside of Canada (low).
2. The data requestor is within Canada, and may share data outside of Canada on a case-by-case basis, but there is no policy in place to prevent this where inappropriate, or such a policy is being developed but is not yet implemented (low).
3. The data requestor is within Canada, and has a policy to not share data, but there is no enforcement of the policy, and remediation is under way (medium).

   OR

   The data requestor is within Canada, and has a policy to not share data, but there is no enforcement of the policy, and the requestor has chosen to accept the risk [with annotations] (medium).
4. The data requestor is within Canada, and has a policy, enforced and audited, to not share data outside of Canada (high).

ii. Records of Agreements [if i.4 is endorsed]
1. The data requestor has records or agreements in place to demonstrate that data have not been shared outside of Canada (high).

References to Standards

■ **Data protection and privacy of personal information** [Section 15.1.4] in ISO/IEC 27002:2005. International Organization for Standardization and International Electrotechnical Commission (2005). Section 15.1.4 states that depending on the nature of legislative and regulatory environments in other jurisdictions, some privacy protecting controls may impose duties on those collecting, processing, and disseminating personal information, and may restrict the transfer of those data to other countries.

■ **Ensure compliance with external requirements** [Section ME3.1] in *COBIT 4.1: Framework, Control Objectives, Management Guidelines, Maturity Models*. IT Governance Institute (2007). Section ME3.1 states the requirement that an organization must identify local and international laws, regulations, and other requirements that must be complied with. Such requirements must be incorporated into the organization's IT policies, standards procedures, and methodologies.

■ **Consistency of privacy policies and procedures with laws and regulations** [Section 1.2.2]. GAPP.

Government of Canada Sources

■ **Step 2.1: laws of foreign jurisdictions** in *Guidance Document: Taking Privacy into Account before Making Contracting Decisions.* Treasury Board of Canada Secretariat (2010). Institutions should consider whether contracts with foreign entities may affect levels of privacy risks. Such risks should be assessed before reaching a final decision.

Government of U.S. Sources

■ **HIPAA Security Rule 45 CFR §164.308(b)(1).**
Standard: business associate contracts and other arrangements. A covered entity must have legal agreements called business associate agreements with contractors and vendors who work for the organization using or creating ePHI.

One of the safeguards under this standard is ensuring that any offshore functions are covered by contracts/agreements (NIST HIPAA Security Rule Toolkit).

Explanations

■ For data disclosures occurring outside Canada, other countries may be substituted. The intention was not to restrict this question to data disclosed only from Canada.

■ The intention is not to prohibit the disclosure of data outside of Canada, but rather to require justifications for disclosures out of Canada. Some questions to consider: (1) Does the jurisdiction that the data will be sent to have equally strong privacy laws that are generally enforced? (2) Will it be possible to enforce a DSA in that jurisdiction (i.e., does it have a relatively effective and efficient judicial system where cases can be brought to court)? (3) Will the custodian spend the money to pursue a breach of contract (for example, if the costs of pursuing someone in that other jurisdiction are so high that the custodian would likely never bother, then there is a big question mark over the meaningfulness of a DSA)? Therefore if data will be disclosed outside of Canada, then an argument should be made in the notes and annotations to this question addressing these three issues.

Data Are Not Disclosed or Shared With Third Parties Without Appropriate Controls or Prior Approval (Low1High2)

This should be self-explanatory. It is normal due diligence for the protection of all parties involved in the DSA.

Response Categories

i. General
1. The data requestor has shared personal information with third parties without appropriate controls (i.e., contractual requirements) (low).
   OR
   The data requestor is unable to determine if personal data have been disclosed to, or shared with, third parties (low).
2. The data requestor does not have a third-party data management policy, or one is being developed and is not yet implemented (low).
3. The data requestor has policies to control the disclosure of information to third parties, but cannot provide appropriate assurances that the policy is being followed regularly, and remediation is under way (medium).
   OR
   The data requestor has policies to control the disclosure of information to third parties, but cannot provide appropriate assurances that the policy is being followed, and the requestor has chosen to accept the risk [with annotations] (medium).
4. The data requestor has policies and processes with enforcement and auditing to control the disclosure or sharing of information with third parties (high).
ii. Records of Sharing [if i.4 is endorsed]
1. The data requestor is able to provide reports to demonstrate compliance with its third-party disclosure rules for the past three years (high).

References to Standards

- **Addressing security in third-party agreements** [Section 6.2.3] in ISO/IEC 27002:2005. International Organization for Standardization and International Electrotechnical Commission (2005). Section 6.2.3 requires that information security should not be diminished by the introduction of a third party. Risks should be assessed and mitigated in such cases.
- **Controlling access and disclosure of personal data: general statement** [Section 8] in *CIHR Best Practices for Protecting Privacy in Health Research* (2005). The statement recommends that there should be strict limits on access to data subject to REB approval and data sharing agreements.
- **Disclosure of personal information** [Section 7.2.1] in *Generally Accepted Privacy Principles* [practitioner version] (2009). American Institute of Certified Public Accountants, Inc. and Canadian Institute of Chartered Accountants. Section 7.2.1 requires that an entity should have procedures in place to prevent the unauthorized disclosure of personal information to third parties and document all disclosures, whether authorized or unauthorized.
- **Supplier risk management** [Section DS 2.3]. COBIT 4.1.

Government of Canada Sources

- *Guidance Document: Taking Privacy into Account before Making Contracting Decisions.* Treasury Board of Canada Secretariat (2010). This guidance document is intended to provide advice to federal government institutions whenever they consider contracting out activities in which personal information is handled or accessed by private sector agencies under contract.
- **Contracts and agreements** [Sections 6.2.10 and 6.2.11] in Policy on Privacy Protection. Treasury Board of Canada Secretariat (2008). Heads of government institutions are responsible for establishing measures and ensuring that appropriate privacy protection clauses are included in contracts or agreements with third parties.
- **Safeguards for use and disclosure** [Section 6.2.20] in Directive on Privacy Practices. Treasury Board of Canada Secretariat (2010). Section 6.2.20 outlines a list of requirements to be met when personal information is being disclosed to another public or private sector institution.

Government of U.S. Sources

- **HIPAA Security Rule 45 CFR §164.314(a)(2)(i)(B).**
  Standard: business associate contracts or other arrangements; implementation specification: business associate contracts. A covered entity's business associate contracts must provide that any agent, including a subcontractor, to whom the business associate provides ePHI, or access to such ePHI, agrees to implement reasonable and appropriate safeguards to protect the ePHI (NIST HIPAA Security Rule Toolkit).

Explanations

- Third parties can be, for example, customers or students of the requestor. The three-year requirement provides a practicable time frame within which to demonstrate consistent compliance with policy and the Limitations Act.

Safeguarding Personal Data

Risk Assessments Have Been Conducted for Information Systems, and These Have Been Conveyed to the Custodian (Low1High2)

A risk assessment for the purposes of security, most commonly known as a threat and risk assessment (TRA), evaluates the vulnerabilities, threats, and controls of an information system so as to determine what the residual risk to confidentiality, integrity, and availability is for that system. A vulnerability assessment is typically a more narrow technical evaluation of a system's security capabilities. A TRA will make recommendations to enable an entity to reduce the risk to its information to an acceptable level for its tolerance for risk.

A privacy impact assessment (PIA) is a similar exercise to identify and make recommendations in respect to the entity's collection, use, and disclosure of personally identifiable information.

Response Categories

   i. Assessments
1. The data requestor has not conducted an internal or external threat and risk assessment (TRA), vulnerability assessment (VA), or privacy impact assessment (PIA) of its information systems or programs (low).
2. The data requestor does not have a TRA or PIA policy or set of practices, or is developing such policies, but they have not yet been implemented (low).
3. TRAs, VAs, or PIAs are conducted on an ad hoc basis, when requested or deemed necessary, and these include systems that will be storing or processing the requested data. The recommendations of these assessments have been or are in the process of being remediated (medium).

      OR

      TRAs, VAs, or PIAs are conducted on an ad hoc basis, when requested or deemed necessary, and these include systems that will be storing or processing the requested data. The requestor has chosen to accept the risk and not take remedial action [with annotations] (medium).
4. There is a TRA and/or PIA policy, TRAs, VAs, and/or PIAs have been conducted as needed, and remediation has been completed or substantially addressed (high).

  ii. Changes [if i.4 is endorsed]
1. There have been no substantial system or program changes since the completion of assessments (high).

 iii. Breaches
1. There has been a security or privacy breach in the last three years, without an investigation and remediation (low).
2. There has been a security or privacy breach in the last three years, resulting in an investigation and systemic remediation (medium).
3. There have been no security or privacy breaches in the last three years (high).

References to Standards

■ **Independent review of information security** [Section 6.1.8] in ISO/IEC 27002:2005. International Organization for Standardization and International Electrotechnical Commission (2005). Section 6.1.8 states that information security should be independently reviewed at planned intervals.

- **Assurance of internal control** [Section ME2.5, p. 158] in *COBIT 4.1: Framework, Control Objectives, Management Guidelines, Maturity Models*. IT Governance Institute (2007). Section ME2.5 states that an entity should ensure comprehensiveness and effectiveness of internal controls through third-party audits or reviews.
- **Security for privacy criteria: testing security safeguards** [Section 8.2.7] in *Generally Accepted Privacy Principles* [practitioner version] (2009). American Institute of Certified Public Accountants, Inc. and Canadian Institute of Chartered Accountants. Section 8.2.7 states that independent audits of security controls (internal or external) should be conducted at least annually.
- **Security measures: organizational safeguards** [Section 7.2.1] in *CIHR Best Practices for Protecting Privacy in Health Research* (2005). Section 7.2.1 suggests that organizations housing research data, including data containing personal information, should implement internal and external reviews and audits.
- **Information security program** [Section 8.2.1]. GAPP.

Government of Canada Sources

- **Directive on Privacy Impact Assessment.** Treasury Board of Canada Secretariat (2010).
- **Harmonized Threat and Risk Assessment (TRA) methodology.** Royal Canadian Mounted Police and Communication Security Establishment (2007).

Government of Ontario Sources

- *Privacy Impact Assessment Guidelines for the Ontario Personal Health Information Protection Act.* Information and Privacy Commissioner/Ontario (2005).

Government of U.S. Sources

- **HIPAA Security Rule 45 CFR §164.308(a)(1)(ii)(A).**
  Standard: security management process; implementation specification: risk analysis. Conduct an accurate and thorough assessment of the potential risks and vulnerabilities to the confidentiality, integrity, and availability of ePHI held by the covered entity.

Explanations

- This question is phrased in the past to reflect current practice with *any* data custodian. However, this may be interpreted as an intention if there is no history.
- A TRA is a threat and risk assessment. The Harmonized Threat and Risk Assessment by the Royal Canadian Mounted Police is one example of this. It is an assessment that focuses on risks to the security of sensitive information,

primarily in the areas of confidentiality of the information, integrity of the information, and availability of the information.

■ A PIA is a privacy impact assessment. The Office of Information and Privacy Commissioner of Ontario has a sample PIA for health data on its site. This is an assessment that focuses on risks to the privacy of personally identifiable information, particularly in the areas of collection, use, disclosure, retention, and disposal.

■ A VA is a vulnerability assessment (for example, penetration testing of an application or an organization's network). Usually a VA does not require a policy, as it is an operational issue that is triggered by a TRA or PIA.

■ One possible explanation for the lack of privacy and security breaches is that the processes and systems in place to detect breaches are not well developed. This issue is addressed in another question. In the context of this question, if TRAs, PIAs, and VAs are performed and there are no breaches, then this is considered a positive indicator.

An Organizational Governance Framework for Privacy, Confidentiality, and Security Is in Place At the Requestor's Site (Low1High2)

Privacy governance is the capability of an organization to set and control priorities to ensure that the organization's objectives for privacy are met. Establishing a minimum program of privacy protection and then only responding to complaints, incidents, and other external factors by making the minimal changes necessary to address those factors is reactive governance. Proactive governance attempts to prevent incidents and complaints by setting and controlling objectives using active controls and feedback mechanisms on the flow of sensitive information. Proactive governance is more likely to engender trust in stakeholders with privacy concerns, including data subjects.

Response Categories

i. General
   1. There is no organizational governance framework for privacy, confidentiality, and security (low).
   2. There is an organizational governance framework for privacy, confidentiality, and security, but enforcement and/or reporting are in reaction to incidents or requests (medium).
   3. There is a proactive organizational governance framework for privacy, confidentiality, and security, with enforcement, that reports regularly to senior management (high).
ii. Operation [if i.3 is endorsed]
   1. The framework has been effectively operational for at least two years (high).

References to Standards

- **Security policy** [Section 5] in ISO/IEC 27002:2005. International Organization for Standardization and International Electrotechnical Commission (2005). An organization should define a policy to clarify its direction of, and support for, information security in an information security policy statement, which should describe the key information security directives and mandates for the entire organization.
- **Provide IT governance** [Section ME4.1] in *COBIT 4.1: Framework, Control Objectives, Management Guidelines, Maturity Models.* IT Governance Institute (2007). An organization should establish the IT governance framework ensuring compliance with laws and regulations.
- **Ensuring accountability and transparency in the management of personal data** [Section 10] in *CIHR Best Practices for Protecting Privacy in Health Research* (2005). Individuals and organizations involved in health research and using personal data are responsible for the proper conduct of such research in accordance with applicable funding policies, and privacy laws/regulations. A suitable framework must be put in place to implement these policies and laws.
- **Establishment of an IT governance framework** [Section ME 4.1]. COBIT 4.1. An organization should establish the IT governance framework ensuring compliance with laws and regulations.
- **Responsibility and accountability for policies** [Section 1.1.2]. GAPP.

Government of Canada Sources

- **Requirements** [Section 6.1.1] in Policy on Government Security. Treasury Board of Canada Secretariat (2009). Section 6.1.1 states that departmental security activities should have a governance structure with defined objectives and are subject to audits.
- **Policy on Privacy Protection**. Treasury Board of Canada Secretariat (2008). The policy requires heads of federal government institutions to establish practices for the management and protection of personal information under their control to ensure that the Privacy Act is administered in a consistent and fair manner.

Government of U.S. Sources

- **HIPAA Security Rule 45 CFR §164.308(a)(2).**
  Standard: assign security responsibility. A covered entity must identify, and name, the security official who is responsible for the development and implementation of the HIPAA security policies and procedures.
- **HIPAA Security Rule 45 CFR §164.308(a)(1)(i).**
  Standard: security management process. A covered entity must implement policies and procedures to prevent, detect, contain, and correct security

violations. Paragraph §164.308(a)(1)(ii) provides the following list of implementation specifications: risk analysis, risk management, sanction policy, and information system activity review.

Organizational Policies for Data Storage, Management, and Access Are in Place At the Requestor Site (Low1High2)

In order to provide assurance that there has not been an unauthorized use or disclosure of personal information, an entity must have positive controls over that personal information. This is captured in policies for the management and storage of data.

Response Categories

i. General
1. The data requestor has no organizational data storage policies, or policies are being developed but are not yet implemented (low).
2. The data requestor does not have an authoritative list of data storage locations and the data that are stored therein (low).
3. The data requestor has organizational data storage policies, but they are not applied to all data resources regularly, and remediation is under way (medium).
   OR
   The data requestor has organizational data storage policies, but they are not applied to all data resources regularly, and the requestor has chosen to accept the risk without remediation [with annotations] (medium).
4. The data requestor has a specific data storage policy with policy enforcement and periodic audits (high).
ii. Compliance [if i.4 is endorsed]
1. The data requestor is able to provide reports about data storage compliance for the last two years (high).

References to Standards

- **Protection of organizational records** [Section 15.1.3] in ISO/IEC 27002:2005. International Organization for Standardization and International Electrotechnical Commission (2005). The system of storage and handling should accommodate the retention, storage, handling, and disposal of records and information.
- **Manage data: storage and retention arrangements** [Section DS11.2] in *COBIT 4.1: Framework, Control Objectives, Management Guidelines, Maturity*

Models. IT Governance Institute (2007). An organization should implement procedures for data storage to meet business objectives, the organization's security policy, and regulatory requirements.

- **Information security policy document** [Section 5.1.1]. ISO/IEC 27002:2005. International Organization for Standardization and International Electrotechnical Commission. (2005)
- **Establishment of an IT governance framework** [Section ME 4.1]. COBIT 4.1.
- **Responsibility and accountability for policies** [Section 1.1.2]. GAPP.

Government of Canada Sources

- **Detailed process description: data flow tables** [Section 5.2.2] in *Privacy Impact Assessment Guidelines: A Framework to Manage Privacy Risks.* Treasury Board of Canada Secretariat (2002). Section 5.2.2 provides a sample of a data flow diagram that includes the following elements: description of personal information, collected by, type or format, purpose of collection, disclosed to, and storage or retention site.

Government of U.S. Sources

- None in Security Rule.

Privacy and Security Policies and Procedures Are Monitored and Enforced (Low1High2)

Self-explanatory

Response Categories

i. General
  1. The data requestor does not have an organized privacy or security program (low).
  2. The data requestor monitors compliance with privacy and security policies by responding to complaints or incidents (medium).
  3. The data requestor compares privacy and security policies and procedures against benchmarks regularly (medium).
  4. The data requestor has a proactive program for monitoring privacy and security policies and procedures (high).
ii. Compliance [if i.4 is endorsed]
  The data requestor has two years of compliance reporting available (high).

References to Standards

- **Review of information security policy** [Section 5.1.2] in ISO/IEC 27002:2005. International Organization for Standardization and International Electrotechnical Commission (2005). Section 5.1.2 states that "the information security policy should be reviewed at planned intervals or if signification changes occur to ensure its continuing suitability, adequacy, and effectiveness."
- **Monitor and evaluate IT performance** [Section ME1] in *COBIT 4.1: Framework, Control Objectives, Management Guidelines, Maturity Models*. IT Governance Institute (2007). Section ME1 provides a full description of evaluating and monitoring methodologies that should be implemented in IT environments.
- **Monitoring and enforcement** [Section 10.0] in *Generally Accepted Privacy Principles* [practitioner version] (2009). American Institute of Certified Public Accountants, Inc. and Canadian Institute of Chartered Accountants. An organization should monitor compliance with its privacy policies and procedures to address privacy-related inquiries, complaints, and disputes.
- **Safeguarding personal data: organizational safeguards** [Section 7.2.1] in *CIHR Best Practices for Protecting Privacy in Health Research* (2005). Institutions housing research projects and archived data should develop, monitor, and enforce privacy and security policies and procedures.

Government of Canada Sources

- **Safeguards for use and disclosure** [Section 6.2.19] in Directive on Privacy Practices. Treasury Board of Canada (2010). Heads of government institutions are responsible for establishing appropriate measures to ensure that access, use, and disclosure of personal information is monitored and documented.
- **Policy statement** [Section 5.1.3] in Policy on Privacy Protection. Treasury Board of Canada Secretariat (2008). One of the objectives of the policy is to ensure effective protection and management of personal information by identifying, assessing, monitoring, and mitigating privacy risks.

Government of U.S. Sources

- **HIPAA Security Rule 45 CFR §164.308(a)(1)(ii)(D).**
  Standard: security management process; implementation specification: information system activity review. A covered entity must implement procedures to regularly review records of information system activity, including audit logs, access reports, security incident reports, and any other documents used by the entity.

Mandatory and Ongoing Privacy, Confidentiality, and Security Training Is Conducted for All Individuals and/or Team Members, Including Those At External Collaborating or Subcontracting Sites (Low1High2)

Providing assurance of privacy depends strongly on the entity instilling a consistent approach to, and awareness of, privacy issues in all staff. Automated data controls are insufficient without a motivated and educated staff to ensure front-line compliance.

Response Categories

i. General
   1. The data requestor does not have a program of training in privacy and/or security for individuals (low).
   2. There is privacy and security training, but individuals request it on a voluntary basis (low).
   3. There is security and privacy training for selected individuals, and the selected individuals include all persons that may have access to the requested data (medium).
   4. There is mandatory security and privacy training for all individuals, but it is not ongoing (medium).
   5. There is mandatory and ongoing privacy, confidentiality, and security training for all individuals (high).
ii. Records [if i.5 is endorsed]
   1. The data requestor maintains records of completion of training to ensure compliance for all individuals (high).

References to Standards

- **Human resources security: information security awareness, education, and training** [Section 8.2.2] in ISO/IEC 27002:2005. International Organization for Standardization and International Electrotechnical Commission (2005). Section 8.2.2 states that employees and third-party IT users should be made aware, educated, and trained in security procedures.
- **Privacy awareness and training** [Section 1.2.10] in *Generally Accepted Privacy Principles* [practitioner version] (2009). American Institute of Certified Public Accountants, Inc. and Canadian Institute of Chartered Accountants. An organization is required to provide in-depth training that covers privacy and relevant security policies and procedures, legal and regulatory considerations, incidence response, and related topics.

- **Ensuring accountability and transparency in the management of personal data** [Section 10] in *CIHR Best Practices for Protecting Privacy in Health Research* (2005). Accountability and transparency practices require communication, education, and privacy protection training.
- **Personnel training** [Section PO 7.4]. COBIT 4.1.

Government of Canada Sources

- **Privacy awareness** [Section 6.2.2] in Policy on Privacy Protection. Treasury Board of Canada Secretariat (2008). Heads of government institutions are responsible for making employees of the government aware of policies, procedures, and legal responsibilities.

Government of U.S. Sources

- **HIPAA Security Rule 45 CFR §164.308(a)(5)(i).**
  Standard: security awareness and training. A covered entity must implement a security awareness and training program for all members of its workforce (including management). For implementation specifications, see §164.308(a)(5)(ii).

Explanations

- Some training would be required for individuals within the requestor site who would not have access to the requested data. The reason is that some of these individuals may still play a role in a breach. For example, an employee may let a stranger into the offices if he or she does not follow policies about providing physical access, or a receptionist may provide useful information, like names of employees or their addresses over the phone, or even credentials to access organizational systems (by an adversary pretending to be someone from IT). Social engineering techniques can be very effective at obtaining access or information from employees. Therefore training would generally be required for all staff. This also enforces a culture of privacy within the organization.

Appropriate Sanctions Are in Place for Breach of Privacy, Confidentiality, or Security, Including Dismissal and/or Loss of Institutional Privileges, and These Have Been Clearly Stipulated in Signed Pledges of Confidentiality (Low1High2)

Self-explanatory

Response Categories

i. General
   1. Sanctions for breach of privacy, confidentiality, or security are applied, if at all, on a case-by-case basis (low).
   2. Sanctions for security or privacy breaches are identified in either security and privacy policies or HR policies, but not both (medium).
   3. Appropriate sanctions are in place in security, privacy, and HR policies (high).
ii. Compliance [if i.3 is endorsed]
   1. There is evidence that sanctions have not been applied, in violation of security or privacy policies (low).
   2. The data custodian is unable to determine whether or not sanctions have been correctly applied (medium).
   3. There is evidence that the sanctions have been applied when warranted (high).

References to Standards

- **Privacy incident and breach management** [Section 1.2.7] in *Generally Accepted Privacy Principles* [practitioner version] (2009). American Institute of Certified Public Accountants, Inc. and Canadian Institute of Chartered Accountants. An entity should implement a privacy incident and breach management program. Section 1.2.7 provides provisions to be included in such a program.
- **Human resources security: disciplinary process** [Section 8.2.2] in ISO/IEC 27002:2005. International Organization for Standardization and International Electrotechnical Commission (2005). An organization should implement disciplinary processes for employees who have committed a security breach.
- **Security measures: organizational safeguards** [Section 7.2.1] in *CIHR Best Practices for Protecting Privacy in Health Research* (2005). Section 7.2.1 stipulates that consequences of breach of confidentiality, including dismissal or loss of institutional privileges, should be clearly specified.
- **Personnel job performance evaluation** [Section PO 7.7]. COBIT 4.1.

Government of Canada Sources

- **Requirements** [Section 6.1.2] in Directive on Privacy Practices. Treasury Board of Canada (2010). Heads of government institutions are responsible for establishing appropriate measures addressing privacy breaches.
- **Guidelines for privacy breaches**. Treasury Board of Canada Secretariat (n.d.).

Government of U.S. Sources

■ **HIPAA Security Rule 45 CFR §164.308(a)(1)(i)(C).**
Standard: security management process; implementation specification: sanction policy. This specification requires that appropriate sanctions be applied against workforce members who fail to comply with the security policies and procedures of the covered entity.

Privacy Officers and/or Data Stewardship Committees Have Been Appointed At the Requestor's Site (Low1High1)

Self-explanatory

Response Categories

i. General
1. The data requestor has not appointed privacy officers and/or a data stewardship committee (low).
2. There is a privacy officer or data stewardship committee at the data requestor, but they are only active in response to incidents or external requests (medium).
3. There is an active privacy officer and/or data stewardship committee, characterized by regular meetings and an active program of activities (high).

References to Standards

■ **Organization of information security: internal organization** [Section 6.1] in ISO/IEC 27002:2005. International Organization for Standardization and International Electrotechnical Commission (2005). Management should assign security roles and coordinate and review the implementation of security across the organization.
■ **Responsibility and accountability for policies** [Section 1.1.2] in *Generally Accepted Privacy Principles* [practitioner version] (2009). American Institute of Certified Public Accountants, Inc. and Canadian Institute of Chartered Accountants. Responsibility and accountability should be assigned to a person or a group for developing, implementing, enforcing, monitoring, and updating the entity's privacy policies.
■ **Security measures: organizational safeguards** [Section 7.2.1] in *CIHR Best Practices for Protecting Privacy in Health Research* (2005). Section 7.2.1 stipulates that institutions housing research projects and data should appoint privacy officers and create data stewardship committees as needed.

- **The security-privacy paradox: issues, misconceptions, and strategies** [pp. 10–11]. Information and Privacy Commissioner (Ontario), Deloitte and Touche (2003).* Organizations that manage personal information should establish a position of chief privacy officer, separate from a chief security officer position.
- **Establishment of an IT governance framework** [Section ME 4.1]. COBIT 4.1.

Government of Canada Sources

- **Delegation under the Privacy Act** [Section 6.1] in Policy on Privacy Protection. Treasury Board of Canada Secretariat (2008). Heads of government institutions may delegate the powers and responsibilities under the act. In such cases, delegates are accountable for any decisions they make. Ultimate responsibility, however, still rests with the head of the institution.

Government of U.S. Sources

- None in Security Rule.

Explanations

- In certain types of organizations, such as large registries, data stewardship committees or data access committees are often created to provide oversight over the disclosure of sensitive information.
- A data management safety board for research purposes may or may not be a data stewardship committee in the sense made here, depending on its terms of reference.

A Breach of Privacy Protocol Is in Place, Including Immediate Written Notification to Custodian (Low1High2)

Privacy breaches are incidents where there are reasonable grounds to assert that there has been an unauthorized collection, use, or disclosure of personally identifiable information. A security incident occurs when there are reasonable grounds to assert that the confidentiality, integrity, or availability objectives for sensitive data have not been met. Most, if not all, privacy breaches are security incidents, but not

---

* A. Cavoukian, Deloitte and Touche. The security-privacy paradox: issues, misconceptions, and strategies, A joint report by Information and Privacy Commissioner/Ontario & Deloitte and Touche, August 2003, Available from: http://www.ipc.on.ca/english/Resources/Discussion-Papers/Discussion-Papers-Summary/?id=248

all security incidents are privacy breaches. The data sets encompassed by security and privacy are different, as are the requirements for protection. There is significant overlap, but neither subsumes the other.

Response Categories

i. General
1. The data requestor has either no or only ad hoc procedures or policies/processes to deal with privacy breaches (low).
2. The data requestor has a specific policy, but it is not always enforced or audited, and remediation is under way (medium).
OR
The data requestor has a specific policy, but it is not always enforced or audited, and the requestor has chosen to accept the risk without remediation [with annotations] (medium).
3. The data requestor has a security breach or critical incident response protocol that will be or has been applied to privacy breaches (medium).
4. There is a privacy and a security breach protocol, with regular test (sand table) exercises (high).

i. Breach [if i.4 is endorsed]
1. A breach has occurred and has been successfully handled and documented in accordance with policy and protocol (high).
OR
No breaches have occurred [with annotations] (high).

References to Standards

■ **Privacy incident and breach management** [Section 1.2.7] in *Generally Accepted Privacy Principles* [practitioner version] (2009). American Institute of Certified Public Accountants, Inc. and Canadian Institute of Chartered Accountants. An entity should implement a privacy incident and breach management program. Section 1.2.7 provides provisions to be included in such a program.
■ **Incident escalation** [Section DS 8.3]. COBIT 4.1.
■ **Information security incident management: responsibilities and procedures** [Section 13.2.1] in ISO/IEC 27002:2005. International Organization for Standardization and International Electrotechnical Commission (2005). Procedures should be established to handle breaches of confidentiality and integrity.
■ **Security measures: organizational safeguards** [Section 7.2.1] in *CIHR Best Practices for Protecting Privacy in Health Research* (2005). Section 7.2.1

stipulates a variety of conditions and practices that should be implemented in order to safeguard personal data.

Government of Canada Sources

- **Guidelines for privacy breaches.** Treasury Board of Canada Secretariat (n.d.).
- **Protection of personal information** [Section 6.6.6.4] in *Guidance on Preparing Information Sharing Agreements Involving Personal Information*. Treasury Board of Canada Secretariat (2010). Safeguard should include any actions that may need to be taken to respond to security or privacy breaches, including the notification of affected parties.

Government of Ontario Sources

- What to do if a privacy breach occurs: *Guidelines for Government Organizations*. Information and Privacy Commissioner (Ontario) (2006).

Government of U.S. Sources

- **HIPAA Security Rule 45 CFR §164.308(a)(6)(ii).**
  Standard: security incident procedure; implementation specification: response and reporting. A covered entity is required to identify and respond to suspected or known security incidents; mitigate, to the extent practicable, harmful effects of security incidents that are known to the covered entity; and document security incidents and their outcomes.

Explanations

- There may be breach notification laws or regulations in effect at the requestor's jurisdiction. However, if the data have a low probability of re-identification, then the requestor would not be in a position to notify the individuals (and may not have the authority to do so anyway). Therefore notification of the custodian would generally be required and the custodian would handle the notifications.
- Considerations of costs of notifications of affected individuals and who should pay for them (requestor or custodian) need to be addressed as part of the DSA.
- It is arguably unlikely that an organization does not have a single privacy and/or security breach (unless it is a new organization, such as a start-up, or has not had access to personal data before). If the organization is not a start-up and has had personal data for some time, then having zero breaches may be a sign that reporting of breaches or the ability to detect breaches is

questionable. Of course, there will be exceptions, but it is generally advised to add some explanations as to why there have been no breaches if that is the response provided in Section ii.

Internal and External Privacy Reviews and Audits Have Been Implemented (Low1High1)

Self-explanatory

Response Categories

i. General
   1. The data requestor has not implemented internal or external privacy reviews or audits (low).
   2. The data requestor conducts internal privacy reviews on an ad hoc basis (medium).
   3. Privacy audits are, or have been, conducted, and identified gaps have been mitigated (medium).
   4. The data requestor regularly conducts both external and internal privacy reviews and audits, and identified gaps are mitigated (high).
   OR
   The data requestor regularly conducts both external and internal privacy reviews and audits, and when identified gaps are not mitigated, the requestor has chosen to accept the risk [with annotations] (high).

References to Standards

- **Independent review of information security** [Section 6.1.8] in ISO/IEC 27002:2005. International Organization for Standardization and International Electrotechnical Commission (2005). Section 6.1.8 states that information security should be independently reviewed at planned intervals.
- **Testing security safeguards** [Section 8.2.7] in *Generally Accepted Privacy Principles* [practitioner version] (2009). American Institute of Certified Public Accountants, Inc. and Canadian Institute of Chartered Accountants. Section 8.2.7 states that independent audits of security controls (internal or external) should be conducted at least annually.
- **Security measures: organizational safeguards** [Section 7.2.1] in *CIHR Best Practices for Protecting Privacy in Health Research* (2005). The section suggests that organizations housing research data, including data containing personal information, should implement internal and external reviews and audits.
- **Infrastructure maintenance** [Section AI 3.3]. COBIT 4.1.
- **Collection limited to identified purpose** [Section 4.2.1]. GAPP.

Government of Canada Sources

- **Departmental IT security assessment and audit** [Section 12.11] in *Operational Security Standard: Management of Information Technology Security (MITS)*. Treasury Board of Canada Secretariat (n.d.). Departments must assess and audit their information technology security and remedy deficiencies where necessary.
- **Privacy protocol for nonadministrative purposes** [Section 6.2.15] in Policy on Privacy Protection. Treasury Board of Canada Secretariat (2008). Heads of government institutions are responsible for establishing privacy protocol within the government institution for audit nonadministrative purposes, including audit and evaluation purposes.

Government of U.S. Sources

- **HIPAA Security Rule 45 CFR §164.312(b).**
  Standard: audit controls. A covered entity is required to implement hardware, software, and/or procedural mechanisms that record and examine activity in information systems that contain or use ePHI.

Explanations

- Reviews tend to be less formal than audits.
- Internal reviews or audits are conducted by the requestor's staff themselves, whereas external ones are performed by an independent third party.

Authentication Measures (Such As Computer Password Protection and Unique Logon Identification) Have Been Implemented to Ensure That Only Authorized Personnel Can Access Computer Systems (Low1High2)

Before a person can access sensitive data, he or she must first be granted access privileges on a computer system, whether that is a personal computer, a centralized system, or a web-based system.

Response Categories

i. Authentication Policy
 1. The data requestor is unable to specify the authentication measures that are in place (low).
 2. Authentication measures are ad hoc or are irregularly applied (low).
 3. Authentication measures are based on policies, but there is limited enforcement or auditing, and remediation is under way (medium).

OR

Authentication measures are based on policies, but there is limited enforcement or auditing, and the requestor has chosen to accept the risk without remediation [with annotations] (medium).

4. Authentication measures are in place and policy based (high).

ii. Authentication Logs

1. Authentication logs are not collected (low).
2. Authentication logs exist and are used for investigations after an incident (medium).
3. Authentication logs are kept and reported on regularly (e.g., through a regular manual analysis process or automated authentication log alerts that have been implemented) (high).
4. Automated authentication log alerts have been implemented (high).

References to Standards

- **Security for privacy criteria: logical access controls** [Section 8.2.2] in *Generally Accepted Privacy Principles* [practitioner version] (2009). American Institute of Certified Public Accountants, Inc. and Canadian Institute of Chartered Accountants. Section 8.2.2 provides a comprehensive list of issues to be addressed by an organization to provide a secure and reliable logical access to personal information.
- **User access management** [Section 11.2] in ISO/IEC 27002:2005. International Organization for Standardization and International Electrotechnical Commission (2005). The allocation of access rights to users should be formally controlled through user registration and administration procedures, including the management of passwords, and regular access rights reviews.
- **Security of network services** [Section 10.6.2] in ISO/IEC 27002:2005. International Organization for Standardization and International Electrotechnical Commission (2005). Security features on network services could be (1) technology applied for security, such as authentication, encryption, and network connection controls; (2) technical parameters required for secured connection; and (3) procedures for the network service usage to restrict access to such services.
- **Ensure systems security** [Section DS5.3] in *COBIT 4.1: Framework, Control Objectives, Management Guidelines, Maturity Models.* IT Governance Institute (2007). An organization should implement authentication mechanisms to ensure all users are uniquely identified.
- **Security measures: technological measures** [Section 7.2.2] in *CIHR Best Practices for Protecting Privacy in Health Research* (2005). Authentication measures should be implemented to ensure that only authorized personnel can access personal data.

Government of Canada Sources

■ **Technological measures to enhance privacy and security** [Section 6] in *Guidance Document: Taking Privacy into Account before Making Contracting Decisions* (2010). Section 6 describes some of the technical measures that apply to the specific privacy considerations. One such measure is the requirement for identification and authentication of users.

■ **Identification and authentication** [Section 16.4.2] in *Operational Security Standard: Management of Information Technology Security (MITS)*. Treasury Board of Canada Secretariat (n.d.). Departments must incorporate identification and authentication safeguards in all their networks and systems, according to the level of risk for the network of the system. If additional security is required, departments can use safeguards such as tokens or biometrics.

Government of U.S. Sources

■ **HIPAA Security Rule 45 CFR §164.312(a)(2)(i).**
Standard: access control; implementation specification: unique user identification. A covered entity must assign each user a unique name or number within the systems/organization.

An organization must uniquely identify and authenticate users and processes acting on behalf of users (NIST HIPAA Security Rule Toolkit).

Authentication Measures (Such As Computer Password Protection and Unique Logon Identification) Have Been Implemented to Ensure That Only Authorized Personnel Can Access Data (Low1High2)

Once a person has gained access to a computer system, access to sensitive data may also be controlled through access control systems for applications and/or databases, thus providing a second layer of authentication and protection. If it is the case that a "single sign-on" system is in place, then standards for protection of passwords and authentication mechanisms must be strong.

Response Categories

i. Authentication Policy
1. The data requestor is unable to specify the authentication measures that are in place (low).
2. Authentication measures are ad hoc or are irregularly applied (low).
3. Authentication measures are based on policies, but there is limited enforcement or auditing, and remediation is under way (medium).
OR

Authentication measures are based on policies, but there is limited enforcement or auditing, and the requestor has chosen to accept the risk without remediation [with annotations] (medium).
  4. Authentication measures are in place and policy based (high).
ii. Authentication Logs
  1. Authentication logs are not collected (low).
  2. Authentication logs exist and are used for investigations after an incident (medium).
  3. Authentication logs are kept and reported on regularly (e.g., through a regular manual analysis process or automated authentication log alerts that have been implemented) (high).
  4. Automated authentication log alerts have been implemented (high).

References to Standards

- **Security of network services** [Section 10.6.2] in ISO/IEC 27002:2005. International Organization for Standardization and International Electrotechnical Commission (2005). Security features on network services could be (1) technology applied for security, such as authentication, encryption, and network connection controls; (2) technical parameters required for secured connection; or (3) procedures for the network service usage to restrict access to such services.
- **Ensure systems security: identity management** [Section DS5.3] in *COBIT 4.1: Framework, Control Objectives, Management Guidelines, Maturity Models.* IT Governance Institute (2007). An organization should implement authentication mechanisms to ensure all users are uniquely identified.
- **Security for privacy criteria: logical access controls** [Section 8.2.2] in *Generally Accepted Privacy Principles* [practitioner version] (2009). American Institute of Certified Public Accountants, Inc. and Canadian Institute of Chartered Accountants. Section 8.2.2 provides a comprehensive list of issues to be addressed by an organization to provide secure and reliable logical access to personal information.

Government of Canada Sources

- **Technological measures to enhance privacy and security** [Section 6] in *Guidance Document: Taking Privacy into Account before Making Contracting Decisions* (2010). Section 6 describes some of the technical measures that apply to the specific privacy considerations. One such measure is the requirement for identification and authentication of users.
- **Identification and authentication** [Section 16.4.2] in *Operational Security Standard: Management of Information Technology Security (MITS).* Treasury Board of Canada Secretariat (n.d.). Departments must incorporate

identification and authentication safeguards in all their networks and systems, according to the level of risk for the network of the system. If additional security is required, departments can use safeguards such as tokens or biometrics.

Government of U.S. Sources

■ **HIPAA Security Rule 45 CFR §164.308(a)(4).**
Standard: information access management. A covered entity must implement policies and procedures for enabling access to ePHI by authorized personnel. This standard is to be implemented by the following specifications: isolating health care clearinghouse functions, access authorization, and access establishment and modification.

Special Protection Has Been Installed for Remote Electronic Access to Data (Low1High2)

Remote access to systems typically means that the "front door" for the system is exposed on the Internet, and is therefore subject to higher levels of protection because of the greater number of threats to such systems.

Response Categories

i. Applicability
  1. The data can be accessed remotely (skip question if not selected).
ii. Remote Access Policy [if i.1. is endorsed]
  1. The data requestor does not have a policy for remote electronic access to data (low).
  2. Remote access to data is handled on an ad hoc or case-by-case basis (low).
  3. The data requestor has a policy for remote electronic access to data but it is not always enforced or audited, and remediation is under way (medium). OR
     The data requestor has a policy for remote electronic access to data, but it is not always enforced or audited, and the requestor has chosen to accept the risk without remediation [with annotations] (medium).
  4. The data requestor enforces a secure remote electronic access policy (high).
ii. Remote Access Logs
  1. Remote access is not logged (low).
  2. Remote access to data is logged, and the logs are used for forensic analysis in the event of an incident (medium).
  3. Remote access to data is logged, and the logs are reviewed on a regular basis, for example, monthly (either through a manual analysis or an automated alerting system in place for remote electronic access to data) (high).

References to Standards

- **User authentication for external connections** [Section 11.4.2] in ISO/IEC 27002:2005. International Organization for Standardization and International Electrotechnical Commission (2005). Access to network services should be controlled. Policy should be defined and remote users (and equipment) should be suitably authenticated.
- **Ensure systems security: exchange of sensitive data** [Section DS5.11] in *COBIT 4.1: Framework, Control Objectives, Management Guidelines, Maturity Models*. IT Governance Institute (2007). Transmission of sensitive data should only take place over trusted path or medium with controls to provide authenticity of content, proof of submission, proof of receipt, and nonrepudiation of origin.
- **Security for privacy criteria: logical access controls** [Section 8.2.2] in *Generally Accepted Privacy Principles* [practitioner version] (2009). American Institute of Certified Public Accountants, Inc. and Canadian Institute of Chartered Accountants. Section 8.2.2 provides a comprehensive list of issues to be addressed by an organization to provide a secure and reliable logical access to personal information.
- **Security measures: technological measures** [Section 7.2.2] in *CIHR Best Practices for Protecting Privacy in Health Research* (2005).

Government of Canada Sources

- **Mobile computing and teleworking** [Section 16.4.7] in *Operational Security Standard: Management of Information Technology Security (MITS)*. Treasury Board of Canada Secretariat (n.d.). To protect the remote computer, the information it contains, and the communications link, departments should use an effective combination of physical protection measures, access controls, encryption, malicious code protection, backups, security configuration settings, identification and authentication safeguards, and network security controls.

Government of U.S. Sources

- **HIPAA Security Rule 45 CFR §164.310(b).**
  Standard: workstation use. Implement policies and procedures that specify the proper functions to be performed, the manner in which those functions are to be performed, and the physical attributes of the surroundings of a specific workstation of a class of workstation that can access ePHI.

  Some of the safeguards under this standard are (1) authorization of remote access to the information system prior to the connection and (2) provision of specifically configured mobile devices to individuals traveling to locations that your organization deems to be of significant risk in accordance with organizational policies and procedures (NIST HIPAA Security Rule Toolkit).

■ **HIPAA Security Rule 45 CFR §164.312(e)(1).**
Standard: transmission security. A covered entity must implement technical security measures to guard against unauthorized access to ePHI that is being transmitted over an electronic communications network.

Virus-Checking and/or Anti-Malware Programs Have Been Implemented (Low1High1)

As part of a "defense in depth" it is insufficient to assume that perimeter and access controls are sufficient. There should be protection at the individual level for each machine that may have access or may contain sensitive information.

Response Categories

i. General
  1. Protective software is not installed on user computers (low).
     OR
     Protective measures are not in place to prevent malware on servers (low).
     OR
     The data requestor does not filter email for viruses, spyware, or other forms of malicious code (low).
  2. Protective programs are in place, but individual users may have the ability to disable antivirus software (low).
  3. Anti-virus and/or anti-spyware programs are in place; users do not have the ability to disable this software, but they are not updated on a regular basis (medium).
  4. The data requestor has a program in place to prevent malicious or mobile code being executed on their servers, workstations, and mobile devices, with regular updates and reports, and users cannot disable these programs (high).

References to Standards

■ **Controls against malicious code** [Section 10.4.1] in ISO/IEC 27002:2005. International Organization for Standardization and International Electrotechnical Commission (2005). Prevention, detection, and recovery controls to protect against malicious code should be put in place. Appropriate user awareness measures should be implemented.

- **Ensure systems security: malicious software prevention, detection, and correction** [Section DS5.9] in *COBIT 4.1: Framework, Control Objectives, Management Guidelines, Maturity Models.* IT Governance Institute (2007). Preventive, detective, and corrective measures should be put in place to protect information systems from malware.
- **Security for privacy criteria: information security program** [Section 8.2.1] in *Generally Accepted Privacy Principles* [practitioner version] (2009). American Institute of Certified Public Accountants, Inc. and Canadian Institute of Chartered Accountants. Section 8.2.1, in its list of illustrative controls and procedures, provides for controls to protect operating system and network software and system files.
- **Security measures: technological measures** [Section 7.2.2] in *CIHR Best Practices for Protecting Privacy in Health Research* (2005). Virus-checking programs and disaster recovery safeguards should be put in place.

Government of Canada Sources

- **Malicious code** [Section 16.4.12] in *Operational Security Standard: Management of Information Technology Security (MITS).* Treasury Board of Canada Secretariat (n.d.). Departments must install, use, and regularly update antivirus software and conduct malicious code scans on all electronic files from external systems. Departments should implement antivirus detection software at several points, including desktop computers, servers, and departmental entry points.

Government of U.S. Sources

- **HIPAA Security Rule 45 CFR §164.308(a)(5)(ii)(B).**
  Standard: security awareness and training; implementation specification: protection from malicious software. A covered entity is required to develop procedures for guarding against, detecting, and reporting malicious software.

A Detailed Monitoring System for Audit Trails Has Been Instituted to Document the Person, Time, and Nature of Data Access, With Flags for Aberrant Use and "Abort" Algorithms to End Questionable or Inappropriate Access (Low1High2)

Audit trails are fundamental for real-time alerting, regular performance reporting, and forensic analysis of systems. The entity must balance the value of auditing against the operational resources available for auditing to achieve an appropriate risk management posture.

Response Categories

i. General

1. The data requestor does not monitor and log access to personal information (low).
2. The data requestor logs access to personal information but only reviews the logs after incidents or in response to queries (medium).
3. The data requestor has implemented a detailed audit/monitoring system to document the person, time, and nature of data access (high).

ii. Aberrant and Inappropriate Uses [if i.3 is endorsed]

1. The data requestor has identified aberrant use conditions and has implemented audit alerts based on them (high).
   OR
   There have been no known cases of aberrant use (high).
2. Inappropriate uses of data have been terminated by automated systems (high).
   OR
   There have been no known cases of or alerts indicating inappropriate uses (high).

References to Standards

- **Network controls** [Section 10.6.1] in ISO/IEC 27002:2005. International Organization for Standardization and International Electrotechnical Commission (2005). Section 10.6.1 outlines secure network management, network security monitoring, and other controls.
- **Acquire and maintain application software: application control and auditability** [Section AI2.3] in *COBIT 4.1: Framework, Control Objectives, Management Guidelines, Maturity Models.* IT Governance Institute (2007). Implement business controls into automated application controls such that processing is accurate, complete, timely, authorized, and auditable.
- **Security for privacy criteria: testing security safeguards** [Section 8.2.7] in *Generally Accepted Privacy Principles* [practitioner version] (2009). American Institute of Certified Public Accountants, Inc. and Canadian Institute of Chartered Accountants. Section 8.2.7 states that independent audits of security controls (internal or external) should be conducted at least annually.
- **Security measures: technological measures** [Section 7.2.2] in *CIHR Best Practices for Protecting Privacy in Health Research* (2005). An audit trail monitoring system should be put in place to document the person, time, and nature of data access, with flags for anomalous use that will trigger the cancelation of questionable or inappropriate access.

■ **Problem tracking and resolution** [Section DS10.2] in *COBIT 4.1: Framework, Control Objectives, Management Guidelines, Maturity Models.* IT Governance Institute (2007). Ensure that the problem management system provides for adequate audit trail facilities that allow tracking, analyzing, and determining the root cause of all reported problems.

Government of U.S. Sources

■ **HIPAA Security Rule 45 CFR §164.308(a)(1)(ii)(D).**
Standard: security management process; implementation specification: information system activity review. The covered entity must implement procedures to regularly review records of information system activity, such as audit logs, access reports, and security incident tracking reports.

■ **HIPAA Security Rule 45 CFR §164.308(a)(5)(ii)(C).**
Standard: security awareness and training; implementation specification: log-in monitoring. The covered entity should implement procedures for monitoring log-in attempts and reporting discrepancies.

■ **HIPAA Security Rule 45 CFR §164.312(b).**
Standard: audit controls. The covered entity must implement hardware, software, and/or procedural mechanisms that record and examine activity in information systems that contain or use ePHI.

If Electronic Transmission of the Data Is Required, an Encrypted Protocol Is Used (Low1High2)

Self-explanatory

Response Categories

i. Applicability
   1. The data may be transmitted electronically (skipQuestionIfNotSelected).
ii. Policies
   1. The data requestor does not have a policy requiring the secure transmission of confidential data (low).
   2. The data requestor has a secure data transmission policy, but the data requestor is unable to determine if there are exceptions, and its application is irregular and ad hoc (medium).
   3. The data requestor has a secure data transmission policy, but it is not applied in all cases, and remediation is under way (medium).
   OR
   The data requestor has a secure data transmission policy, but it is not applied in all cases, and remediation is under way (medium) and the

requestor has chosen to accept the risk without remediation [with annotations] (medium).

4. The data requestor has a secure data transmission policy, with detection mechanisms and enforcement (high).

iii. Systems

1. The data requestor does not have a valid SSL certificate for its website (where web transmission of data, including email, is possible) (low).

2. The data requestor allows unencrypted transmission of data (i.e., users may inadvertently send data "in the clear") (low).

3. The data requestor is aware of cases where insecure transmission of confidential data has occurred, and remediation is under way or complete (medium).

OR

The data requestor is aware of cases where insecure transmission of confidential data has occurred, and the requestor has chosen to accept the risk without remediation [with annotations] (medium).

4. The data requestor is not aware of any instances where insecure transmission of confidential data has occurred, and takes reasonable precautions to prevent such transmission from occurring (high).

5. The data requestor has a system in place to detect the insecure transmission of confidential data, with automatic alerting enabled (high).

References to Standards

- **Information exchange policies and procedures** [Section 10.8.1] in ISO/IEC 27002:2005. International Organization for Standardization and International Electrotechnical Commission (2005). Formal exchange policies, procedures, and controls should be in place to protect the exchange of information. One of the recommended measures is the use of cryptographic techniques to protect the confidentiality, integrity, and authenticity of information.

- **Data classification scheme** [Section PO2] in *COBIT 4.1: Framework, Control Objectives, Management Guidelines, Maturity Models.* IT Governance Institute (2007). Data classification scheme should be used as the basis for applying controls such as access controls, archiving, or encryption.

- **Security for privacy criteria: transmitted personal information** [Section 8.2.5] in *Generally Accepted Privacy Principles* [practitioner version] (2009). American Institute of Certified Public Accountants, Inc. and Canadian Institute of Chartered Accountants. Personal information collected and transmitted over the Internet or other insecure networks, including wireless networks, must be protected by deploying industry standard encryption technology for transferring and receiving personal information.

■ **Security measures: technological measures** [Section 7.2.2] in *CIHR Best Practices for Protecting Privacy in Health Research* (2005). Encryption, scrambling of data, and other methods intended to reduce the potential of a privacy breach should be put in place.

Government of Ontario Sources

■ **The information highway: access and privacy principles** [Section 6]. Office of Information and Privacy Commissioner, Ontario (1994). Personal information should not be collected, used, or disclosed through information technologies and services that do not have an appropriate level of security. Serious consideration should be given to the encryption of sensitive personal information or information that is at great risk of being improperly accessed.

Government of Canada Sources

■ **Technological measures to enhance privacy and security: segregation using encryption** [Section 6] in *Guidance Document: Taking Privacy into Account before Making Contracting Decisions* (2010). Encryption is an important measure that can be used to protect sensitive information, and it should be used for transmission over insecure networks and for storage devices that are at risk of loss of theft. Cryptography must be properly implemented and the keys must be securely managed.

■ **Protection of personal information** [Section 6.6.6.4] in *Guidance on Preparing Information Sharing Agreements Involving Personal Information*. Treasury Board of Canada Secretariat (2010). Methods of protecting personal information can include the following technical measures: passwords, audit trails, encryption, and firewalls.

Government of U.S. Sources

■ **HIPAA Security Rule 45 CFR §164.312(e)(2)(ii).**
Standard: transmission security; implementation specification: encryption. The covered entity must implement a mechanism to encrypt ePHI whenever deemed appropriate.

Computers and Files That Hold the Disclosed Information Are Housed in Secure Settings in Rooms Protected by Such Methods As Combination Lock Doors or Smart Card Door Entry, With Paper Files Stored in Locked Storage Cabinets (Low1High2)

Self-explanatory

Response Categories

i. General
1. The data requestor does not have a physical security policy or regularly followed processes (low).
   OR
   Individuals have paper files in unsecured filing cabinets or desk drawers (low).
   OR
   The data requestor is aware of incidents where physical files have been unsecured (low).
2. The data requestor has a physical security policy, but it is not always followed, and remediation is under way (medium).
   OR
   The data requestor has a physical security policy, but it is not always followed, and the requestor has chosen to accept the risk without remediation [with annotations] (medium).
3. The data requestor has a physical security policy and has processes in place to implement the policies (medium).
4. The data requestor has a physical security policy and has processes in place to implement the policies and audit compliance (high).
ii. Compliance and Audits [if i.4 is endorsed]
1. The data requestor uses a third party (i.e., a security company) to conduct regular checks of its physical security, including clean desks, locked doors, and locked cabinets (high).

References to Standards

■ **Secure areas** [Section 9.1.2] in ISO/IEC 27002:2005. International Organization for Standardization and International Electrotechnical Commission (2005). Section 9.1.2 states that secure areas should be protected by appropriate entry control to prevent unauthorized access to these facilities.
■ **Physical security measures** [Section DS12.2] in *COBIT 4.1: Framework, Control Objectives, Management Guidelines, Maturity Models.* IT Governance Institute (2007). Physical security measures must be capable of effectively preventing, detecting, and mitigating risks relating to theft, temperature, fire, smoke, water, vibration, terror, vandalism, power outages, chemicals, or explosives.
■ **Security for privacy criteria: physical access controls** [Section 8.2.3] in *Generally Accepted Privacy Principles* [practitioner version] (2009). American Institute of Certified Public Accountants, Inc. and Canadian Institute of Chartered Accountants. Physical safeguards must be put in place. They may include the use of locked files, card access systems, or other systems to control

access to offices, data centers, and other locations where personal data are processed or stored.

■ **Security measures: physical security** [Section 7.2.3] in *CIHR Best Practices for Protecting Privacy in Health Research* (2005). Electronic equipment and files with personal information should be placed in secure settings properly protected (e.g., combination locks, smart card door entry, etc.).

■ **Security measures: physical security** [Section 7.2.3] in *CIHR Best Practices for Protecting Privacy in Health Research* (2005). Electronic equipment and files with personal information should be placed in secure settings and properly protected (e.g., combination locks, smart card door entry, etc.).

■ **Physical security perimeter** [Section 9.1.1]. ISO/IEC 27002:2005. International Organization for Standardization and International Electrotechnical Commission (2005).

■ **IT security plan** [Section DS 5.2]. COBIT 4.1.

Government of Canada Sources

■ **Security** [Section 3] in *Policy Framework for Information Technology*. Treasury Board of Canada Secretariat (2007). Effective security of information requires a systematic approach that identifies and categorizes information, assesses risks, and implements appropriate personnel, physical, and IT safeguards.

■ **Methods to control access** [Section 6, p. 5] in *Physical Security Guide (G1-024): Control of Access*. Royal Canadian Mounted Police (2004). Common methods of physical access control include personal recognition, access badges, doors and locks, and card access systems. Often a combination of strategies is used.

■ **Policy on government security.** Treasury Board of Canada Secretariat (2009).

Government of U.S. Sources

■ **HIPAA Security Rule 45 CFR §164.310(a)(1).**
Standard: facility access controls. The covered entity must implement policies and procedures to limit physical access to its electronic information systems and the facility or facilities in which they are housed while ensuring that properly authorized access is allowed. A facility is defined in the rule as the physical premises and the interior and exterior of the building(s). The implementation specifications for this rule include the following: contingency operations, facility security plan, access control and validation procedures, and maintenance records (§164.310(a)(2)).

One of the safeguards under this standard is the provision of secure keys, combinations, and other physical access devices (NIST HIPAA Security Rule Toolkit).

Staff Have Been Provided With Photo Identification or Coded Card Swipe (Low1High2)

Self-explanatory

Response Categories

   i. Identification Policy
1. Staff have not been provided with photo identification or coded card swipe (low).
2. The regular practice of the data requestor is to not carry or wear the supplied photo identification or card swipe (low).
3. The data requestor has a policy requiring the wearing of photo identification and/or card swipes (medium).
4. The data requestor has a policy requiring the wearing of photo identification and/or card swipes, with penalties that are enforced (high).

   ii. Inappropriate Use [if i.4 is endorsed]
1. Data requestor staff are trained not to lend each other their photo identification or swipe cards, with enforced consequences if they are found to have done so (high).

   iii. Access Logs
1. Access to the data requestor's facility is allowed without carrying or wearing supplied photo identification and/or card swipes, and access is not logged (low).
2. No access to the data requestor's facility is allowed without carrying or wearing supplied photo identification and/or card swipes, but access is not logged (medium).
3. There are access logs of the facilities identifying entry and exit of all individuals, which are checked after an incident has occurred (medium).
4. There are access logs of the facilities identifying entry and exit of all individuals, which are reviewed regularly (high).

References to Standards

- **Physical entry controls** [Section 9.1.2c] in ISO/IEC 27002:2005. International Organization for Standardization and International Electrotechnical Commission (2005). Section 9.1.2c states that all employees and third-party users (including visitors) should be required to wear some form of visible identification.
- **Security for privacy criteria: physical access controls** [Section 8.2.3] in *Generally Accepted Privacy Principles* [practitioner version] (2009). American Institute of Certified Public Accountants, Inc. and Canadian Institute of Chartered Accountants. Physical safeguards must be put in place. They may

include the use of locked files, card access systems, or other systems to control access to offices, data centers, and other locations where personal data are processed or stored.

- **Identity management** [Section DS 5.3]. COBIT 4.1.
- **Identification cards** [Section 7.6.1]. TB:OSSPS. All government employees must be issued an identification card that, as a minimum, includes the name of the department/organization, the bearer's name and photo, a unique card number, and expiry date.

Government of Canada Sources

- **Scope and application** [Section 2] in *Physical Security Guide (G1-024): Control of Access.* Royal Canadian Mounted Police (2004). All government employees must be issued an identification card that, as a minimum, includes the name of the department/organization, the bearer's name and photo, a unique card number, and expiry date. This requirement is also stated in the *Operational Security Standard on Physical Security* document published by Treasury Board of Canada Secretariat [Section 7.6.1—Identification Cards].

Government of U.S. Sources

- **HIPAA Security Rule 45 CFR §164.310(a)(1).**
  Standard: facility access controls. A covered entity must implement policies and procedures to limit access to its electronic information systems and the facility or facilities in which they are housed while ensuring that properly authorized access is allowed.

  One of the safeguards under this section is the provision of authorization credentials, such as badges, identification cards, and smart cards, for the facility where the information system resides (NIST HIPAA Security Rule Toolkit).

Visitors Are Screened and Supervised (Low1High2)

While this may be impracticable in a clinical, research, or academic setting for the entire entity, it is a reasonable requirement for data centers, laboratories, and offices that contain, or may reasonably contain, personal health information. For the purposes of this section a "visitor" is a person who has not signed an NDA or CA that applies to the data covered by a DSA.

Response Categories

i. Policy
   1. The data requestor does not screen or supervise visitors (low).
   2. There is a policy for visitor screening, but it has not been implemented (low).

3. The data requestor has a visitor screening policy (i.e., reception sign-in is required), but it is applied irregularly, and remediation is under way (medium).
OR
The data requestor has a visitor screening policy (i.e., reception sign-in is required), but it is applied irregularly, and the requestor has chosen to accept the risk without remediation [with annotations] (medium).
4. The data requestor has a visitor screening policy (i.e., reception sign-in is required) that is regularly applied (high).

ii. Incidents [if i.4 is endorsed]
1. There has been a security or privacy incident involving a visitor and an investigation has occurred and remediation has been implemented (medium).
OR
There have been no known security or privacy incidents involving a visitor (medium).

iii. Records
1. The data requestor does not keep a record of all visitors (low).
2. The data requestor keeps a record of all visitors (medium).
3. The data requestor keeps a record of all visitors, and regularly audits the log (i.e., spot checks visitors to ensure that they are supervised and in the sign-in book) (high).

References to Standards

- **Physical entry controls** [Section 9.1.2c] in ISO/IEC 27002:2005. International Organization for Standardization and International Electrotechnical Commission (2005). Section 9.1.2c states that all employees and third-party users (including visitors) should be required to wear some form of visible identification.
- **Ensure systems security** [Section DS5.3] in *COBIT 4.1: Framework, Control Objectives, Management Guidelines, Maturity Models.* IT Governance Institute (2007). An organization should implement authentication mechanisms to ensure all users are uniquely identified.
- **Identity management** [Section DS 5.3]. COBIT 4.1. An organization should implement authentication mechanisms to ensure all users are uniquely identified.
- **Physical access controls** [Section 8.2.3]. GAPP.

Government of Canada Sources

- **Who should be granted access** [Section 4, p. 2] in *Physical Security Guide (G1-024): Control of Access.* Royal Canadian Mounted Police (2004). Visitors and contractors must be subject to the appropriate security screening.

Visitors may be granted access, but they should be appropriately escorted. Departments should have procedures to follow, such as sign-in and issuance of temporary passes when access is provided to visitors.
■ **Access badges** [Section 7.6.2] in *Operational Security Standard on Physical Security*. Treasury Board of Canada Secretariat (n.d.). Access badges indicate authorized employees and visitors. Access badge must be issued to all visitors, which clearly identifies them as a non-employee.

Government of U.S. Sources

■ **HIPAA Security Rule 45 CFR §164.310(a)(2)(iii).**
Standard: facility access controls; implementation specification: access control and validation procedures. A covered entity needs procedures to screen and validate every person's entry to its facilities, including visitors.

Some of the safeguards under this specification are (1) control physical access to the information system by authenticating visitors before authorizing access to the facility where the information system resides, (2) maintain visitor access records to the facility where the information system resides, and (3) periodically review visitor access records (NIST HIPAA Security Rule Toolkit).

Alarm Systems Are in Place (Low1High2)

Self-explanatory

Response Categories

i. General
 1. The data requestor does not have an alarm system in place (low).
 2. The data requestor's alarm system is not activated on a regular basis (low).
 3. The data requestor has an activated alarm system, but no one is notified if the alarm system is tripped (low).
 4. The data requestor has an alarm system, which is turned on regularly, and which notifies a security company when it is tripped (medium).
 5. The data requestor has an alarm system, which is turned on regularly, and which notifies a security company when it is tripped.
 AND
 The data requestor uses staff roles to assign access levels to the alarm system (i.e., only staff with a job requirement for after hours or weekend access to facilities are able to disarm/arm the alarm after hours or on weekends) (high).
ii. Testing [if i.3, i.4, or i.5 is endorsed]
 1. The data requestor regularly conducts tests of the alarm system, including staff training in how to respond to alarm conditions (high).

iii. Logging

    1. There is no logging of alarm system events (low).

    2. The data requestor has an electronic log of alarm system events, which is reviewed in the event of an incident (medium).

    3. The data requestor reviews alarm system logs regularly (e.g., monthly) (high).

References to Standards

■ **Physical security perimeter** [Section 9.1.1f] in ISO/IEC 27002:2005. International Organization for Standardization and International Electrotechnical Commission (2005). Section 9.1.2f states that suitable intruder detection systems should be installed and regularly tested.

■ **Ensure systems security** [Section DS12.2] in *COBIT 4.1: Framework, Control Objectives, Management Guidelines, Maturity Models.* IT Governance Institute (2007). Section DS12.2 states that physical security measures must be capable of effectively preventing, detecting, and mitigating risks relating to theft, temperature, fire, smoke, water, vibration, terror, vandalism, power outages, chemicals, or explosives.

■ **Security for privacy criteria: physical access controls** [Section 8.2.3] in *Generally Accepted Privacy Principles* [practitioner version] (2009). American Institute of Certified Public Accountants, Inc. and Canadian Institute of Chartered Accountants. Physical safeguards must be put in place. They may include the use of locked files, card access systems, or other systems to control access to offices, data centers, and other locations where personal data are processed or stored.

Government of Canada Sources

■ **Physical security within the IT security environment** [Section 16.1] in *Operational Security Standard: Management of Information Technology Security (MITS).* Treasury Board of Canada Secretariat (n.d.). Physical security measures, e.g., locks and alarm systems, reduce the risk of unauthorized access to information and IT assets. Physical security can also protect information and IT assets from fire, flood, earthquakes, power failures, etc.

Government of U.S. Sources

■ **HIPAA Security Rule 45 CFR §164.308(a)(1)(ii)(D).**
Standard: security management process; implementation specification: information system activity review. Implement procedures to regularly review records of information system activity, such as audit logs, access reports, and security incident tracking reports.

Some of the safeguards under this specification are the deployment of monitoring devices (1) strategically within the information system to collect organization-determined essential information, and (2) at ad hoc locations within the system to track specific types of transactions of interest to your organization (NIST HIPAA Security Rule Toolkit).

■ **HIPAA Security Rule 45 CFR §164.310(a)(1).**
Standard: facility access controls. The covered entity must implement policies and procedures to limit physical access to its electronic information systems and the facility or facilities in which they are housed while ensuring that properly authorized access is allowed. A facility is defined in the rule as the physical premises and the interior and exterior of the building(s). The implementation specifications for this rule include the following: contingency operations, facility security plan, access control and validation procedures, and maintenance records (§164.310(a)(2)).

One of the safeguards under this standard is the provision of locks and cameras in nonpublic areas (NIST HIPAA Security Rule Toolkit).

The Number of Locations in Which Personal Information Is Stored Has Been Minimized, and These Locations Can Be Specified in Advance (Low1High2)

Self-explanatory

Response Categories

i. Policy
1. The data requestor does not have a policy to restrict the locations where personal information may be stored (low).
2. The requestor has a policy to restrict the locations where personal information may be stored, but it has not been implemented (low).
3. The data requestor has a policy specifying the locations where personal information may be stored, but it is applied irregularly, and remediation is on the way (medium).
   OR
   The data requestor has a policy specifying the locations where personal information may be stored, and the requestor has chosen to accept the risk without remediation [with annotations] (medium).
4. The data requestor has a policy that specifies the locations where personal information may be stored, it is regularly followed, and it restricts such storage to the minimal number of locations required for processing of the data (high).

  ii. Implementation

    1. The data requestor cannot specify in advance where personal information may be stored (low).

    2. The data requestor trains its staff to ensure that personal data are stored in specified locations (medium).

    3. The data requestor trains its staff and implements technical means to ensure that personal data are stored in specified locations (high).

References to Standards

- **Equipment siting and protection** [Sections 9.2.1b and 9.2.1c] in ISO/IEC 27002:2005. International Organization for Standardization and International Electrotechnical Commission (2005). Sections 9.2.1b and 9.2.1c state that facilities handling sensitive data should be positioned in ways reducing the risk of information being viewed by unauthorized persons. Equipment requiring special safeguarding should be isolated to reduce the general level of protection.
- **Security measures: physical security** [Section 7.2.3] in *CIHR Best Practices for Protecting Privacy in Health Research* (2005). The number of locations in which personal information is stored should be minimized.
- **Security requirements for data management** [Section DS 11.6]. COBIT 4.1.
- **Use of personal information** [Section 5.2.1]. GAPP.

Government of U.S. Sources

- None in Security Rule.

Architectural Space Precludes Public Access to Areas Where Sensitive Data Are Held (Low1High1)

This is the corollary to the requirement for access cards and/or photographic identification.

Response Categories

  i. General

    1. The data requestor's architectural space allows public access to areas where sensitive data may be held (low).
    OR
    The data requestor is aware of incidents where members of the public have been found in areas where sensitive data are held (low).

2. The data requestor's facilities present reasonable physical barriers to public entry (i.e., reception desks, locked doors, and so on) (medium).
3. The data requestor's facilities present highly secure physical barriers to public entry (i.e., permanently staffed security desks, man trap doors, and so on) (high).

References to Standards

- **Equipment siting and protection** [Sections 9.2.1b and 9.2.1c] in ISO/IEC 27002:2005. International Organization for Standardization and International Electrotechnical Commission (2005). Sections 9.2.1b and 9.2.1c state that facilities handling sensitive data should be positioned in ways reducing the risk of information being viewed by unauthorized persons. Equipment requiring special safeguarding should be isolated to reduce the general level of protection.
- **Security for privacy criteria: physical access controls** [Section 8.2.3] in *Generally Accepted Privacy Principles* [practitioner version] (2009). American Institute of Certified Public Accountants, Inc. and Canadian Institute of Chartered Accountants. Physical safeguards must be put in place. They may include the use of locked files, card access systems, or other systems to control access to offices, data centers, and other locations where personal data are processed or stored.
- **Security measures: physical security** [Section 7.2.3] in *CIHR Best Practices for Protecting Privacy in Health Research* (2005). Architectural space should be designed to preclude public access to areas where sensitive data are held.
- **Physical access** [Section DS 12.3]. COBIT 4.1.

Government of Canada Sources

- **Demarcation** [Appendix A, Section 1.3] in *Physical Security Guide (G1-024): Control of Access.* Royal Canadian Mounted Police (2004). Provide physical barriers around each separate area to which access is controlled. Identify each area with appropriate signs.

Government of U.S. Sources

- **HIPAA Security Rule 45 CFR §164.310(a)(1).**
  Standard: facility access controls. The covered entity must implement policies and procedures to limit physical access to its electronic information systems and the facility or facilities in which they are housed while ensuring that properly authorized access is allowed. A facility is defined in the rule as the physical premises and the interior and exterior of the building(s).

One of the safeguards under this standard is the provision that all workstations should be protected from public access and viewing (NIST HIPAA Security Rule Toolkit).

Routine Video Surveillance of Premises Is Conducted (Low1High1)

Employee and contractor privacy should be respected in the siting of the video surveillance, particularly in terms of respecting individual workspaces and normally private areas such as washrooms and lunchrooms. The purpose of the surveillance should be conveyed as for the reduction of risk to both staff and entity.

Response Categories

i. General
   1. The data requestor does not conduct video surveillance of its premises (low).
   2. The data requestor conducts surveillance but does not have a policy governing the use of surveillance (low).
   3. The data requestor conducts surveillance of its premises (public spaces, entry/exit, and security areas) based on a policy and with public notice of video surveillance (medium).
   4. Surveillance is not monitored, but recordings are used for investigations and/or proceedings (medium).
   5. The data requestor has live monitoring by security personnel of the premises using surveillance equipment (high).

References to Standards

- **Physical security perimeter** [Section 9.1.1f] in ISO/IEC 27002:2005. International Organization for Standardization and International Electrotechnical Commission (2005). Section 9.1.2f states that suitable intruder detection systems should be installed and regularly tested.
- **Ensure systems security** [Section DS12.2] in *COBIT 4.1: Framework, Control Objectives, Management Guidelines, Maturity Models*. IT Governance Institute (2007). Section DS12.2 states that physical security measures must be capable of effectively preventing, detecting, and mitigating risks relating to theft, temperature, fire, smoke, water, vibration, terror, vandalism, power outages, chemicals, or explosives.
- **Security for privacy criteria: physical access controls** [Section 8.2.3] in *Generally Accepted Privacy Principles* [practitioner version] (2009). American Institute of Certified Public Accountants, Inc. and Canadian Institute of Chartered Accountants. Physical safeguards must be put in place. They may

include the use of locked files, card access systems, or other systems to control access to offices, data centers, and other locations where personal data are processed or stored.

■ **Security measures: physical security** [Section 7.2.3] in *CIHR Best Practices for Protecting Privacy in Health Research* (2005).

Government of Canada Sources

■ **Closed-circuit video equipment** (CCVE) [Section 7.6.4] in *Operational Security Standard on Physical Security*. Treasury Board of Canada Secretariat (n.d.). CCVE may assist a department in providing appropriate monitoring of access to its facility.

Government of U.S. Sources

■ **HIPAA Security Rule 45 CFR §164.310(a)(1).**
Standard: facility access controls. The covered entity must implement policies and procedures to limit physical access to its electronic information systems and the facility or facilities in which they are housed while ensuring that properly authorized access is allowed. A facility is defined in the rule as the physical premises and the interior and exterior of the building(s).

One of the safeguards under this standard is the provision of locks and cameras in nonpublic areas (NIST HIPAA Security Rule Toolkit).

Physical Security Measures Are in Place to Protect Data From Hazards Such As Floods or Fire (Low1High1)

Self-explanatory

Response Categories

i. General
1. The data requestor does not have physical security measures to protect data (low).
2. The data requestor has implemented physical security measures to prevent damage to data due to hazards such as floods or fire (medium).
3. The data requestor has a business continuity or disaster recovery policy, with mechanisms in place, to ensure that physical threats will not destroy data (medium).
4. The data requestor has implemented highly available systems with off-site redundancy to ensure ongoing operations in the event of an environmental threat such as a flood or fire (high).

References to Standards

- **Physical security perimeter** [Section 9.1.1e] in ISO/IEC 27002:2005. International Organization for Standardization and International Electrotechnical Commission (2005). Section 9.1.2e states that "all fire doors on a security perimeter should be alarmed, monitored, and tested in conjunction with the walls to establish the required level of resistance in accordance to suitable regional, national, and international standards; they should operate in accordance with local fire code in a failsafe manner."
- **Physical security measures** [Section DS12.2] in *COBIT 4.1: Framework, Control Objectives, Management Guidelines, Maturity Models.* IT Governance Institute (2007). Physical security measures must be capable of effectively preventing, detecting, and mitigating risks relating to theft, temperature, fire, smoke, water, vibration, terror, vandalism, power outages, chemicals, or explosives.
- **Security for privacy criteria: environmental safeguards** [Section 8.2.4] in *Generally Accepted Privacy Principles* [practitioner version] (2009). American Institute of Certified Public Accountants, Inc. and Canadian Institute of Chartered Accountants. Personal information, in all forms, must be protected against accidental disclosure due to natural disasters and environmental hazards.
- **Security measures: physical security** [Section 7.2.3] in *CIHR Best Practices for Protecting Privacy in Health Research* (2005). Physical security measures must be implemented to protect information from hazards such as flood, fire, etc.

Government of Canada Sources

- **Physical security within the IT security environment** [Section 16.1] in *Operational Security Standard: Management of Information Technology Security (MITS).* Treasury Board of Canada Secretariat (n.d.). Physical security measures, e.g., locks and alarm systems, reduce the risk of unauthorized access to information and IT assets. Physical security can also protect information and IT assets from fire, flood, earthquakes, power failures, etc.

Government of U.S. Sources

- **HIPAA Security Rule 45 CFR §164.308(a)(7)(i).**
  Standard: contingency plan. Establish (and implement as needed) policies and procedures for responding to an emergency or other occurrence (for example, fire, vandalism, system failure, and natural disaster) that damages systems that contain ePHI. The implementation specifications for this standard include the following: (1) data backup plan, (2) disaster recovery plan, (3) emergency mode operation plan, (4) testing and revision procedures, and (5) application and data criticality analysis. §164.308(a)(7)(ii).

- **HIPAA Security Rule 45 CFR §164.310(a)(2)(i).**
  Standard: facility access controls; implementation specification: contingency operations. Establish (and implement as needed) procedures that allow facility access in support of restoration of lost data under the disaster recovery plan and emergency mode operations plan in the event of an emergency.

  The contingency plan should be appropriate for all types of potential disasters, such as fire, flood, or earthquake (NIST HIPAA Security Rule Toolkit).

Ensuring Accountability and Transparency in the Management of Personal Data

Contact Information and Titles of Senior Individuals Who Are Accountable for Privacy, Confidentiality, and Security of Data Have Been Provided to the Custodian, and the Requestor Will Notify the Custodian of Any Changes to This Information (Low1High1)

Self-explanatory

Response Categories

  i. Designated Individuals
1. The data requestor has not designated senior individuals to be accountable for privacy and security (low).
   OR
   The data requestor has designated staff to be responsible for privacy and security that are junior or are untrained about security and privacy matters (medium).
2. The data requestor has designated senior individuals to be accountable for privacy and security (high).

  ii. Policies
1. The data requestor does not have transparency and governance policies that require the appointment of senior individuals to be accountable for privacy and security (low).
2. The data requestor has transparency and governance policies that require the appointment of senior individuals to be accountable for privacy and security, and the names of these individuals have been communicated by the data requestor (medium).
3. The data requestor has transparency and governance policies that require the appointment of senior individuals to be accountable for privacy and

security, and regularly updates the custodian on the names of the senior individuals that are accountable for privacy and security (medium).

4. The data requestor has transparency and governance policies that require the appointment of senior individuals to be accountable for privacy and security, and the contact information for these individuals, or their roles, is publicly available (high).

References to Standards

■ **Responsibility for risk, security, and compliance** [Section PO4.8] in *COBIT 4.1: Framework, Control Objectives, Management Guidelines, Maturity Models.* IT Governance Institute (2007). An organization should establish ownership and responsibility for IT-related risks within the business at an appropriate senior level. Define and assign roles critical for managing IT risks, including the specific responsibility for information security, physical security, and compliance.

■ **Establishment of roles and responsibilities** [Section PO4.6] in *COBIT 4.1: Framework, Control Objectives, Management Guidelines, Maturity Models.* IT Governance Institute (2007). An organization should establish and communicate roles and responsibilities for IT personnel and end users that delineate between IT personnel and end user authority, responsibilities, and accountability for meeting the organization's needs.

■ **Management criteria: responsibility and accountability for policies** [Section 1.1.2] in *Generally Accepted Privacy Principles* [practitioner version] (2009). American Institute of Certified Public Accountants, Inc. and Canadian Institute of Chartered Accountants. An organization should assign responsibility for privacy policies to a designated person (this responsibility may be different from those assigned for other policies, such as security). The responsibility, authority, and accountability of the designated person should be clearly documented, and the names of persons responsible for privacy are communicated to internal personnel.

■ **Accountability: academic and other affiliated or hosting institutions** [Section 10.2.1] in *CIHR Best Practices for Protecting Privacy in Health Research* (2005). An organization is responsible for designating an individual who is accountable for the institution's compliance with privacy policies and procedures.

Government of Canada Sources

■ **Delegation under the Privacy Act** [Section 6.1] in Policy on Privacy Protection. Treasury Board of Canada Secretariat (2008). Heads of government institutions may delegate the powers and responsibilities under the act. In such cases, delegates are accountable for any decisions they make. Ultimate responsibility, however, still rests with the head of the institution.

Government of U.S. Sources

■ **HIPAA Security Rule 45 CFR §164.308(a)(2).**
Standard: assigned security responsibility. A covered entity must identify, and name, the security official who is responsible for the development and implementation of HIPAA security policies and procedures.

Explanations

■ It is assumed in these items that the individuals who are accountable for privacy and security in general would also be accountable for privacy and security of the data that have been requested.
■ Public availability of information means that, for example, it is posted on a website or in publicly available pamphlets.

Contact Information and Title(s) of Senior Individual(S) Who Are Accountable for Employees and Subcontractors Have Been Provided to Custodian, and the Requestor Will Notify the Custodian of Any Changes to This Information (Low1High1)

When it is the case that data are for a long-term study, or where there may be high turnover in the data requestor's collaborators, it is critical that the obligations are maintained.

Response Categories

i. Designated Individuals
  1. The data requestor has not designated senior individuals to be accountable for employees and subcontractors (low).
     OR
     The data requestor has designated junior staff to be responsible for employees and subcontractors that are untrained about security and privacy matters (medium).
  2. The data requestor has designated senior individuals to be accountable for employees and subcontractors (high).
ii. Policies
  1. The data requestor does not have transparency and governance policies that require the appointment of senior individuals to be accountable for employees and subcontractors (low).
  2. The data requestor has transparency and governance policies that require the appointment of senior individuals to be accountable for employees

and subcontractors, and the names of these individuals have been communicated by the data requestor (medium).

3. The data requestor has transparency and governance policies that require the appointment of senior individuals to be accountable for employees and subcontractors, and regularly updates the custodian on the names of the senior individuals that are accountable for employees and subcontractors (medium).

4. The data requestor has transparency and governance policies that require the appointment of senior individuals to be accountable for employees and subcontractors, and the contact information for these individuals, or their roles, is publicly available (high).

OR

The data requestor has transparency and governance policies that require the appointment of senior individuals to be accountable for employees and subcontractors, and regularly updates the custodian on the names of the senior individuals that are accountable for employees and subcontractors, but for security or other business reasons is not making that information public (high).

References to Standards

■ **Supervision** [Section PO4.10] in *COBIT 4.1: Framework, Control Objectives, Management Guidelines, Maturity Models.* IT Governance Institute (2007). An institution should implement adequate supervisory practices in the IT function to ensure that roles and responsibilities are properly exercised, and to assess whether all personnel have sufficient authority and resources to execute their roles and responsibilities.

■ **Responsibility for risk, security, and compliance** [Section PO4.8] in *COBIT 4.1: Framework, Control Objectives, Management Guidelines, Maturity Models.* IT Governance Institute (2007). An organization should establish ownership and responsibility for IT-related risks within the business at an appropriate senior level. Define and assign roles critical for managing IT risks, including the specific responsibility for information security, physical security, and compliance.

■ **Establishment of roles and responsibilities** [Section PO4.6] in *COBIT 4.1: Framework, Control Objectives, Management Guidelines, Maturity Models.* IT Governance Institute (2007). An organization should establish and communicate roles and responsibilities for IT personnel and end users that delineate between IT personnel and end user authority, responsibilities, and accountability for meeting the organization's needs.

■ **Responsibility and accountability for policies** [Section 1.1.2] in *Generally Accepted Privacy Principles* [practitioner version] (2009). American Institute of Certified Public Accountants, Inc. and Canadian Institute of Chartered Accountants. An organization should assign responsibility for privacy policies to a designated person (this responsibility may be different from those assigned for other policies, such as security). The responsibility, authority, and accountability of the designated person should be clearly documented, and the names of persons responsible for privacy are communicated to internal personnel.

■ **Accountability: academic and other affiliated or hosting institutions** [Section 10.2.1] in *CIHR Best Practices for Protecting Privacy in Health Research* (2005). An organization is responsible for designating an individual who is accountable for the institution's compliance with privacy policies and procedures.

Government of Canada Sources

■ **Delegation under the Privacy Act** [Section 6.1] in Policy on Privacy Protection. Treasury Board of Canada Secretariat (2008). Heads of government institutions may delegate the powers and responsibilities under the act. In such cases, delegates are accountable for any decisions they make. Ultimate responsibility, however, still rests with the head of the institution.

Government of U.S. Sources

■ **HIPAA Security Rule 45 CFR §164.308(a)(2).**
   Standard: assigned security responsibility. A covered entity must identify, and name, the security official who is responsible for the development and implementation of HIPAA security policies and procedures.

Explanations

■ These may be different from the individuals responsible for privacy and security at the custodian site, and are responsible for the conduct of individuals handling the requested data at the requestor site.

An Organizational Transparency and Public Notification Plan Is in Place At the Data Requestor Site and the Requestor Is Open about Collection, Use, or Disclosure of Information, Analysis Objectives, and Privacy Policy and Practices (Low1High1)

Self-explanatory

Response Categories

i. General
1. The data requestor is not open about the collection, use, or disclosure of personal information (for example, the data requestor does not publish its objectives or privacy policies for the data it collects) (low).
2. The data requestor is open about the collection, use, or disclosure of personal information (e.g., makes that information available on demand) but does not have a public notification plan (low).
3. The data requestor has a transparency and public notification policy in place, but does not have enforcement or audit mechanisms (medium).
4. The data requestor publishes and keeps up-to-date information about the collection and disclosure of information, including objectives and privacy policies and procedures (medium).
5. The data requestor has a transparency and public notification policy in place, with enforcement and audit mechanisms (high).

References to Standards

■ **Notice criteria** [Sections 2.0 and 2.2.1] in *Generally Accepted Privacy Principles* [practitioner version] (2009). American Institute of Certified Public Accountants, Inc. and Canadian Institute of Chartered Accountants. An organization should provide notice about its privacy policies and procedures and identify the purposes for which personal information is collected, used, retained, and disclosed. The notice is easily accessible and available when personal information is first collected from the individual.
■ **Transparency** [Section 10.1] in *CIHR Best Practices for Protecting Privacy in Health Research* (2005). Individuals and organizations engaged in the conduct and evaluation of health research should be open to the public with respect to the objectives of the research and about the policies and practices relating to the protection of personal data used in the research.

Government of Canada Sources

■ **Privacy notice** [Section 6.2.9] in Directive on Privacy Practices. Treasury Board of Canada Secretariat (2010). Executives and senior officials who manage programs or activities involving the creation, collection, or handling of personal information are responsible for notifying the individual whose personal information is collected directly of the following: (1) the purpose and authority for the collection, (2) any uses or disclosures that are consistent with the original purpose, (3) any uses or disclosures that are not relevant to the original purpose, (4) any legal or administrative consequences for refusing to provide the personal information, and (5) the rights of access to, correction of, and protection of personal information under the Privacy Act.

Government of U.S. Sources

- None.

The Requestor's Site Has Procedures in Place to Receive and Respond to Public Complaints or Inquiries about Its Policies and Practices Related to the Handling of Personal Data, and Complaint Procedures Are Easily Accessible and Simple to Use (Low1High2)

Self-explanatory

Response Categories

i. Policy
1. The data requestor does not, or is not able to, respond to public complaints or inquiries (low).
2. The data requestor has identified an individual or group to deal with public complaints or inquiries, but there are no policies that include openness and transparency clauses (low).
3. The data requestor has identified an individual or group to deal with public complaints or inquiries, and a policy for dealing with complaints or inquiries exists or is being developed, but it is irregularly applied, and remediation is on the way (medium).
   OR
   The data requestor has identified an individual or group to deal with public complaints or inquiries, and a policy for dealing with complaints or inquiries exists or is being developed, but it is irregularly applied, and the requestor has chosen to accept the risk without remediation [with annotations] (medium).
4. The data requestor has a policy-based system for dealing with complaints and inquiries, including metrics and audits (high).

ii. Implementation [if i.4 is endorsed]
1. The data requestor has documentation showing that complaints or inquiries have been dealt with in an open and transparent manner (high).
   OR
   There have been no known complaints or inquiries (high).

References to Standards

- **Monitoring and enforcement criteria** [Section 10.0] in *Generally Accepted Privacy Principles* [practitioner version] (2009). American Institute of Certified Public Accountants, Inc. and Canadian Institute of Chartered Accountants. An organization should monitor compliance with its privacy policies and practices and have procedures to address privacy-related inquiries, complaints, and disputes.
- **Accountability** [Section 10.2] in *CIHR Best Practices for Protecting Privacy in Health Research* (2005). It is a responsibility of entities (individuals or institutions) engaged in publicly funded health research to provide a mechanism to handle queries and complaints from participants about privacy aspects of the research.

Government of Canada Sources

- **Processing requests** [Sections 6.2.4 and 6.2.5] in Policy on Privacy Protection. Treasury Board of Canada Secretariat (2008). Heads of government institutions are responsible for (1) directing employees to provide accurate, timely, and complete responses to requests under the Privacy Act, and (2) implementing processes and practices to ensure that every effort is made to help requestors receive proper responses.

Government of U.S. Sources

- None in Security Rule.

Explanations

- This question can also be interpreted to pertain to customers of the requestor (if it is a business) as the "public."

An Independent Authority (e.g., a Research Ethics Board) Has Approved the Proposal for Secondary Use of Data (Low1High1)

If the data custodian is unfamiliar with the independent authority, it would not be unreasonable to exercise due diligence in ensuring that the independent authority is reputable and that its members have appropriate skills and knowledge for the evaluation that is asked of them.

Response Categories

    i. General

        1. The data requestor has not received approval from a research ethics board (REB) or equivalent body for the use of the requested data (low).

        2. The data requestor does not have a plan for the use of data (e.g., a research plan) or will not share the plan (low).

        3. The data requestor has REB approval for a research plan for the use of personal information (medium).

        4. The data requestor has REB approval for a research plan for the use of personal information, and the plan includes processes for monitoring and reporting compliance with REB requirements (high).

References to Standards

- **Use of personal information** [Section 5.2.1] in *Generally Accepted Privacy Principles* [practitioner version] (2009). American Institute of Certified Public Accountants, Inc. and Canadian Institute of Chartered Accountants. Personal information is used only for the purposes identified in the notice and with the individual's consent, unless a law or regulation specifically requires otherwise.
- **Secondary use** [Section 3.3] in *CIHR Best Practices for Protecting Privacy in Health Research* (2005). When personal data are to be collected from sources other than the individuals to whom the data relate, consent should be obtained from those individuals unless a research ethics board determines that a waiver of consent is appropriate in the specified circumstances. These circumstances should include that a waiver of the consent requirement is permitted by law.

Government of Canada Sources

- **Data matching** [Section 9] in *Use and Disclosure of Personal Information.* Treasury Board of Canada Secretariat (1993). A data matching program must be approved only by the head of the government institutions or an official specifically delegated this authority by the head. Note: Included in the definition of data matching is data linkage, also known as data profiling.

Government of U.S. Sources

- None in Security Rule.

Explanations

- The purpose of this question is to have an independent entity that would take the interests of the individuals whose data are being disclosed into account, and advise the requestor accordingly.
- If the requestor does not perform research, then this independent authority may be a data access committee staffed with external experts that works with the privacy officer of the organization, for example. Alternatives that may be more appropriate given the business of the requestor can be used as long as they meet the intended purpose of independent oversight. For instance, in a commercial context, instead of an REB/institutional review board (IRB)/equivalent, this entity may be the privacy officer of the custodian.
- To simplify the wording of the questions and response categories and to make it concrete, the acronym *REB* is used, but it should be understood that this can be substituted for another appropriate entity.
- Note that if the purpose of the data disclosure is research, there may be legislated requirements for a research plan and a review by an REB or equivalent body. Therefore the interpretation of this question should take into account relevant legislation.

Internal and External Audit and Monitoring Mechanisms Are in Place As Appropriate (Low1High2)

Self-explanatory

Response Categories

i. Auditing
   1. The data requestor does not have data use or disclosure audit mechanisms in place (low).
   2. The data requestor conducts audits of data use and disclosure from time to time, normally in response to external requirements or incidents (medium).
   3. The data requestor conducts regular audits of data use and disclosure, and remediates identified issues (high).
ii. Monitoring
   1. The data requestor does not have data use or disclosure monitoring mechanisms in place (low).
   2. The data requestor has systems or processes to monitor and report on the use or disclosure of information that are applied on a discretionary basis (medium).

3. The data requestor has systems or processes to monitor and report on the use or disclosure of information, with automated alerting and response plans (high).

References to Standards

■ **Acquire and maintain application software: application control and auditability** [Section AI2.3] in *COBIT 4.1: Framework, Control Objectives, Management Guidelines, Maturity Models*. IT Governance Institute (2007). Implement business controls into automated application controls such that processing is accurate, complete, timely, authorized, and auditable.

■ **Independent review of information security** [Section 6.1.8] in ISO/IEC 27002:2005. International Organization for Standardization and International Electrotechnical Commission (2005). Section 6.1.8 states that information security should be independently reviewed at planned intervals.

■ **Testing security safeguards** [Section 8.2.7] in *Generally Accepted Privacy Principles* [practitioner version] (2009). American Institute of Certified Public Accountants, Inc. and Canadian Institute of Chartered Accountants. Section 8.2.7 states that independent audits of security controls (internal or external) should be conducted at least annually.

■ **Security measures: organizational safeguards** [Section 7.2.1] in *CIHR Best Practices for Protecting Privacy in Health Research* (2005). The section suggests that organizations housing research data, including data containing personal information, should implement internal and external reviews and audits.

Government of Canada Sources

■ **Departmental IT security assessment and audit** [Section 12.11] in *Operational Security Standard: Management of Information Technology Security (MITS)*. Treasury Board of Canada Secretariat (n.d.). Departments must assess and audit their information technology security and remedy deficiencies where necessary.

■ **Requirements: monitoring and reporting requirements** [Section 6.3] in Policy on Government Security. Treasury Board of Canada Secretariat (2009). Deputy heads are responsible for ensuring that period reviews are conducted to assess whether the departmental security program is effective, whether the goals, strategic objectives, and control objectives detailed in their departmental security plan were achieved, and whether their departmental security plan remains appropriate to the needs of the department and the government as a whole.

■ **Monitoring and reporting requirements** [Section 6.3] in Policy on Privacy Protection. Treasury Board of Canada Secretariat (2008). Heads or their delegates are responsible for monitoring compliance with the Policy on Privacy Protection as it relates to the administration of the Privacy Act.

Government of U.S. Sources

■ **HIPAA Security Rule 45 CFR §164.308(a)(1)(ii)(D).**
Standard: security management process; implementation specification: information system activity review. An organization must implement procedures to regularly review its records of information system activity, including audit logs, access reports, security incident reports, and any other documents used by the organization.

■ **HIPAA Security Rule 45 CFR §164.312(b).**
Standard: audit controls. Implement hardware, software, and/or procedural mechanisms that record and examine activity in information systems that contain or use ePHI.

An Independent Advisory or Data Stewardship Committee Serves in a Data Oversight Capacity (e.g., As an Advisory Committee for Defining the Scope and Strategic Priorities of Research Studies) (Low1High1)

A data safety management board (DSMB) may or may not fulfill this role depending on its terms of reference. In particular, a DSMB's terms of reference must include reference to, and appropriate weight to, the protection of data subject autonomy and data subject privacy.

Response Categories

  i. General
    1. The data requestor does not have data oversight mechanisms in place (low).
    2. There are data oversight mechanisms in place, but they may not be applied to the requested data (low).
    3. The data requestor has a data oversight policy with mechanisms in place to implement the policies (medium).
      OR
      The data requestor will put in place data oversight mechanisms with respect to the requested data (medium).
    4. The data requestor has a data oversight policy with mechanisms in place to implement the policies, as well as monitoring and audit processes (high).

References to Standards

- **Independent review of information security** [Section 6.1.8] in ISO/IEC 27002:2005. International Organization for Standardization and International Electrotechnical Commission (2005). The organizational management of information security should be reviewed independently.
- **Independent assurance** [Section ME4.7] in *COBIT 4.1: Framework, Control Objectives, Management Guidelines, Maturity Models*. IT Governance Institute (2007). An organization should obtain independent assurance about the conformance of information technologies with relevant laws and regulations; the organization's policies, standards, and procedures; and generally accepted practices.
- **Review and approval** [Section 1.2.1] in *Generally Accepted Privacy Principles* [practitioner version] (2009). American Institute of Certified Public Accountants, Inc. and Canadian Institute of Chartered Accountants. Section 1.2.1 states that privacy policies and procedures should be reviewed and approved by senior management or a management committee.
- **Risk assessment** [Section 1.2.4] in *Generally Accepted Privacy Principles* [practitioner version] (2009). American Institute of Certified Public Accountants, Inc. and Canadian Institute of Chartered Accountants. Section 1.2.4 states that the board or a committee of the board should provide oversight of the privacy risk assessment.
- **Security measures: organizational safeguards** [Section 10] in *CIHR Best Practices for Protecting Privacy in Health Research* (2005). Roles and responsibilities of all those involved in the conduct and evaluation of research should be clearly defined and understood, including those of researchers, their employing institutions, REBs, any data stewardship committees, privacy commissioners, and other legally designated privacy oversight agencies. Their concerted efforts should aim to provide a coherent governance structure for effective and efficient data stewardship.
- **Independent data stewardship committees** [Section 10.2.4] in *CIHR Best Practices for Protecting Privacy in Health Research* (2005). When a database containing personal information is created for multiple purposes or across multiple sites or jurisdictions, a centralized data stewardship committee could be put in place to authorize future uses of the database in accordance with research objectives and REB approval.

Government of Canada Sources

- **Privacy protocol for nonadministrative purposes** [Section 6.2.15] in Policy on Privacy Protection. Treasury Board of Canada Secretariat (2008). Heads of government institutions are responsible for establishing a privacy protocol within a government institution for collection, use, or disclosure of personal information for nonadministrative purposes, including audit and evaluation purposes.

Government of U.S. Sources

- None in Security Rule.

Chapter 28

Assessing the Motives and Capacity Construct

The objective of this chapter is to define a way to measure the motives and capacity construct. This construct assumes that the custodian is disclosing/using data that have gone through some kind of de-identification. Therefore we are concerned with the motives and capacity of the data requestor to re-identify these data.

This construct has two dimensions: "motives" and "capacity." Since "motives" pertain to individuals, the motives dimension can be considered in terms of the staff, collaborators, or employees of the data requestor entity. The motive to re-identify the data implies an intentional re-identification. The capacity dimension evaluates whether the data requestor is able to re-identify the data, irrespective of whether the re-identification is intentional or not.

The custodian is expected to be able to respond to/assess all of the items below. In some cases the custodian may have to exercise his or her best judgment in order to respond, as some of the items are subjective.

Data	The data are assumed to have gone through some kind of de-identification before they are disclosed/used. The amount of de-identification will vary depending on the specifics of the disclosure/use.
Purpose	This is the purpose for which the data requestor has requested the data.

Dimensions

The motives and capacity construct has two dimensions:

Motives to re-identify the data
Capacity to re-identify the data

Motives to Re-Identify the Data

A1	The data requestor has directly or indirectly worked/collaborated with the custodian in the past without incident.
	This item assumes that this collaboration has not resulted in any incidents where the data requestor processed the data in an inappropriate way or attempted to re-identify the data (i.e., it was perceived to be a successful collaboration). If the custodian has worked with the data requestor before, then there is an empirical trust that has been built up, suggesting that the data requestor is trustworthy.
Precondition: None.	
Response categories: Yes/no (yes = fewer motives to re-identify; no = greater motives to re-identify).	
A2	**The data requestor can potentially gain financially from re-identifying the data.**
	The first consideration is whether the data requestor is in financial distress, although this may be difficult to assess in practice.
	Consider if the data requestor or his/her family/employees/collaborators may receive financial benefits from processing identifiable data. For example, a pharmaceutical company may want to contact the data subjects directly for marketing purposes or to recruit them in a study.
	Another consideration is if the data, once re-identified, can be useful for committing financial fraud or identity theft (e.g., the database has dates of birth and mother's maiden name).
Precondition: None.	
Response categories: Yes/no (yes = greater motives to re-identify; no = fewer motives to re-identify).	

A3 **There is possibly a nonfinancial reason for the data requestor to try to re-identify the data.**

For example, there may a reason that the data requestor may want to embarrass the custodian by demonstrating that re-identification is possible, or say a reporter wants to do a story about a specific identifiable person in the data or a famous person known to be in the data. Also, a disgruntled employee may wish to adversely affect the custodian's reputation by re-identifying a data subject and making that public.

Precondition: None.

Response categories: Yes/no (yes = greater motives to re-identify; no = fewer motives to re-identify).

Capacity to Re-Identify the Data

B1 **The data requestor has the technical expertise to attempt to re-identify the data.**

Re-identification requires some basic database and statistical expertise. However, in real data sets there are missing data and data errors that would also have to be accounted for in terms of expertise. Of course an incorrect re-identification can also be problematic, but we are only concerned with a correct re-identification here.

Precondition: None.

Response categories: Yes/no (yes = greater capacity to re-identify; no – less capacity to re-identify).

B2 **The data requestor has the financial resources to attempt to re-identify the data.**

Some types of re-identification require funds to get data sets to link with. Also, gathering background information about a data subject in the data who is a target of re-identification can be costly.

Precondition: None.

Response categories: Yes/no (yes = greater capacity to re-identify; no = less capacity to re-identify).

B3   The data requestor has access to other private databases that can be linked with the data to re-identify data subjects.

Such private databases would only be useful if they contain the identity information about the data subjects. Then linkage with the de-identified database could reveal the identity of one or more data subjects in the data.

Some data that can be used for linking and re-identification could be publicly available. In such a case we would consider item B2 on the financial resources of the data requestor. This item pertains to private databases.

A data requestor may obtain such private databases from previous disclosures by the custodian. For example, the custodian may have disclosed a particular data set to a researcher last year, and this year the same researcher wants another data set that can be linked to the earlier one. The data requestor may also obtain a private database by colluding with someone else. For example, the researcher may arrange to link a new administrative data set from the custodian with another researcher who has obtained a different clinical data set from the same custodian (and the custodian would not approve for the two data sets to be linked).

An agent can also have access to data useful for linking. For example, in hospitals many staff members have access to administrative data but not to clinical data. An employee can get a de-identified clinical data set and link it with the readily available administrative data set to re-identify data subjects in the clinical data set.

Precondition: None.

Response categories: Yes/no (yes = greater capacity to re-identify; no = less capacity to re-identify).

Index

Printed and bound by CPI Group (UK) Ltd, Croydon, CR0 4YY

24/10/2024

01778283-0013